Neuro-ophthalmology

Symposium of the University of Miami and the Bascom Palmer Eye Institute

VOLUME VIII

Neuro-ophthalmology

Symposium of the University of Miami and the Bascom Palmer Eye Institute

Edited by

JOEL S. GLASER, M.D.

Assistant Professor of Ophthalmology and Neurological Surgery,
Bascom Palmer Eye Institute, Department of Ophthalmology,
University of Miami School of Medicine, Miami, Florida

J. LAWTON SMITH, M.D.

Professor of Ophthalmology, Bascom Palmer Eye Institute,
Department of Ophthalmology, University of Miami School of Medicine,
Miami, Florida

with 259 illustrations,
including 2 four-color plates

The C. V. Mosby Company

Saint Louis 1975

VOLUME VIII

Printed in the United States of America

International Standard Book Number 0-8016-1846-0

Library of Congress Catalog Card Number 64-18729

Distributed in Great Britain by Henry Kimpton, London

CB/CB/B 9 8 7 6 5 4 3 2 1

Contributors

ROY D. ALTMAN, M.D.

Assistant Professor of Medicine, University of Miami School of Medicine, Miami, Florida

DOUGLAS R. ANDERSON, M.D.

Associate Professor of Ophthalmology, Bascom Palmer Eye Institute, Department of Ophthalmology, University of Miami School of Medicine, Miami, Florida

JAMES E. BIRKETT, B.A.

Department of Neurology, University of Miami School of Medicine and Veterans Administration Hospital, Miami, Florida

RONALD M. BURDE, M.D.

Professor of Ophthalmology and Neurology, Washington University School of Medicine, St. Louis, Missouri

HENRY M. CLAYMAN, M.D.

Clinical Instructor in Ophthalmology, University of Miami School of Medicine, Miami, Florida

JAMES J. CORBETT, M.D.

Clinical Instructor, Neurology, Thomas Jefferson Medical College; Assistant Neurologist, Wills Eye Hospital, Philadelphia, Pennsylvania

ROBERT B. DAROFF, M.D.

Professor of Neurology, University of Miami School of Medicine and Veterans Administration Hospital, Miami, Florida

NOBLE J. DAVID, M.D.

Professor of Neurology and Associate Professor of Ophthalmology, University of Miami School of Medicine; Chief, Neurology Service, Veterans Administration Hospital, Miami, Florida

FREDIE P. GARGANO, M.D.

Professor of Radiology, University of Miami School of Medicine, Miami, Florida

JOEL S. GLASER, M.D.

Assistant Professor of Ophthalmology and Neurological Surgery, Bascom Palmer Eye Institute, Department of Ophthalmology, University of Miami School of Medicine, Miami, Florida

BAIRD S. GRIMSON, M.D.

Department of Ophthalmology, University of Iowa College of Medicine, Iowa City, Iowa

JAMES M. HENRY, M.D., LTC, MC, USA

Chief, Division of Neuropathology, Armed Forces Institute of Pathology, Washington, D.C.

JOHN C. JOHNSON, M.D.

Assistant Professor of Radiology, The Ohio State University College of Medicine, Columbus, Ohio

JOSEPH S. KARP, M.D.

Resident in Ophthalmology, Washington University School of Medicine, St. Louis, Missouri

K. FRANCIS LEE, M.D., Sc.D.

Professor of Radiology, Thomas Jefferson Medical College, Philadelphia, Pennsylvania

SIMMONS LESSELL, M.D.

Professor of Ophthalmology and Associate Professor of Neurology, Boston University School of Medicine; Director, Ophthalmology Service, Boston City Hospital, Boston, Massachusetts

STEPHEN LICHTENSTEIN, M.D.

Intern, Department of Neurology, Thomas Jefferson University Hospital, Philadelphia, Pennsylvania

MARTIN LUBOW, M.D.

Associate Professor of Ophthalmology and Neurology, The Ohio State University College of Medicine, Columbus, Ohio

JOHN A. McCRARY, III, M.D.

Associate Professor of Ophthalmology, Baylor College of Medicine, Houston, Texas

SYDNEY F. J. PILLEY, M.B., F.R.C.S.

Department of Ophthalmology, University of Iowa College of Medicine, Iowa City, Iowa

JOEL S. SANDBERG, M.D.

University of Miami School of Medicine, Miami, Florida

PETER J. SAVINO, M.D.

Clinical Instructor, Ophthalmology, Thomas Jefferson Medical College; Assistant Neurologist, Wills Eye Hospital, Philadelphia, Pennsylvania

NORMAN J. SCHATZ, M.D.

Associate Professor of Neurology and Clinical Assistant Professor of Ophthalmology, Thomas Jefferson Medical College; Associate Director of Neurology, Wills Eye Hospital, Philadelphia, Pennsylvania

JAMES A. SHARPE, M.D.

Assistant Professor, Division of Neurology, Toronto Western Hospital, Department of Medicine, University of Toronto, Toronto, Ontario, Canada

J. L. SILVERSIDES, M.D.

Professor, Division of Neurology, Toronto Western Hospital, Department of Medicine, University of Toronto, Toronto, Ontario, Canada

ROBERT H. SPECTOR, M.D.

Fellow in Neuro-ophthalmology, University of Miami School of Medicine, Miami, Florida

JOHN O. SUSAC, M.D., LTC, MC, USA

Neuro-ophthalmology, Walter Reed Army Medical Center, Washington, D.C.

H. STANLEY THOMPSON, M.D.

Associate Professor of Ophthalmology, Department of Ophthalmology, University of Iowa College of Medicine, Iowa City, Iowa

FRANK B. WALSH, M.D.

Professor Emeritus of Ophthalmology, The Wilmer Ophthalmological Institute, The Johns Hopkins University School of Medicine, The Johns Hopkins Hospital, Baltimore, Maryland

Preface

This series serves to provide an ongoing forum for the presentation of new topics related to neuro-ophthalmology, as well as for ventilation of old subjects through up-to-date reviews. For the most part, the papers included are elaborations of lectures presented at the University of Miami Neuro-ophthalmology Course, and the present volume includes material from the January meetings of 1974 and 1975. In addition, several vital topics to be covered in the 1976 course are previewed. The variety of subjects encompassed by the hybrid discipline of neuro-ophthalmology is reflected in the diversity of issues currently discussed in these symposia. I would like to underscore several of the more important topics.

For several years Douglas Anderson has meticulously studied the micro-anatomy of the optic nerve, and that material is admirably brought up to date (Chapter 3), along with a discussion of mechanisms in the production of optic nerve disease (Chapter 4).

Chapter 9 is a republication of the McLean Memorial Lecture by Frank B. Walsh, dealing with orbital and canalicular meningiomas that involve the optic nerve. Dr. Walsh stresses that such meningiomas in youth do not behave like similar tumors in adulthood.

Although the overwhelming majority of cases of chiasmal syndrome are produced by pituitary and parasellar tumors, Norman J. Schatz and co-workers discuss two *nonneoplastic causes of visual loss,* ischemic chiasmal disease (with K. Francis Lee in Chapter 6) and delayed radionecrosis in the anterior visual pathways (Chapter 7). As a companion piece—regarding another parachiasmal syndrome most celebrated by incorrect or delayed diagnosis—Noble J. David and associates reflect on personal experience with so-called pituitary apoplexy (Chapter 8), elaborating the more atypical aspects of symptomatology accompanying *acute* changes in pituitary adenomas. Johnson and Lubow provide an innovative neuroradiologic technique for investigation of the optic nerves and chiasm (Chapter 5).

The higher integration of visual function, beyond the primary visual cortex, is a confusing subject to anatomist and clinician alike. Simmons Lessell succeeds in elucidating this difficult area in terms with which any clinician may feel at ease (Chapters 1 and 2). The peripheral ocular motor system is the subject of essays by Burde and Karp (Chapter 10) and Lessell (Chapter 11), and John McCrary provides an outline for assessment of the pupil (Chapter 12).

The final section of the volume is comprised of free papers presented at the January, 1975, course (Chapter 13).

The contributors to the symposia are thoughtful and experienced clinicians who bring considerable expertise to bear on their selected topics. The reader will sense the pragmatism that pervades the discussions, whether an elegant essay on the fine structure of the optic nerve or a what-to-do approach to the patient with diplopia. Hopefully, both the beginner and the accomplished will find this material instructional and applicable.

Joel S. Glaser

Contents

COLOR PLATES

Neuro-ophthalmology

Symposium of the University of Miami and the Bascom Palmer Eye Institute

Chapter 1

Higher disorders of visual function: negative phenomena

Simmons Lessell

Patients with so-called disorders of higher function may manifest a variety of visual symptoms and signs. At one extreme are patients with geniculocalcarine blindness, who cannot see despite having normal eyes. At the other extreme are instances of visual hallucinations in which blind patients see things that are not there. In between are intermediate levels of dysfunction. The agnostic patient cannot recognize objects, the prosopagnostic cannot recognize faces, and the alexic cannot read. The patient with paliopsia has abnormal persistence of vision and continues to see objects after they have been removed from view. In the descriptions that follow, I have limited myself to these manifestations of disease. Many manifestations that are not included are interesting and important, but there is not sufficient space to include them.

In the interests of clarity and simplicity, I use the word *seeing* to indicate that the patient claims to see something or that one can be certain from his behavior that he sees something. *Recognition* indicates that the subject claims to know or appears to know what it is that he sees.

GENICULOCALCARINE BLINDNESS

Geniculocalcarine blindness refers to subnormal visual acuity due to bilateral lesions in the geniculocalcarine pathway. Classically, geniculocalcarine blindness is characterized by total loss of vision in both eyes in the presence of normal fundi and normal pupillary responses to light stimulation. Patients with this disorder may have any degree of visual loss, but both

Table 1. Causes of geniculocalcarine blindness

Migraine	? Methanol
Ischemia	Ethanol
Anoxia	Lead
Ictal	Mercury
Postictal	Tansy tea
Posttraumatic	Postpump oxygenator
Brain swelling	Tumor
Congenital malformations of brain	Postventriculography
Hydrocephalus (congenital)	Postcerebral angiography
Schilder's disease	Jakob-Creutzfeldt disease
Subacute sclerosing panencephalitis	

eyes have the same level of vision unless there are additional unilateral or asymmetric, anterior visual system lesions. The causes of geniculocalcarine blindness are listed in Table 1. It is sufficiently common that one can expect to encounter it in practice. Therefore, one must be prepared to recognize it. Unfortunately it is difficult to diagnose. Problems in the recognition and differential diagnosis of geniculocalcarine blindness include the following:

1. Coexistent anterior visual pathway lesions may mask geniculocalcarine lesions that are the actual cause of a patient's defective vision.

2. Unilateral or asymmetric anterior visual system pathway lesions may produce unequal visual acuities in the two eyes, thereby deterring the physician from considering a geniculocalcarine lesion.

3. Early in life, geniculocalcarine lesions may cause retrograde, transsynaptic degeneration in the visual system.[1] As a result, the patient's discs may be pale. One may reach the false conclusion that the defect in vision in these cases is due primarily to an optic neuropathy.

4. In the early stages of some chiasmal and bilateral retrobulbar nerve lesions, the fundi may be normal and the pupils may show light responses. One may falsely conclude that the patient has geniculocalcarine blindness.

5. Struggling, crying infants may develop miosis when the physician tries to pry open the lids in order to test the pupillary responses. This may mislead the examiner into believing that pupillary light reflexes exist. Hippus may also be confused with a light response. Patients may also respond with miosis in attempting to attend to the activity near them—a "psychic near response." This may also mislead the examiner into believing that pupillary reactions are present when they are not. In all of these circumstances, in a patient with blindness, the examiner will be led to the false conclusion that geniculocalcarine blindness exists.

6. Geniculocalcarine blindness may coexist with motor, intellectual, psychiatric, and language disorders sufficient to prevent the recognition of the blindness.

7. Hysterical or malingered blindness can be hard to differentiate from geniculocalcarine blindness. In all these the patient claims to be blind but has normal eyes and normal pupillary responses. To establish the factitious basis of hysterical or malingered blindness, the examiner must demonstrate that the patient sees more than he claims to see. If the patient claims to be totally blind, the task is easy. One can use opticokinetic stimuli to produce nystagmus. I have also had success with presenting to the allegedly blind patient a large card on which are written obscenities. Some patients with factitious blindness cannot suppress their amusement or indignation and thus give away the presence of vision. Another device that I have used is a ball on a string. I conceal the ball in my hand, with the string attached to one of my fingers. I then throw the ball towards the patient's face, being careful to stand farther away from the patient than the length of the string. The malingering or hysterical patient will attempt to protect himself and catch the ball despite his alleged visual disability. Electric testing may be helpful in these patients also. The visual evoked response measured over the scalp and averaged by a computer can demonstrate that a signal is reaching the brain. Unfortunately, it is possible to record a visual evoked response in the presence of occipital lesions, at least in monkeys.[2] Absence of the visual evoked response is probably quite significant.

In patients with factitious blindness who claim to have some vision, more refined clinical and electric testing may be helpful. The only limitations are the ingenuity of the examiner and the sophistication of the patient. In many hysterics who claim to be unable to read the small letters on the chart, reassurance and encouragement during the reading, with the examiner virtually cheerleading the reading of the Snellen chart, may establish the factitious nature of the visual deficit. In other instances, one may be absolutely unable to distinguish between true geniculocalcarine visual impairment and factitious visual impairment. In these cases, electric testing may be helpful, depending upon the age and cooperation of the patient and the alleged level of visual failure. Patterned responses in a patient who claims only light perception may indicate that the patient's assessment of his own visual acuity is inaccurate.

8. Patients with geniculocalcarine blindness not only may not call attention to their problem, they may deny or minimize it. Such a patient behaves as an "inverse hysteric." Denial of blindness (Anton's syndrome) is usually considered in association with geniculocalcarine blindness. This stems from the early descriptions of von Monakow,[3] Dejerine and Vailet,[4] and Anton.[5] It is seen in a large majority of patients with geniculocalcarine blindness, but it can also occur with any kind of blindness. One may encounter denial of blindness in patients blind from cataracts, retinopathies, or optic atrophy. Some patients who deny blindness at the outset of their illness subsequently stop denying without their having been any change

in the nature of the blindness. Conversely, some patients with blindness and no denial may develop denial years later! The denial may be explicit—the patient actively claiming that he can see—or implicit—the patient acting as if he can see and not complaining about his blindness. In both instances the physician may be misled into believing that the patient can see. The patient may make intricate excuses and explanations for his difficulty. Some of these are patently ridiculous, but others may be plausible enough to contribute to confusion in diagnosis.

What is responsible for denial? There are several theories, and each probably explains some of the cases. According to Geschwind,[6] patients with denial commonly have an alteration in emotional reactivity. The alteration may be similar to that encountered in some patients with frontal lobe syndromes and in some cases of metabolic disorders and congestive heart failure where there is an acute confusional state. These patients have been described by Geschwind as having an "irritable, euphoric apathy." Their emotions are said to be coarse and shallow. Patients with right hemisphere lesions, who predominate in series of cases of denial syndromes of all kinds, may have the same symptoms as patients with frontal lobe lesions. The right hemisphere seems responsible for the finer aspects of emotional behavior, and right hemisphere lesions seem particularly apt to alter the emotional state of the patient in such a way as to predispose him to denial. Psychiatric denial probably exists as well, and it may be an accentuation of a common response to illness. In psychiatric denial, the denial seems implicit in the behavior of the patient. His activity and speech content lead the doctor to believe that the patient wishes his illness were just not there. He does not want to face up to his problem, and his denial may seem quite plausible. By contrast, patients with neurologic denial tend to have a less plausible picture. They tend to be very explicit in their denial. Their responses are very crude, and they may deny that there is any problem at all when there obviously is one. In a few instances, denial may reflect a memory disorder, as in Korsakoff's syndrome, in which the patient simply cannot remember from moment to moment that he is blind. This must be exceedingly uncommon. Finally, it is possible that patients with lesions that involve not only the geniculocalcarine pathway but also areas of the brain responsible for the recognition and interpretation of what the visual cortex is receiving may become blind to their blindness. The area of the brain capable of telling them what is going on visually is not operative. All this suggests that in many instances denial depends on the existence of abnormalities apart from those in the primary visual pathway. Certainly this seems true in patients with neurologic denial. Support for this comes from the observation that in one large series of cases of geniculocalcarine blindness due to penetrating wounds in which the damage seemed limited to primary visual pathways, denial was conspicuously absent.[7]

Ictal blindness

Geniculocalcarine blindness may follow seizures and then persist for relatively long periods.[8, 9] It may occur even when the seizures do not appear to have arisen from a focus within the visual system. The seizures are usually severe and prolonged, and they are often associated with fever and a period of postictal coma. This blindness is probably not due to exhaustion of cells in the visual cortex from seizure discharges. The concept of cell exhaustion, as in Todd's paralysis, is questionable. For example, it has been observed that patients may get a Todd's paralysis of a limb that did not participate in a convulsion. It is more likely that the blindness that follows seizures represents cortical anoxia due to the combined effects of brain swelling and heightened metabolic needs. True inhibitory seizures do occur in the visual system. In contrast to the ictal blindness described above, this type of ictal blindness occurs at the outset of the seizure and may constitute the greater part of the episode. I saw my first two cases within the past year.

Inhibitory visual seizures were described many years ago by Gowers,[10] who found that in 1000 personally collected cases of seizures, 26 had loss of sight that preceded loss of consciousness. He apparently knew of a patient in whom loss of sight persisted for an hour and was followed by an hour's sleep. According to Gowers, the loss of vision was always preceded by a flash of light.

Teuber and co-workers[11] reported a patient who suffered a gunshot wound of the brain in World War I. It left him with a bilateral inferior altitudinal heminanopia. In the 39 years that elapsed between his injury and their observations, he had seizures several times a year, heralded by photisms in the blind portion of his field, followed by complete blindness.

In the study of traumatic epilepsy by Russell and Whitty,[12] negative visual phenomena were seen in two of nine patients with calcarine injuries, 6 of 21 with injuries of the radiation, and 16 of 30 with lesions in higher visual areas. One patient had no persistent visual difficulty between episodes. In the others, the blurring extended from hemianopic field into previously functioning field. These negative phenomena, including visual loss, were sometimes of very brief duration.

In 1970 Kooi[13] reported three examples of ictal blindness as a late effect of head injury. The first patient, a 20-year-old man, had incurred a compound, depressed left, occipital fracture in a fall. Prior to surgery he had a right homonymous hemianopia. The defect cleared, and the patient was asymptomatic for almost five years. Then he had attacks of bilateral blindness without other significant abnormalities. The episodes lasted less than a minute. On several occasions he fell down but regained control immediately. Evaluation showed a normal physical exam, and his episodes responded to Dilantin. His visual evoked responses were abnormal.

The second patient was a 24-year-old woman, who four years before had developed unconsciousness after an auto accident. She had continuing visual difficulty and episodes of fading vision. On two occasions she had clonic movements of the extremities, altered consciousness, weakness, and confusion. The episodes of visual impairment lasted several minutes. Her visual evoked responses were normal.

The third patient was a 16-year-old boy who six years previously had suffered an epidural hematoma after head trauma. Surgery included evacuation of the clot, elevation of a depressed skull fracture, and brain debridement. He had a stormy course but when ultimately discharged had no visual difficulty. Five years later, he began to have episodes of total blindness lasting 10 to 15 seconds. On one occasion the patient became rigid. The episodes occurred several times a month. He was not out of contact with the environment during the episodes. He had intact visual fields but his visual evoked responses were abnormal.

Kooi believed these cases were "examples of visual epilepsy manifested by paroxysmal, negative visual phenomena." He thought the episodes were due to cortical inhibition.

There may be other mechanisms by which visual impairment may occur during seizures. Electroretinograms were recorded in monkeys before and after spike and wave electroencephalographic patterns were induced by intravenous administration of chlorambucil. During the seizure activity, the electroretinogram was reduced or abolished. This effect could be abolished by cutting the optic nerve.[14] Perhaps during seizures inhibitory potentials pass from the brain to the eyes through the optic nerves and suppress vision at a retinal level.

Recovery from geniculocalcarine blindness

One striking feature of geniculocalcarine blindness is the tendency for affected individuals to regain vision. The pattern of visual recovery tends to be such that light- and movement-sense return first. Sense of form and color return later, if at all. Sometimes many months elapse before recovery begins, and an interval of visual agnosia may intervene between the return of some vision and the return of good function. Patients who do not recover are likely to have diffuse brain disease, tumor, or a progressive, degenerative disorder of the brain such as Schilder's disease.

Why does the visual system show such a capacity for recovery? In some cases recovery can be explained by the healing of cells in the geniculocalcarine pathway that at the time of the insult were not totally destroyed. However, recovery is sometimes recorded in patients whose visual systems appear to have suffered permanent damage. Furthermore, there is now abundant evidence in subhuman primates of recovery of vision after complete ablations of the visual cortex.[15-17] One must conclude that there is a degree of plasticity in the visual system sufficient to permit accessory visual systems to assume some of the function that was lost. Pasik and Pasik[18, 19] have been systematically investigating these back-up systems in primates. At least in monkeys, it seems that the tectum cannot account for the visual recovery. It may be that a mesencephalic nucleus (the paralemniscal nucleus) in which the accessory optic tract ends is responsible for the retention of visual discrimination in monkeys with ablations of striate cortex. In the intact animal, this nucleus may be inhibited by connections from the striate cortex. With the loss of synaptic terminals from the cells in the visual cortex, there may be morphologic adaptation; that is, additional terminals may arise from direct retinomesencephalic or geniculomesencephalic sources in a manner analogous to the morphologic adaptation shown in rat forebrain by Raisman.[20] The importance of back-up visual systems is obvious. In a patient with one of the common varieties of geniculocalcarine blindness (after an anoxic episode, stroke, and angiography) one can predict some return of visual function, even when the patient has been totally blind for days or weeks. Evolution has provided us not only with two eyes but also with multiple visual systems. Vision is apparently too valuable for the survival of the individual and the species to be left to a single unit.

VISUAL AGNOSIA

Visual agnosia is a rare disorder characterized by the patient's failure to recognize objects that he can see. Almost from the earliest description of visual agnosia, the concept has been questioned by critics. Recently, however, cases of visual agnosia have been described whose features leave no doubt as to the existence of this entity. A review of the history of visual agnosia may help put these cases into perspective.

In 1877 the German physiologist Munk[21] reported the effects of partial ablation of the occipital cortices in dogs. He noted that although these dogs behaved as if they could see, they seemed unable to recognize the objects around them. Munk called this mind blindness (Seelenblindheit). Twelve years later, Lissauer[22] encountered an elderly man who had suffered a stroke and had great difficulty in recognizing objects and faces in addition to having a right hemianopia and alexia without agraphia. As soon as the man was given nonvisual clues, he was readily able to make the identifications. Lissauer realized that his patient manifested a syndrome similar to that which Munk's dogs had demonstrated. He suggested that mind blindness could occur in human brain diseases. Lissauer furthermore indicated that mind blindness could come about in two ways. In the first type, which he called *aperceptive,* the patient's image of an object was in some way imperfect or distorted and therefore could not be recognized. In the second type, which he called *associative,* the image was clear, but connections to association cortex were impaired, preventing recognition. Subsequent studies appear to have proved Lissauer correct in all details. A year later Sigmund Freud[23] coined the word *agnosia* and applied the term *visual agnosia* to the entity that had been described by Lissauer. Tragically, Lassauer died a year later at the age of 30. After Lissauer's death, the patient whom he had described died, and the brain was examined pathologically. The lesions were limited to the left occipital lobe and the splenium of the corpus callosum.

Subsequent critics of the concept of visual agnosia have been particularly dubious about the existence of an associative type. Among the critics have been such authorities as Bay,[24] Bender,[25] and Critchley.[26] A recent publication by Bender and Feldman[27] has emphasized this contrary point of view. All the patients they saw who seemed to have what others would consider visual object agnosia also had "some of the following disturbances: (a) subtle or marked defects in the field of vision; (b) mild or severe organic mental syndrome; (c) with or without impairment of communication abilities (partial aphasia); (d) defects in perceptual interactions between same and different modalities especially visual." Bender apparently believes that the cases that present with visual agnosia have some combination of mental deficit and defect in visual function. Included within this would be patients with severe mental disturbance and mild visual field defects, patients with moderate defects in both, and patients with mild mental difficulty and severe visual field defects. Another explanation, championed by Luria,[28] is that patients with visual agnosia actually have difficulty in seeing several parts of a scene simultaneously, perhaps because of a motor defect. This has been called *simultanagnosia.* Critchley[26] commented that clinical experience has not shown clear-cut cases of pure agnostic defect where objects are "sensed clearly but remain devoid of meaning" in a patient who does not have significant language or intellectual disorders. Teuber[29] is in agreement with this view.

In the late 1960s two patients were seen at the Aphasia Research Unit of the Boston Veterans Administration Hospital by Dr. Frank Benson and his colleagues. These patients manifested the two varieties of visual agnosia described or predicted by Lissauer. These cases have been reported in exquisite detail[30, 31] and should be read by all ophthalmologists and neurologists. The descriptions are models of clarity and completeness. I was fortunate to have the opportunity to examine both these patients, and through the courtesy of Dr. Benson will recount their histories here.

Case 1. This patient, a 25-year-old soldier who was accidentally asphyxiated, is thought to be an example of the aperceptive variety of visual agnosia. The asphyxiation left him drowsy and confused for two days. He then went into a coma and had decerebrate rigidity. He survived the episode of coma and was admitted to the Boston Veterans Administration Hospital. He was said to be blind, and to have a diffuse encephalopathy. Indeed, he behaved as if he were blind, but to everyone's surprise, it was found that he could name colors. He had an extrapyramidal syndrome but was intellectually intact and had no disturbance of language. Vision was present, and by an objective measure, a graded series of optokinetic targets, his visual acuity was found to be at least 20/200. He not only could identify colors but also differences in tint. He could tell where things were and recognize changes in illumination. He could tell the directions of lines. He could not tell form or faces unless he was given ancillary clues. When given nonvisual clues he could recognize objects and people readily. Thus, he seemed to have a visual form agnosia or aperceptive visual agnosia. He could not integrate the angles necessary to make forms from the lines that he saw. One might suspect that he could do what Hubel and Wiesel have shown that the primary visual cortex can do. He could tell lines and how they were oriented. He could tell about movements. He just couldn't put it all together. He could not process primary visual sensory data in a manner that gave him images sufficient for recognition. It was clear from his other behavior, particularly his ability to recognize things by hearing or touch, that there was no language disturbance, anomia, or lack of comprehension, and that there was no intellectual deficit that would prevent recognition. There was good evidence of visual function, at least in a very rudimentary sense, that extended to his ability to differentiate tints. Whether this constitutes visual agnosia as described by Lissauer or fails to qualify on the basis of the objections of many subsequent investigators really seems to hinge on semantic issues. Since it admittedly involves some defects in seeing, it may not be a truly agnostic disorder. But it is not a primary problem in seeing; it is something more complex.

Case 2. This patient had associative visual agnosia, and his symptoms and signs leave no doubt as to the existence of this entity. It has been primarily this form of agnosia that has been questioned by critics. The patient was a 47-year-old, right-handed, chronic alcoholic who was admitted to the hospital for convalescence after an episode of coma. A year earlier he had been found unconscious, with urinary incontinence and a left hemiparesis. These all cleared readily. At one point in the preceding year he had been admitted to a hospital because of alcoholism and malnutrition. On a second admission to a psychiatric hospital, he had been depressed and potentially suicidal. A month prior to admission he had been found unconscious and had vomited. It was discovered that he might have ingested chloral hydrate, because 20 tablets were missing from a bottle located near him. At the time of admission he was apneic, unresponsive, and had large, fixed, dilated pupils. He was hypotensive and required intubation, support with artificial respiration, and vasopressive drugs. He responded after a period of three hours, and a day later he was awake. He had hyperreflexia and an extensor plantar response on the right. For ten days he was disoriented, confused, and incontinent of urine. He thought that there was something wrong with his eyes and kept them closed. A pneumoencephalogram showed an enlarged left lateral ventricle. Bilateral carotid arteriograms were normal. Several weeks later, at another hospital, he was discovered to have a right homonymous hemianopsia, visual acuity of 20/30 in each eye, and alexia without agraphia. He also could not name objects that he was shown, and his memory was impaired. On admission to the Aphasia Unit at the Boston Veterans Administration Hospital, his vital signs were normal. He had a right homonymous hemianopia with splitting of fixation and a tiny left homonymous wedge defect adjoining the midline superiorly. The visual acuity was 20/30 in each eye. Intellectual function was normal. His digit span was 7 forward and 5 backward. He could recall four unrelated words after five minutes. He did have difficulty remembering names of individuals, but he was not aphasic. Deep tendon reflexes were slightly greater in his right arm than in his left. His right plantar response was neutral, while the left plantar response was flexor. He had no apraxia and no right-left disorientation. He had no difficulty in locating directions and could draw maps and clocks normally. He could draw well on command. Copying was quite accurate, but he could not identify objects that he was able to copy. His writing was normal. He could not name colors correctly but could correctly sort chips of various colors into piles of the same color. He had no difficulty with the pseudoisochromatic plates. He could not recognize anyone's face, including his own, although he could tell if a face that was shown to him was correctly oriented. It was also possible for him to consistently describe the type of expression on faces that he was shown. His defect in the recognition of faces was so severe that he never learned to recognize the faces of physicians who saw him daily for many months. However, as soon as he could hear their voices he would identify them. He had difficulty in reading, but his visual memory was good.

This patient clearly could see, because he could copy drawings in great detail. He also did not seem to have difficulty in seeing all parts of things at once. Yet he had tremendous difficulty in recognizing what it was that he saw. His disability later improved to the point where he approached nearly normal performance for naming real objects. He did well on about half of the line drawings that he was shown and in color naming. He ultimately learned to read rapidly but had some difficulty with technical material. He never was able to learn to recognize faces again. Three years later the patient died. Autopsy showed lesions in the left occipital lobe and the splenium of the corpus callosum. In addition, there was a small lesion in the inferior occipitotemporal region on the right nicking the visual radiations and inferior longitudenal bundle.[32]

There is no doubt in my mind that both types of visual agnosia exist. Certainly the associative type is a true agnosia by anyone's definition. In the patient with the aperceptive variety, one can only guess at the nature of the lesion. He probably had involvement in the preoccipital cortex bilaterally, although there is no means of being certain. The second patient had the lesions of alexia without agraphia (see below) as well as an additional lesion in the right hemisphere interrupting occipital-limbic connections. For an individual to put a name on an object, and perhaps to recognize it, its image must make connection in the left hemisphere in right-handed individuals. No direct input to the left hemisphere was possible in the second patient because the left occipital lobe was destroyed. Material coming from the right hemisphere must pass across the corpus callosum, and apparently in this patient the area or one of the areas in which the patient carried object information was interrupted.

ALEXIA

Alexia is loss of the ability to understand written words. In the discussion that follows I will confine myself to alexia so defined and not deal with dyslexia. *Dyslexia,* or developmental dyslexia as it is frequently called, designates a specific disability in learning to read. The patients I will discuss in this section have alexia; they have already learned to read, but an acquired lesion of the central nervous system has deprived them of that ability. I have borrowed heavily in the preparation of this material from the published and unpublished ideas of Dr. Norman Geschwind. It would be worthwhile for the interested physician to read Dr. Geschwind's original publications in this area. They range from material suitable for the informed layman *(Scientific American)*[33] to a series of scholarly reports *(Brain)* on the disconnection syndromes.[34, 35] He and Benson have recently reviewed the alexias.[36]

What events take place when an individual learns to read? He sees a particular set of letters, which he is taught to associate both with a specific

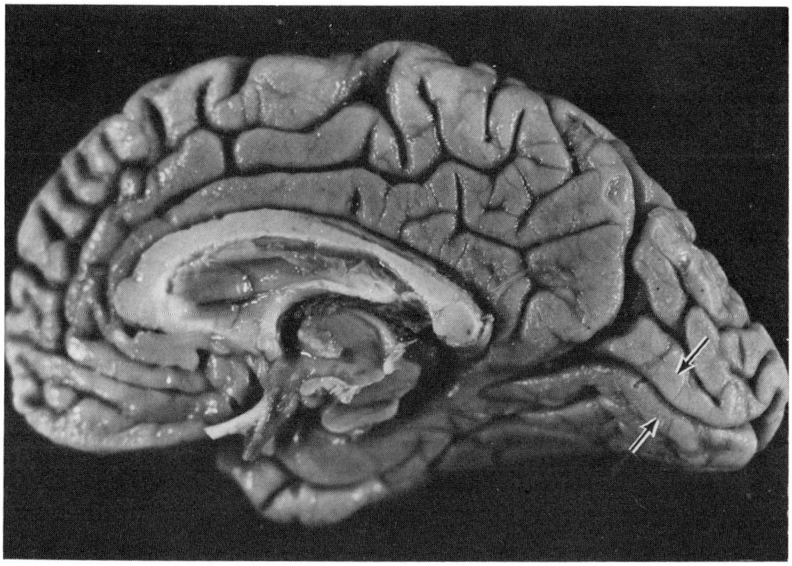

Fig. 1-1. Medial aspect of a bisected brain, showing primary visual area of right hemisphere (arrows).

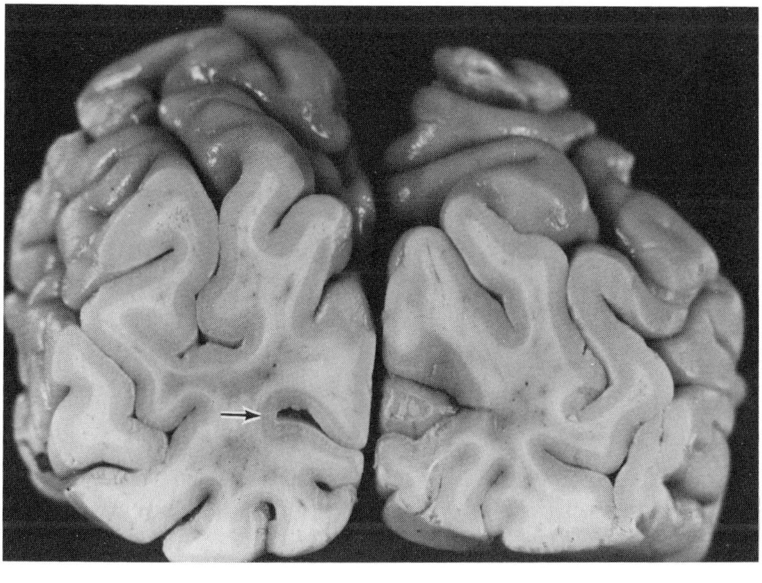

Fig. 1-2. Coronal section through occipital lobes of the brain, showing striate cortex (arrow).

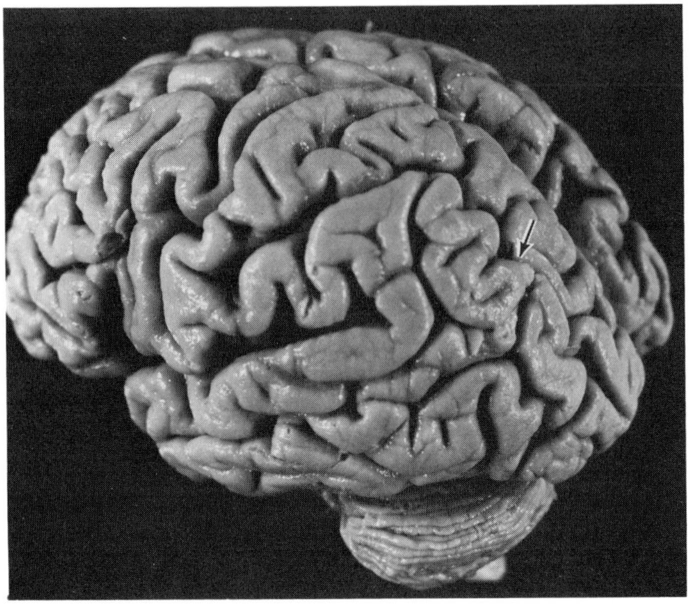

Fig. 1-3. View of left side of the brain, showing angular gyrus (arrow).

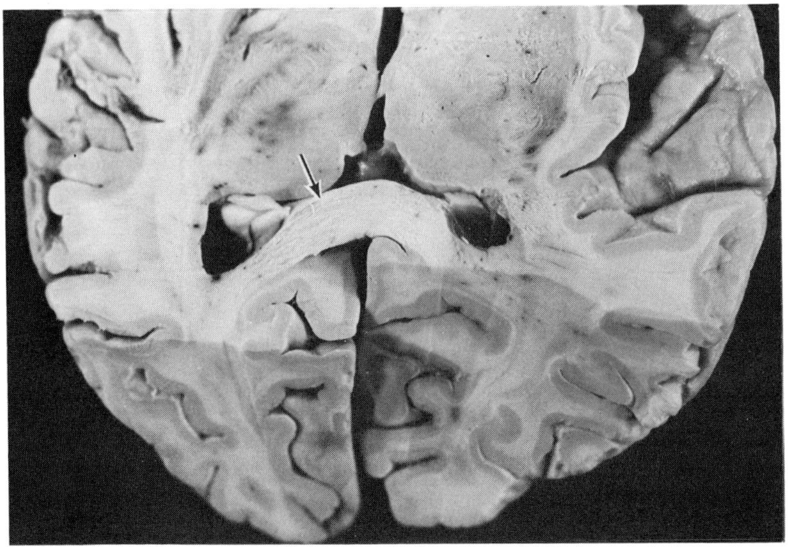

Fig. 1-4. Brain dissected to show the splenium of the corpus callosum (arrow). Occipital lobes are at bottom.

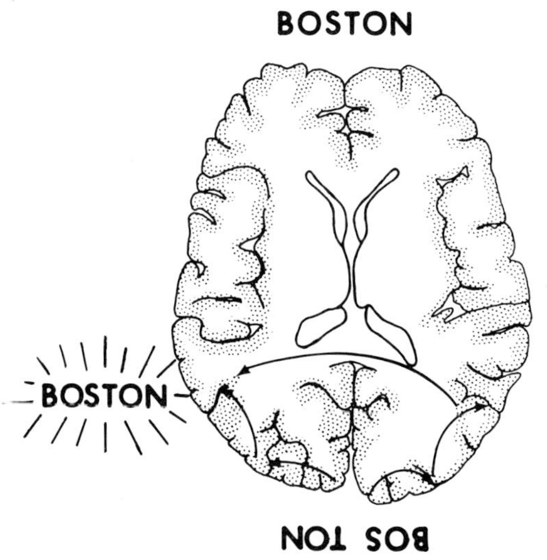

Fig. 1-5. Diagram showing pathways concerned with comprehension of written language.

sound and frequently with an image. The picture of the word is transmitted from the retinas to the striate cortices (Figs. 1-1 and 1-2). In turn, it is processed in both occipital lobes in areas 18 and 19. In right-handed individuals, the next way station is an area of association cortex at the confluence of the left temporal, parietal, and occipital lobes. This area of cortex, the angular gyrus (Fig. 1-3), receives input from both occipital lobes. The connections from the left occipital cortex are quite direct. Those from the right occipital cortex must traverse the splenium of the corpus callosum in order to reach the angular gyrus on the left side (Figs. 1-4 and 1-5). The angular gyrus appears to contain the rules that transform word pictures into an auditory form and probably those for the reverse operation as well. The use of written language is limited to man, and the angular gyrus apparently has developed late in phylogeny. The angular gyrus is present only in rudimentary form in some subhuman primates. Geschwind[6] points out that features suggesting its late development include variability in gyral structure, late myelination, and the paucity of inputs from thalamus to angular gyrus. Once reading has been learned, an individual confronted with a word must pass the image of this word through the angular gyrus of his dominant hemisphere in order to understand the word. Since it apparently is necessary for at least an internal audition of the word to occur, the individual must be able to evoke the auditory equivalent as well. Therefore, the adjacent auditory association cortex (Wernicke's area) must be intact or reading will fail because the auditory equivalent cannot be released. An intact occipital lobe does not appear to be required for the act of writing, but the angular gyrus is necessary. It permits the individual to obtain an internal image of the word he wishes to write.

The angular gyrus, then, is an association cortex that has inputs from other association cortices. Of particular importance with regard to reading and writing are the inputs from the auditory association cortex and the visual association cortex of both sides. It is the programming of the angular gyrus during one's education that makes one literate. Regardless of one's previous education, a lesion that destroys the angular gyrus renders one illiterate, as if one had never learned to read and write.

Pseudoalexia

It would be best to begin this section on pseudoalexia with a comment about pseudonormality. The ability to read is frequently tested by asking the patient to read aloud. Sometimes patients can read aloud but cannot comprehend what they read. Geschwind has seen two such cases. One of the patients had been deaf since late childhood. These patients may have lesions of Wernicke's area, but for some reason they do not have to go through Wernicke's area in order to be able to read aloud.

One category of pseudoalexia that should not be overlooked is the primary illiterate patient, the patient who has never learned to read or write. I have seen several patients advertised as alexic who actually had never learned to read or write. This category includes patients who are educationally deprived as well as patients with developmental dyslexia who have remained dyslexic into adult life. Both types of illiterates are likely to be ashamed of their disability and may not admit that they never learned to read.

Another group of patients who will appear alexic when they are not are patients with hemianopias. The patient with a right hemianopia is less likely to have reading difficulties than the patient with a left heminanopia; however, some patients with macula-splitting, right hemianopias compensate poorly for the defect in seeing the letters that follow the ones they are looking directly at. This is relatively uncommon but can cause trouble with reading. Patients with a left hemianopia have trouble getting to the beginning of the next line of text, and this is likely to be troublesome. Some of them may also have features of visual neglect to the left, and this may contribute to the pseudoalexia.

Some patients with Broca's aphasia appear to have difficulty in reading individual letters or words aloud. Here one has the reverse of the pseudonormal patient. A patient with Broca's aphasia usually can understand the words he reads aloud, even though he reads them aloud incorrectly.

Another type of aphasia that may produce a pseudoalexia is conduction aphasia. In this form of aphasia a lesion interrupts the connection between Wernicke's and Broca's areas. The lesion is usually in the parietal operculum.

Speech is fluent and comprehension is intact, but the patient has a severe disturbance in repetition and cannot read aloud. The limitations of testing for alexia by reading aloud should be obvious in light of the aphasic pseudo-alexias.

Aphasic alexia

True alexia due to aphasia is common. Wernicke's aphasia is probably the most prevalent aphasia associated with alexia. Wernicke's aphasia is characterized by fluent speech, impaired repetition, and poor comprehension. It is due to a lesion in the auditory association area of the dominant hemisphere. True alexia is also found in the syndrome of isolation of the speech area. In this syndrome, lesions surround Wernicke's and Broca's areas as well as the interconnecting arcuate fasciculus. There is intact repetition of material without any comprehension. The patient understands no written or spoken language because he does not have access to Wernicke's area. These lesions also tend to involve the angular gyrus.

Alexia with agraphia

Alexia with agraphia results from a lesion in the angular gyrus of the dominant hemisphere (Fig. 1-6), as was shown conclusively by Dejerine.[37] As noted above, the patient loses the ability to evoke the sound of words that he sees. A functional angular gyrus is necessary for the individual to remain literate. A lesion within it makes the patient unable to read or write.

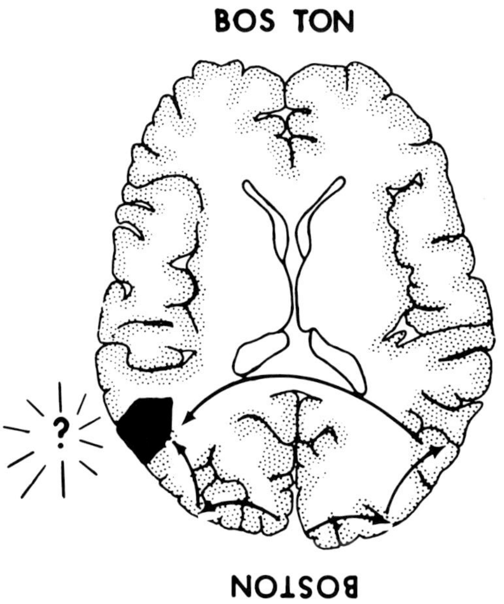

Fig. 1-6. Diagram showing the lesion in the syndrome of alexia with agraphia.

Previously familiar languages seem like foreign languages. If you ask the patient to spell a word, he will not be able to do so. If you spell a word to him, he will not be able to tell you what the word was. Like illiterates, these patients perform flawlessly with spoken language. Only when required to read or write do they manifest their difficulty. They cannot interpret word pictures and they cannot evoke the images of words in order to write them down. If the lesion is superficial in the angular gyrus, there will not be a hemianopia, but if the lesion is deep, a hemianopia may be present. Lesions in this region may also produce left-right disorientation, problems in calculating, finger agnosia, and word-finding difficulty.

Alexia without agraphia (pure word blindness)

Alexia without agraphia is less common than alexia with agraphia, but it is by no means rare. Patients with this syndrome cannot read but they can write. An understanding of this syndrome is of central importance in understanding some of the brain mechanisms that underlie other visual disorders of higher function. There is some disagreement as to who first described alexia without agraphia, but certainly the most important early contribution was that of Dejerine.[38] The patient he described was an elderly man who had had a stroke that had left him unable to read but had not affected his ability to write. He had no difficulty with spoken language. He had a right hemianopia. Dejerine suggested that the patient not only had a lesion in the left occipital lobe, which would prevent any input of visual material to the angular gyrus from the left hemisphere, but also a lesion in the corpus callosum, which would impair the transfer of information from the right visual cortex to the left side (Fig. 1-7). When this patient died and was autopsied just such lesions were found. Patients with alexia without agraphia do not become illiterate. While they do not understand written words, they can recognize words that are spelled to them, and they can spell words that they are requested to spell. In contrast to their inability to read words and a lesser problem in reading individual letters and Roman numerals, these patients generally do well with Arabic numerals. It may be that in learning numerals as a child, one forms many nonvisual associations (for example, counting with the fingers). Therefore, information about numbers may cross the corpus callosum further "upstream." Some patients with alexia without agraphia also cannot name colors. Such defects are the commonest form of cerebral defects in color vision in patients who still have some retention of primary visual function. Patients with color naming defects cannot match the correct name of a color to the color, but they can see the colors, as can be shown by having them place pieces of paper of the same color in piles. They perform flawlessly. They also read the pseudoisochromatic charts normally. They simply do not know what name to associate with a particular color.[39] In rare instances patients with alexia without agraphia may manifest prosopagnosia (see below) or visual object agnosia. Some patients lose the ability to read music although they do not have difficulty in learning new tunes by ear.

The pathologic lesions found in Dejerine's case have been present in the majority of cases of alexia without agraphia. However, patients have been reported in whom there was no right homonymous hemianopia. Such cases may be due to involvement of the splenium of the corpus callosum and the left visual association cortex or its connections. Conceivably, single subcortical lesions in the angular gyrus, critically placed, could have the same effect. A patient described by Geschwind for which no autopsy data were available had a left hemianopia. It was due to a right occipital cortex lesion that rendered the patient alexic. He previously had had a vascular accident, probably in the left posterior parietal region. Therefore, he had no input from the right because the right visual cortex was destroyed, and he could not get into the angular gyrus from his intact left occipital lobe because the connections between it and the angular gyrus were destroyed.

After left occipital lobectomies, patients frequently have a transient syndrome of alexia without agraphia.[40] The duration is usually too long to be explained by edema impairing transcallosal transmission. The phenomenon probably results from the existence of a pathway from right visual association cortex that crosses the corpus callosum to reach the left visual association areas. It only then proceeds to the left angular gyrus. The main pathway is probably directly from right angular gyrus across to the left angular gyrus.

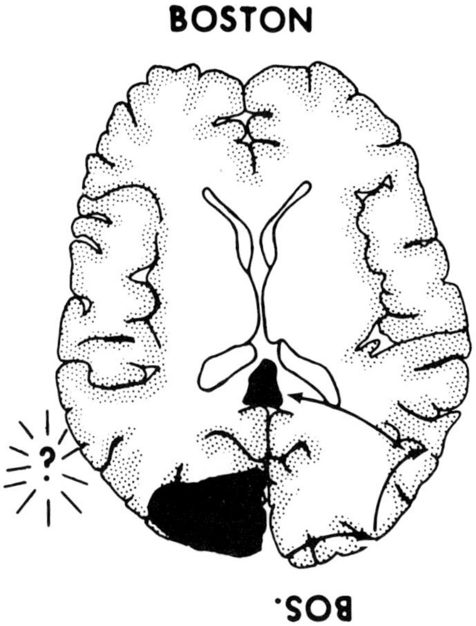

Fig. 1-7. Diagram showing the lesions that produce the syndrome of alexia without agraphia.

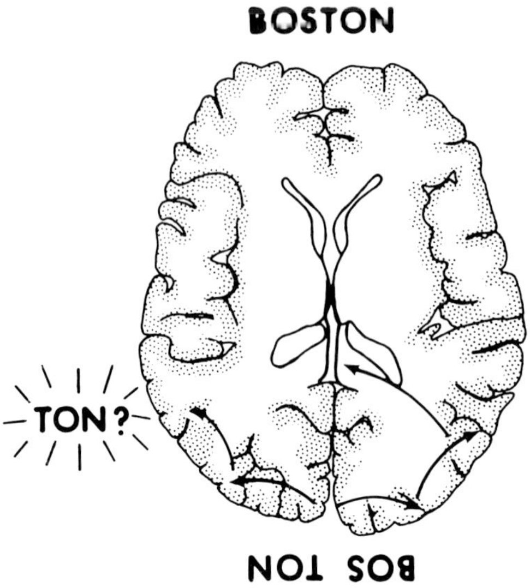

Fig. 1-8. Diagram showing how a lesion in the splenium of the corpus callosum produces a left hemialexia.

In the occipital lobectomy patients, this pathway ultimately takes over. Geschwind[6] has pointed out that there may be some permanent effects of the lesions in the alternate pathway, since David and co-workers[40] have indicated that patients with left occipital lobectomies do not like to read. The The importance of the splenium seems well established. After surgical procedures in which the splenium of the corpus callosum is sectioned, such as in the direct surgical attack upon lesions within the third ventricle, alexia develops, but only in the left visual field (Fig. 1-8).[41] In such postoperative hemialexics, information from the left occipital lobe is unimpeded in reaching the angular gyrus for interpretation, but nothing from the right will cross over. The defect is permanent. More anterior transsections of the corpus callosum fail to produce this syndrome.[42]

Some cases of alexia without agraphia are due to tumor, but the syndrome seems to be exceedingly rare after trauma. This is probably because one would be unlikely to get the appropriate concordance of lesions after an injury. Certainly the vast majority of cases of pure alexia are due to vascular disease. The majority of these are occlusions of the left posterior cerebral artery. It is important to look for alexia in patients with right homonymous hemianopia. Among uncomplaining patients and those with vague visual complaints one will find some with the syndrome of alexia without agraphia. These patients manufacture all kinds of excuses to explain their reading difficulty. They may say, for example, that they really need a change in glasses or that it is their field defect that makes them unable to read. Don't be fooled into believing that it is the hemianopia per se. It may be possible to demonstrate conclusively that the patient really can see well by showing that he can read off a long line of Arabic numerals that are written quite small when he is unable to read large letters comprising simple words, regardless of their orientation.

The third type of true, nonaphasic dyslexia

Recently Dr. Martin Albert and associates[43] at the Aphasia Unit of the Boston Veterans Administration Hospital have called attention to a third variety of true, nonaphasic alexia. Like the other true, nonaphasic alexias, it was described many years ago by Dejerine. In 1904 Dejerine and Thomas[44] reported an example of alexia with agraphia in which the patient was able to spell requested words and recognize words spelled to him. In contrast to other cases of alexia with agraphia, this patient was not illiterate. Dejerine and Thomas suggested that the patient had the same lesions as those found in alexia without agraphia but that there was an additional lesion that disconnected the angular gyrus from the area subserving control of the left hand. Only the left hand could be tested because the patient had a severe right hemiplegia. The patient described by Albert and associates was a 57-year-old, right-handed man who had a left tempero-occipital glioma removed in January, 1971. He had a residual right homonymous hemianopia. Eleven months later, he developed right-sided motor seizures and had headaches, vomiting, and abnormal gait. He had some word-finding difficulty. He could not read and was severely agraphic, but he could spell orally and understood words that were spelled to him. Despite his inability to read, special testing showed that the patient had a considerable ability to understand written words. For example, he was given lists of three words that resembled a test word, either phonemically or semantically. He did quite well in identifying the correct word. When shown a single written word and asked to select one of three pictures named by that word, he performed quite well. He did well on an odd-word-out test; given a series of five words, four of which belonged to the same semantic category, he could pick out the word that did not belong. In another test, he was shown a series of words and asked to select from the list words of a particular semantic category, such as parts of the body. He did very well on these. As Albert and associates pointed out, "he was able to extract much more information from the written word than his performance on clinical reading tests would indicate." He was also asked to inspect words and see if they were in their correct form. The words were doctored in various ways, including inversion, reversal, and replacement of a letter. Nonsense words and foreign words were also included. He was able to tell whether the words were English and what errors were present. Albert and associates commented that "in the light of these results, the conclusion seems justified that the patient's perception and semantic comprehension of written letters or words are to all intents and purposes intact." They indicate that reading is not a single capacity but has components that may be differentially affected by lesions. In this patient they suggest that *phonemic* reading ability was lost, but *semantic* reading ability was preserved to some extent. The authors suggest that this is a third and distinct category of alexia, or more exactly, of nonaphasic, true alexia, but they failed to demonstrate the mechanism. The patients underlying lesion was undoubtedly a recurrence of a malignant glioma.

PROSOPAGNOSIA

Prosopagnosia refers to the circumstance in which a patient cannot recognize faces with which he was previously familiar. It is most strikingly manifested in the patient who cannot recognize his own face in the mirror. Charcot,[45] was probably the first to describe this disorder, which Bodamer[46] named prosopagnosia in 1947. One might expect that recognition of faces would not be affected differentially from the recognition of objects. Nevertheless, while most instances of prosopagnosia do occur in the setting of visual agnosia, there are instances of visual agnosia in which faces can be recognized but not objects, and instances of prosopagnosia in which there is no defect in the recognition of objects. If one considers the behavior of infants, the special importance of facial recognition and its fundamental value in the socialization of the individual become obvious. The first thing that the infant studies intently is the face of his mother. This face contact is present at 2 to 3 months of age. At this juncture, the infant will smile at a human face. The components of the face that the infant responds to have been studied in detail.[47] To respond appropriately, the child must see two eyes. The eyes may be the main area of the face upon which the infant concentrates. The child also responds to a mask until 3 or 4 months old. Thereafter he becomes capable of making the appropriate discrimination. This chronologic sequence is remarkably consistent in all societies regardless of the mode of rearing the child. By the time the child is 8 months old, the faces of unfamiliar persons elicit an unpleasant response. Also, instead of responding to a mask with a smile, the child now responds to the mask as if it were the face of a stranger. Ellinwood[48] has made an interesting analogy to imprinting. He comments "the smiling response is but a more sophisticated and prolonged anlage of imprinting. Both are initiated by perceptual configurations that are responded to and, in the process, the perceptual unit becomes the most significant general attachment the infant will have for the rest of his life." The conversion from a friendly to a fearful response when confronted with a strange face occurs at a characteristic age in each species. The time of this conversion apparently coincides with the beginning of ambulation. Thus, the prosopagnostic patient has lost what probably was his first visual recognition function, the ability to recognize faces of other human beings and differentiate between them.

In some patients with prosopagnosia, including Bodamer's original case, there is difficulty in recognizing animal faces or the difference between animals. Some patients cannot tell the difference between human faces and animal faces. In one case a patient who was adept at bird watching was unable to differentiate between birds when she lost her ability to recognize human faces.[49] The two faculties returned together when she recovered. In another instance,[50] a 50-year-old farmer who previously had an outstanding ability to recognize individual animals in large herds lost this ability. The underlying lesion was a stroke. He developed a left homonymous hemianopia with good retention of eye movements, visual acuity, memory, judgement, orientation, and language. He could read and write, and he had no difficulty with colors. There was agnosia for objects. He had severe prosopagnosia, not only for people but also for animals. When he returned to his farm from the hospital two weeks after the stroke, he was unable to recognize individual animals that he had been able to recognize previously. He did not know how he had previously been able to do it, but he had certainly lost the ability. Eighteen months later, he had improved considerably with regard to both animal and human face recognition.

How does failure of facial recognition come about in neurologic disease? In some patients it is simply an additional category of failure of recognition, no different from that of the recognition of words, objects, or colors, and must share the same mechanism. In the cases in which it occurs in circumscribed form, various explanations have been proposed. Bay[24] has suggested that constriction of the visual field to an effective field of less than 5° is responsible for most cases. When the field is so constricted, the patient allegedly cannot survey the entire face at once and therefore loses the gestalt of the face. That defect alone should not be a problem, since patients with visual fields absolutely constricted to less than 5° have been known to be able to recognize faces. Another explanation that has been offered is that recognition of faces is lost as a result of *simultanagnosia* in which the affected person is allegedly unable to synthesize all the features in an array. This concept, introduced by Wolpert[51] in 1924 and emphasized by Luria,[28] has been offered as the explanation for other visual agnostic problems. Whether the limitation in simultanagnosia is primarily sensory or motor is unclear. Balint's syndrome[52] probably represents an example of this. Balint's original patient is particularly important because he could recognize single objects regardless of their size. If the problem were fundamentally sensory, one wouldn't expect that type of performance. In his detailed analysis of a case of Balint's syndrome, Tyler[53] found a difference between the way in which his patient explored a picture and the way in which normals explored them. Normals exploring a picture fixate a few highly informative areas. Tyler's patient did not look at objects in a reproducible fashion. She could not go to the places in a picture that would give her the most information. This would impair the synthesis necessary for the interpretation of what it was that she was seeing. Tyler reported that "it seemed as though she would visually explore in detail any areas she saw and did not or could not make visual relating movements to other areas. She often 'lost' the object, usually when her very restricted, effective field of vision left the area." The eye movements of the patient were abnormal in that the longer eye movements, which are thought to help in relating bits of visual information to one another,[54] were abnormal. Could such a motor or sensory defect, including real or effective field constriction, explain a defect in the recognition of faces? I think not. With a single fixation of a small picture corresponding to about 5° normals can recognize a face. Perhaps the patient's effective field constriction or defective exploration of scenes would result in defective recognition only when there was in addition some defect in intellect or memory. If a normal scans a complex object bit by bit by moving a small aperture over the object, he usually is able to identify the object. By comparison, Tyler's patient said the following when confronted with an American flag: "I see a lot of lines, now I see some stars. When I see things like this, I see a lot of parts. It's like you have one part here and one part there, and you put them together to see what they make." Faced with these clues, most would make a reasonable guess that they were dealing with a flag. Simply because a patient sees only one small part of an object at a time does not in and of itself preclude recognition.

Weigl[55] has questioned several of Wolpert's concepts of defects in recognition based upon so-called simultanagnosia. Weigl believes that in cases where details were perceived but not the meaning as a whole, there is evidence of defective recognition of the individual details. Those details with characteristic cues, which should in themselves alert the subject, have apparently lost their cognitive value. As Weigl states, "the perception of the picture does not come about only on the basis of gnostic processes, but with the participation of cognitive ones." He thinks there are automated processes that are defective in the brain. Certain individuals with brain disease cannot reactivate stored-up optical stereotypes. Weigl thus brings a Pavlovian interpretation to these problems in recognition.

In contrast to the view that the exploration of the entire face is necessary for recognition, and important in light of what I have mentioned regarding the development of facial recognition in children, is the emphasis by Bodamer[46] on the eyes. Bodamer said that the ocula, the area composed of the eyes and root of the nose, was the important area of focus in the recognition of faces. Gloning and co-workers[56] found that some patients with prosopagnosia had difficulty in matching fragments of faces that included the eye region with the corresponding full faces. If this is true, it certainly does not characterize all cases of prosopagnosia, since this has not been demonstrated in patients evaluated by DeRenzi and colleagues.[57] In some instances there may be a defect in the revisualization of faces that causes the defect in recognition. In the process of recognizing a face one probably compares it in one's mind to those seen before. The very term recognition emphasizes that fact. It is also possible that in some cases there is a subtle defect in visual function. Benton and Gordon[58] showed that there was a relationship between facial discrimination and the discrimination of differential brightness patterns. In some cases there may be distortion of faces that causes the failure of recognition. These cases represent a kind of aperceptive prosopagnosia. Tyler[53] has suggested that facial recognition is of a different order of difficulty than object recognition because it calls for "more fine recognition of details, relation of lines and shadows and shadings, than for example, recognizing an object as a cup or a vase."[59] I do not disagree. Clearly we know many scores of faces and can discriminate and recognize them on the basis of remarkably subtle differences. We readily recognize faces that we are unable to describe in detail. But sensory defects alone are unlikely to be a common cause for prosopagnosia because many patients with prosopagnosia are able to match pictures of unfamiliar persons. There isn't good correlation between the occurrence of prosopagnosia, the inability to recognize familiar faces, and the discrimination of unfamiliar faces. Many individuals with right hemisphere lesions have some difficulty in the discriminating of unfamiliar faces,[60] but few of these patients have clinical prosopagnosia. As far as I know, there is only one well studied case in which there was prosopagnosia as well as a defect in the discrimination of unfamiliar faces.[58] In the other cases of prosopagnosia in which facial recognition was tested for unfamiliar faces, discrimination of unfamiliar faces was intact. The defect in many cases is thus one of disturbed memory for faces. It has been suggested that prosopagnosia may be a circumscribed form of amnesia. Meadows[61] points out that if this is the case, it is surprising that faces learned in the remote past are not recognized in prosopagnosia. In patients with more generalized amnestic syndromes, faces that were learned in the distant past can still be recognized. It is only new faces that cannot be memorized in such cases. I am inclined to think that there may be both an associative and an aperceptive type of facial agnosia or prosopagnosia. The evidence seems to parallel that for both object agnosia and the recognition of colors. The necessary pathologic condition for all these is probably bilateral posterior hemispheric disease or unilateral disease with the additional involvement of the corpus callosum or other commisural tract.

Meadows[61] has made some valuable observations regarding the lesions in prosopagnosia. He has shown that there is not only a preponderance of right-sided lesions in reported cases but also a tendency for the lesions to be inferior. This is reflected by involvement of the left upper visual field in a high proportion of cases. In 14 of 15 cases of bilateral homonymous hemianopia and in 19 of 19 cases of left homonymous hemianopias, the upper quadrant was involved. In four cases there was a right hemianopia only; however, two of the patients subsequently were autopsied and had right occipitotemporal lesions. In all autopsied cases of prosopagnosia reviewed by Meadows there were bilateral lesions. In all of them the right occipitotemporal area was involved. The left-sided lesions have been posterior, and the majority were occipitotemporal. Meadows suggests that damage to the inferior longitudinal fasciculus near its occipitotemporal origin may disconnect an area of occipitotemporal cortex specialized for facial recognition from temporal lobes. Similar lesions in monkeys are known to affect visual discrimination.

SUMMARY

With the exception of geniculocalcarine blindness, all the conditions described above involve so-called higher functions, levels of neural integration that go beyond simple seeing. Geniculocalcarine blindness has relevance, not only because it sometimes precedes or follows other higher disorders of visual function, but because patients with geniculocalcarine blindness may deny their blindness as a result of other nervous system dysfunction.

Some physicians deny localizing value to many of the higher functions. Specifically, they doubt some of the pathologic-clinical relationships I have discussed in this report. It is tempting to throw one's hands up in despair when confronted by the meager data available on many of the behavioral syndromes and disorders of higher function. Much of the requisite neuroanatomy, -physiology, -pharmacology, -pathology, and -chemistry are not yet available. But I believe that these syndromes are as amenable to interpretation on the basis of focal brain lesions as are primary sensory and motor disorders. The disorders of higher function provide an especially tempting challenge to the clinician in practice because he can make meaningful contributions based on single cases. By recognizing patients with these disorders, carefully recording their symptoms and signs, and meticulously examining the brain, he can provide data that will help in understanding cerebral function. No technology, no matter how sophisticated, can substitute for such clinical-pathologic correlations. It is a chance to return to the discipline of clinical observation that began with Charcot and Jackson and their contemporaries in English and European ophthalmology and neurology and that is our professional heritage.

REFERENCES

1. Hoyt, W. F., Rios-Montenegro, E. N., Behrens, M. M., Eckelhoff, R. J.: Homonymous hemioptic hypoplasia. Its funduscopic features in standard and red free illumination in three patients with congenital hemiplegia, Br. J. Ophthalmol. **56:**537-545, 1972.
2. Cohn, R.: Visual evoked responses in the brain injured monkey, Arch. Neurol. **21:**321-329, 1969.
3. Von Monakow, A.: Experimentelle und pathologish-anatomische Untersuchungen uber die Beziehungen der sogennanten Sehspare zu den infracorticalen Opticus-

centrem und zum Nervus opticus, Arch. Psychiatr. Nervenkr. **16**:151-199, 1885.
4. Dejerine, J. and Vailet,: Sur un cas de cecite corticole, Compt. Rendu. Soc. De Biol. **4**:983-987, 1893.
5. Anton, G.: Uber die Selbstwahrnehmung der Herderkrankungen des Gehirns durch den Kranken bie Rindenblindheit und Rindentaubheit, Arch. Psychiatr. Nervenkr. **32**:86, 1899.
6. Geschwind, N.: Unpublished lectures on behavioral neurology given at Harvard University Medical School, 1973.
7. Teuber, H., Battersby, W. S., and Bender, M. D.: Visual field defects after penetrating missile wounds of the brain, Cambridge, Mass., 1960, Harvard University Press, p. 88.
8. Pritchard, E.: Case of amaurosis following violent convulsions, Proc. R. Soc. Med. **11**:1-2, 1917-1918.
9. Ashby, H., and Stephenson, S.: Acute amaurosis following infantile convulsions, Lancet **1**:1294-1296, 1903.
10. Gowers, W. R.: Epilepsy and other convulsive diseases, Lancet **1**:1295, 1903. Cited in Ashby and Stephenson.[9]
11. Teuber, H., Battersby, W. S., and Bender, M. D.: Visual field defects after penetrating missile wounds of the brain, Cambridge, Mass., 1960, Harvard University Press, p. 103.
12. Russell, W. R., and Whitty, C. W. M.: Studies in traumatic epilepsy. III. Visual fits, J. Neurol. Neurosurg. Psychiatry **18**:79-96, 1955.
13. Kooi, K. A.: Episodic blindness as a late effect of head trauma. Electrophysiological study of 3 cases, Neurology (Minneap.) **20**:569-573, 1970.
14. Mirsky, A. F., Bloch, S., Tecce, J. J., Lessell, S., and Marcus, E.: Visual evoked potentials during experimentally induced spike-wave activity in monkeys, Electroencephalogr. Clin. Neurophysiol. **34**:25-37, 1973.
15. Humphrey, N. K.: What the frog's eye tells the monkey's brain, Brain Behav. Evol. **3**:324-337, 1970.
16. Pasik, T., and Pasik, P.: The visual world of monkeys deprived of striate cortex: Effective stimulus parameters and the importance of the accessory optic system, Vision Res. **13**(suppl. 3):419-435, 1973.
17. Schilder, P., Pasik, T. and Pasik, P.: Extrageniculostriate vision in the monkey II. Demonstration of brightness discrimination, Brain Res. **32**:383-398, 1973.
18. Pasik, T. and Pasik, P.: Extrageniculostriate vision in the monkey. IV. Critical structures for light vs. no-light discrimination, Brain Res. **56**:165-82, 1973.
19. Pasik, P. and Pasik, T.: Extrageniculostriate vision in the monkey. V. Role of accessory optic system, J. Neurophysiol. **36**:450-457, 1973.
20. Raisman, G.: Neuronal plasticity in the septal nuclei of the adult rat, Brain Res. **14**:25-48, 1969.
21. Munk, M.: Erfahrungen zu Gunsten der Localization, Verh. Physiol. Ges. Berl. 16 (March 30), 1887.
22. Lissauer, H.: Ein Fall von Seelenblindheit nebst einem Beltrage zur Theorie derselben, Arch. Psychiatr. and Nervenkr. **21**:2-50, 1889.
23. Freud, S.: Zur Auffassung der Aphasien, Deuticke (Leipzig), 1891.
24. Bay, E.: Disturbances of visual perception and their examination, Brain **76**: 515-550, 1953.
25. Bender, M. D.: Neuro-ophthalmology. In Baker, A. B., editor: Clinical neurology, New York, 1962, Paul B. Hoeber, Inc., pp. 275-347.
26. Critchley, M.: The problem of visual agonsia, J. Neurol. Sci. **1**:274-290, 1964.
27. Bender, M. D., and Feldman, M.: The so-called "visual agnosias," Brain **95**: 173-186, 1972.
28. Luria, A. R.: Disorders of "simultaneous perception" in a case of bilateral occipito-parietal brain injury, Brain **82**:437-449, 1959.
29. Teuber, H. L.: Alteration of perception and memory in man. In Weiskrantz, L., editor: Analysis of behavioral change, New York, 1968, Harper & Row, Publishers.
30. Benson, D. F., and Greenberg, J. P.: Visual form agnosia. A specific defect in visual discrimination, Arch. Neurol. **20**:82-89, 1969.
31. Rubens, A. B., and Benson, D. F.: Associative visual agnosia, Arch. Neurol. **24**:305-316, 1971.
32. Benson, D. F., Segarra, J., and Albert, M. L.: Visual agnosia-prosopagnosia: A

clinical pathological correlation, Arch. Neurol. **30:**307-310, 1974
33. Geschwind, N.: Language and the brain, Sci. Am. **226:**76-83, 1972.
34. Geschwind, N.: Disconnexion syndromes in animals and man. I, Brain **88:**237-294, 1965.
35. Geschwind, N.: Disconnexion syndromes in animals and man. II, Brain **88:**585-644, 1965.
36. Benson, D. F., and Geschwind, N.: The alexias. In Vinken, P. J., and Bruyn, G. W., editors: Handbook of clinical neurology, Amsterdam, 1969, North-Holland Publishing Co., vol. 4, pp. 112-140.
37. Dejerine, J.: Sur un cas de cecite verbale avec agraphie, suivi d'autopsie, Mem. Soc. Biol. **3:**197-201, 1891.
38. Dejerine, J.: Des differentes varietes de cecite verbale, Mem. Soc. Biol. **4:**61-90, 1892.
39. Geschwind, N., and Fusillo, M.: Color-naming defects in association with alexia, Arch. Neurol. **15:**137-146, 1966.
40. David, M., Hecaen, H., Angelergues, R., and Magis, C.: Les tumeurs occipitales, Neuro-chirurgie **1:**85-108, 1955.
41. Trescher, J. H., and Ford, F. R.: Colloid cyst of the third ventricle. Report of a case: Operative removal with section of corpus callosum, Arch. Neurol. Psych. **37:**959-973, 1937.
42. Gazzaniga, M. S., and Freedman, H.: Observations on visual processes after posterior callosal section, Neurology (Minneap.) **23:**1126-1130, 1973.
43. Albert, M. L., Yamadori, A., Gardner, H., and Howes, D.: Comprehension in alexia, Brain **96:**317-328, 1973.
44. Dejerine, J., and Thomas, A.: Un cas de cecite verbale avec agraphie suivi d' autopsie, Rev. Neurol. (Paris) **12:**655-664, 1904.
45. Charcot, J. M.: Un cas de supression brusque et isolee de la vision mentale des signes et des objects (formes et couleurs), Prog. Med. **11:**508-582, 1883.
46. Bodamer, J.: Die Prosop-agnosie, Arch. Psychiatr. Nervenkr. **179:**6-53, 1947.
47. Spitz, R.: The first year of life, New York, 1965, International Universities Press.
48. Ellinwood, E. H.: Perception of faces, Psychiatr. **43:**622-646, 1969.
49. Bornstein, B.: Prosopagnosia. In Halpern, L., editor: Problems of dynamic neurology, New York, 1963, Grune & Stratton, Inc.
50. Bornstein, B., Sroka, H., and Munitz, H.: Prosopagnosia with animal face agnosia, Cortex **5:**164-169, 1969.
51. Wolpert, I.: Die Simultanagnosia. II, Ges. Neurol. Psychiat. **93:**397-415, 1924.
52. Balint, R.: Seelenlahmung des Schauens', optische Ataxie, raumliche Storung der Aufmerksamkeit, Monat. Psychiat. Neurol. **25:**51-81, 1909.
53. Tyler, H. R.: Abnormalities of perception with defective eye movements (Balint's syndrome), Cortex **4:**154-171, 1968.
54. Mackworth, J. F., and Bruner, J. S.: Selecting visual information during recognition by adults and children. Publication Harvard University Center For Cognitive Studies, July 1966.
55. Weigl, E.: Some critical remarks concerning the problem of so-called simultanagnosia, Neuropsychologia **2:**189-207, 1964.
56. Gloning, I., Gloning, K., Hoff, H., and Tschabitscher, H.: Zur Prosopagnosie, Neuropsychologia **4:**113-131, 1966.
57. DeRenzi, E., Faglioni, P., and Spinnler, H.: The performance of patients with unilateral brain damage on face recognition tasks, Cortex **4:**17-34, 1968.
58. Benton, A. L., and Gordon, M. C.: Correlates of facial recognition, Trans. Am. Neurol. Assoc. **96:**146-150, 1971.
59. Tyler, H.: Cerebral disorders of vision. In Smith, J. L., editor: Neuro-ophthalmology, vol. 4, St. Louis, 1968, The C. V. Mosby Co., pp. 266-281.
60. Yin, R. K.: Face of recognition by brain-injured patients: A dissociable ability? Neuropsychologia **8:**395-502, 1970.
61. Meadows, J. C.: The anatomical basis of prosopagnosia, J. Neurol. Neurosurg. Psychiatry **37:**489-501, 1974.

Chapter 2

Higher disorders of visual function: positive phenomena

Simmons Lessell

In Chapter 1 I described and discussed disorders of higher function that alter seeing and recognizing. Those disorders are manifested by a lack of function—impaired recognition of faces or objects, impaired vision, and impaired ability to read. This chapter is concerned with two symptoms of disorders of higher function in which too much is seen. These symptoms are paliopsia and visual hallucinations. They are probably closely related pathogenetically, but I will discuss them separately.

PALIOPSIA

MacDonald Critchley[1] introduced the term *paliopsia.* He indicated that it was a phenomenon of "visual perseveration in time." Patients with paliopsia continue to see objects after they have left their field of vision. The terms *paliopia, paliopsia, palinopsia,* and *palinopia* are synonymous. The following case report describes a patient with paliopsia.

Case report. A previously healthy 36-year-old man fell from the fourth story of a building while at work. He incurred a cervical fracture and was left with a quadriparesis and a sensory level at the sixth cervical segment. For a period of six months thereafter while hospitalized in a rehabilitation setting, he had a fever with spikes of temperature as high as 104.6° F. This fever defied explanation by an army of consultants and a plethora of laboratory tests. It failed to respond to a variety of antibiotics. Seven months after the accident, in the midst of this same siege of fever, the patient suddenly developed a severe right-sided headache and vomited. Examination by a physician a few minutes later showed that he was having a left focal seizure and had a left hemiparesis and left hemianopia. Later in the day the examiner found a bilateral homonymous hemianopia. An electroencephalogram showed spike waves in the right occipital region. Skull x-rays, brain scan, and lumbar puncture were uninformative. In the course of the next few weeks the hemianopias apparently cleared. The patient continued to have intermittent attacks that were presumed to be seizures. Approximately nine months after his injury he began to complain of some difficulty in the right field of vision. Examination at that time showed a right homonymous inferior quadrantanopia that was congruous and did not extend to the periphery. Opticokinetic testing showed poor responses when targets were rotated towards his right side; on forced closure, the eyes deviated to his left. Subsequently, the character of his focal seizures changed in that there would be deviation of the eyes to the left. Several months later neuro-ophthalmic reexamination was sought because of intermittent visual blurring. This was associated with headache and seemed related to obstruction of a urethral catheter. At that time, for the first time, he admitted that for a period of six weeks he had been experiencing a peculiar visual phenomenon. When he looked at a face or an object he might continue to see it for a period of many minutes. It sometimes annoyed him, and it made it difficult for him to watch television. But he had not been sufficiently disturbed by the illusions to request help from his doctors. In fact, he amused himself by placing the palioptic image of one doctor's beard on the faces of the nurses. He showed off his trick by literally rereading the Snellen chart from his perseverated image 20 minutes after he left the examining room. The palioptic images might be in any part of his visual field. Onset of the illusion was contiguous in time with his last view of the object. There was no interval during which the object disappeared. His paliopsia continued for two years and then abated. At no point did he experience geniculocalcarine visual loss, visual agnosia, metamorphopsia, or any visual distortions. The cause of his bilateral cerebral hemispheric disease and fever were never identified.

Paliopsia is a rare symptom. I personally have recognized it only three times in my own patients. Despite its rarity, there is an abundance of literature on the subject, possibly because of the intriguing, quasiparapsychologic nature of the symptom. Paliopsia was most recently reviewed by Bender and associates,[2] who also described a group of their own patients. Their observations and those of others have indicated the following about paliopsia:

1. Paliopsia is almost never an isolated visual symptom. Among the other symptoms that are commonly present are visual hallucinations in the traditional sense and hemianopias. Some patients with paliopsia also experience a spread of the visual image into surrounding space. This can result in distortions (metamorphopsia). These distortions may occur only in certain directions and may effect only certain portions of the image. Critchley[1] calls this "visual perseveration in space" or "illusory visual spread." There may also be visual allesthesia, in which objects appear displaced from their true position in space. Some patients with paliopsia may have monocular diplopia or polyopia on a cerebral basis. Bender and co-workers[2] have suggested that some patients with cerebral monocular diplopia or polyopia may actually be seeing the extra objects as a manifestation of the paliopsia.

2. Perseveration of other sensations may occur. One of my patient's had both auditory and visual perseveration. The auditory perseveration made it sound to her as if there were an echo, and this interfered with her ability to understand conversation.

3. Paliopsia tends to occur in evolving lesions. It is compatible with a variety of lesions, including neoplastic, vascular, and traumatic types and

toxic disorders, and sometimes occurs as an ictal phenomenon. The only major category in which I have not found it described is in degenerative diseases of the brain. Quite possibly I have overlooked examples of paliopsia in degenerative disorders in my review of the literature.

Hallucinogenic drugs such as mescaline and lysergic acid diethylamide (LSD) can produce paliopsia. In Critchley's original paper[1] there is a description of a woman who had used mescal. While waiting for a bus in Picadilly Circus, she saw several camels appear in the stream of traffic. She assumed that this was an effect of the mescal. The entire scene then changed to a desert, and when a bus arrived, the conductor appeared to be an Arab. At intervals thereafter, any place at which she steadily looked appeared to turn into a desert "peopled with camels and Arabs." This continued for hours. The next day she learned that while she had been standing in Picadilly Circus a group of camels had actually paraded through!

4. Palioptic images can be seen in any part of the field of vision. However, there is a tendency for them to occur in the half fields in which there is impaired acuity.

5. There is usually little or no interval between the exposure to the stimulus and the onset of the perseverated image. Once it appears, the image may intrude on the patient's vision for a period of minutes or, less commonly, hours or days. In general, paliopsia occurs only as a transitory phenomenon that persists for a period of weeks or days. But there are patients in whom it goes on for years.

6. A review of cases of paliopsia suggests that the symptom can arise from lesions in many loci and that the lesion need not involve the primary visual pathways. The majority of the patients have had lesions in the right cerebral hemisphere. In the series of Bender and co-workers,[2] 11 of 12 patients had lesions in the right hemisphere. The only consistent feature in patients with paliopsia in whom there has been a focal lesion has been involvement of the posterior half of one or both of the cerebral hemispheres.

In contemplating the mechanisms by which paliopsia might occur, one would do well to consider the characteristics of the physiologic afterimage (Table 2). What is the relationship between the afterimage that normals experience and paliopsia? Bender and co-workers[2] found no alteration of the physiologic afterimage in their own cases of paliopsia. Palioptic images usually do not have the characteristics of the normal afterimage. Exception can be found in the patients reported by Kinsbourne and Warrington.[3] They suggested that the normal afterimage somehow becomes enhanced in patients with paliopsia.

If a single mechanism is to explain paliopsia, it must involve something other than the accentuation of the physiologic afterimage and be capable of resulting from lesions in either or both hemispheres and from lesions that do not directly involve the primary visual pathway. I think of paliopsia as in-

Table 2. Characteristics of afterimage*

Intensity and duration is related to intensity and duration of original stimulus
Apparent size increases with distance to surface on which it is projected
Against dark background image is same color as stimulus. Against light background the colors are complimentary
Blinking or flashing light helps elicit it
Sequential images may be seen concurrently
Seen by both eyes if only one eye is stimulated
Image moves in same direction as active eye movement. With passive eye movement, image either appears immobile or moves in opposite direction

*Modified from Bender, M. B., Feldman, M., and Sobin, A. J.: Palinopsia, Brain **91:** 321-338, 1968.

voluntary visual memory, limited to the most recent events. It could represent the release of a circuit between areas of visual memory and visual association such that a recurrent sequence of storage and retrieval occurs. Thus paliopsia would be due to an uninhibited reverberating circuit.

VISUAL HALLUCINATIONS

Esquirol[4] introduced the term *hallucinations* at the beginning of the nineteenth century. He defined hallucinations as false sensory impressions not due to disease of the sense organs. For reasons that will be apparent, this definition is no longer entirely suitable. Perhaps a better operational definition of a visual hallucination would be a symptom in which the patient claims to see something or behaves as if he sees something that the observer cannot see. This definition would include a dream. Dreams will be treated only in relation to insights that they provide into the mechanisms by which other visual hallucinations occur.

It should be emphasized that it is impossible to verify a patient's contention that he is having hallucinations. It is also impossible to distinguish between the willed visual images that imaginative people can conjure and visual hallucinations.

Unformed visual hallucinations in disorders of the peripheral visual apparatus

Unformed visual hallucinations (sparks, flashes, blobs of light, spots, pointlike scintillations, and so on) can occur in normals and in patients with local eye and optic nerve lesions. For example, normal individuals may become aware of their own retinal circulation, as in Scheerer's phenomenon.[5] They see moving points of light, particularly when looking at the sky or at a bright field of snow. The moving objects appear to travel in arcs or lines and then disappear. The images may represent white blood cells as they travel through retinal capillaries. Many normal adults have opacities in the vitreous of the eye whose images may be projected into the environment. The images may drift or move when the subject's eye moves. If there is bleeding from the retina into the vitreous, the patient may see clouds of such spots. The sudden appearance of a shower of floaters is therefore an indication for careful ophthalmoscopy. It is well known that mechanical stimulation of the retina may produce sensations of light, demonstrated, for example, by the phenomenon of seeing stars when punched in the eye. Traction of the vitreous upon the underlying retina may give rise to sensations of light that are called phosphenes. There are several such phosphenes, the most typical and common of which is Moore's lightening streaks.[6] These are seen in the temporal field and appear vertical. They may occur in one or both eyes and tend to occur in dim illumination. Although Moore believed that they disappeared after a period of months, they can remain with patients for years. Similarly, traction on the retina in the posterior pole may give rise to phosphenes on quick eye motion.[7] According to Nebel[7] this "flick phosphene" is best observed in the dark-adapted, well-rested eye. When the eyes are flicked with the lids closed, the patient may briefly observe a bright pattern. This hallucination is described as lines arcing temporally to fixation in the central portion of the visual field. Retinal detachment may also produce phosphenes.

The phosphenes of ocular origin may be mistaken for symptoms of brain disease. Other positive visual symptoms that originate in the eye can mislead the physician into believing that there is a brain lesion. For example, metamorphopsia is characteristic of certain maculopathies. Even in a neuro-ophthalmic practice the great majority of cases of metamorphopsia I have seen have been due to retinal lesions rather than secondary to cerebral lesions. Monocular diplopia and polyopia, which can occur with cerebral disease, are more commonly due to refractive errors, early cataracts, or other local ocular problems. In certain disorders of the retina and optic nerve there may be unformed visual hallucinations at the outset of the illness. I have seen this in central retinal artery occlusions, ischemic optic neuropathies, optic neuritis, and compressive lesions of the optic nerve. It should be noted that an early theory concerning the origin of visual hallucinations held that they all originated in the eye.[8] This type of thinking has not entirely disappeared. Oster[9] suggested that the visual hallucinations of LSD intoxication are due to an increased state of awareness of stimuli that are always there but are not seen. For example, the image of the meshwork of the nerves and blood vessels in the retina is alleged to be the nucleus for the development of hallucinations. Macley and Guttman believe that mescaline-induced hallucinations in artists may have the same foundation.[10]

Visual hallucinations in normal people

Formed visual hallucinations, in which actual objects or people are seen, can occur in healthy people. Among children, formed visual hallucinations are quite common and may become extensively systematized so that the child has imaginary human or animal companions.[11] Estimates of the frequency with which this occurs vary, but imaginary companions are seen most often by pre-school-aged children. These children frequently believe in their companions and may show considerable interaction with the imaginary friend. Such hallucinations are not only entirely normal but may in some way be helpful to the psychologic development of the child. Other normal children may experience isolated episodes of visual hallucinations. The images are usually of animals or people, and the child believes in their existence. These visual hallucinations do not occur in relation to any physical illness or ongoing psychopathology. Some adults, whose psychiatric status may not be entirely normal, may fantasy imaginary sexual partners. It is difficult to decide if these are hallucinations; this will be discussed further in the section on hallucinations in psychiatric disease.

The commonest forms of visual hallucination in psychiatrically and physically healthy adults are hypnagogic and hypnopompic.[12] The former are hallucinations that occur on going to sleep, and the latter are those that occur on awakening. These hallucinations occur in the twilight between sleep and wakefulness, consist of very realistic visions, and rarely have an auditory component. They are not under voluntary control. In fact, if the person attempts to concentrate upon them they may vanish. The images may be formed or unformed, and they can be frightening or pleasant. Some patients seem able to will them simply by closing their eyes. In a casual survey of professional friends, about one-fifth admitted to such hallucinations. Several of them find them so entertaining and satisfying that they look forward to them and may even go so far as to use techniques to prevent falling asleep. One person keeps his television set on for a long period of time so that he can witness the visual display that occurs almost every night. In at least one disease state, narcolepsy, similar hallucinations may occur.

Visual hallucinations in psychiatric illness

Among children with behavioral problems related to psychoneurosis and social deprivation who come to the attention of psychiatrists, visual hallucinations appear common. The hallucinations they describe seem to be very rich in content related to the patient's social circumstances and psychopathology. Auditory accompaniments are frequently present. Whereas auditory hallucinations are uncommon in nonschizophrenic adults, they commonly occur in nonschizophrenic children with behavioral problems and neuroses. Doctor Loretta Bender[13] found auditory hallucinations in 10% of such children and visual hallucinations in 5%. Lukianowicz[14] found that almost 12% of a large group of nonpsychotic children with psychiatric problems had hallucinations, most frequently encountered under extreme stress as a manifestation of anxiety. They were more often visual than auditory but occasionally were both auditory and visual. The hallucinations in these children seemed to involve wish fulfillment, exterior displacement of anxiety, expressions of hostility, guilt, fear, or punishment, and a reliving of traumatic events. The relationship of the hallucinatory content to the patient's life situation was quite obvious. For example, one of the boys described by Lukianowicz felt guilty because he masturbated and would hallucinate the face and "all seeing eye of God" whenever he wanted to masturbate. Unlike in adults, whose hypnagogic hallucinations are generally unrelated to their life stresses and experiences, emotionally loaded material may color the content of hypnagogic hallucinations in children. Hysterical hallucinations also may occur in children; they are likely to be quite obviously related to the patient's situational stress. Such hysterical hallucinations tend to be multisensorial, involving hearing, vision, and touch, and engender a great emotional response. Children are more likely than adults to believe that their hallucinated images are real.

I mentioned earlier the occurrence of imaginery sex partners among adults. A great many adults with such histories actually began to have imaginary sex partners when they masturbated in childhood.[15] Many of the patients with imaginary sexual partners, heterosexual or homosexual, have significant associated psychopathology. The imaginary sex partners always seem to fill a need. Heterosexual individuals always have heterosexual imaginary sex partners, and homosexual patients have appropriate companions. The patient's particular fetishes may be reflected in what he sees. The psychopathology manifested by these patients encompasses the entire gamut of inpatient psychiatric diagnosis.

Auditory hallucinations, particularly when there is voice content, are most characteristic of schizophrenia. Pure visual hallucinations are rarely encountered among schizophrenics. Pure visual hallucinations in the presence of disease occur overwhelmingly in structural and toxic disorders of the central nervous system. Isolated hallucinations of voices are decidely rare among people with structural and toxic diseases of the nervous system. In sharp contrast to this view stands a recent report by Goodwin and associates[16] in which they indicate that visual hallucinations may be more common in psychotic patients than has been previously suggested. Psychotic patients are said to be more likely to believe in their hallucinations and to interact with them than are patients with structural brain disease. I have personally seen sufficient exceptions to that generalization to make me dubious about its use as a diagnostic feature in differentiating between so-called functional disorders and structural disorders.

Sensory deprivation hallucinations

Sensory deprivation can potentiate hallucinations.[17] Visual hallucinations may occur even when visual deprivation is not a prominent feature.[18] It has happened in isolated prisoners of war, people who are lost, and individuals on long automobile rides and airplane flights. Similarly, visual deprivation due to patching of the eyes after cataract extraction and the visual loss after unilateral enucleation are recognized causes of visual hallucinations. These varieties seem more common in elderly patients. While some of the patients find them pleasant, others find them exceedingly unpleasant. The majority of these patients experience complex visions—people, animals, and less commonly, objects. Sleep deprivation may also induce visual hallucinations. In his book on hallucinations, Lhermitte[19] tells of his own experiences in this regard.

Loss of vision also seems to potentiate visual hallucinations. Following the onset of blindness, patients not only have enhancement of the visual imagery in their dreams, which become more vivid with more intense colors, but while awake many of them have "visual experiences seemingly out of their control."[20] These visual hallucinations in the recently blind are generally unformed but occasionally are formed. They are most common shortly after visual loss has occurred. I have had personal experience with patients who had similar symptoms in the presence of unilateral or partial loss of vision. One was a 78-year-old woman recovering from ligation of the carotid artery for an aneurysm of the left posterior communicating artery. The vision in her left eye suddenly decreased from 20/20 to counting fingers while in the hospital, and I saw her within minutes. For the first two hours after her central retinal artery occlusion she experienced formed visual hallucinations. They consisted of bright, silver and gold fleur-de-lis that vibrated and scintillated. She saw them only if the involved eye was kept open. Visual information from the uninvolved eye apparently made no difference, since the hallucinations occurred whether it was opened or closed. In another patient who had bilateral disciform degeneration of the macula but still retained 20/400 visual acuity, the loss of vision was accompanied by constant visual hallucinations of fields of brightly colored violets that covered everything she looked at. While they were not threatening to her, they were very annoying. They covered her entire field of vision, although her scotoma involved only the central 10° in both eyes.

Lhermitte[21] stated that while the onset of an ophthalmopathy may bring on hallucinations, particularly in the elderly, there is usually some other contributing factor. He believed that this had often led him to discover unsuspected focal brain lesions. I have *not* discovered any unsuspected cerebral lesions among the patients I have evaluated for visual hallucinations associated with blindness.

What mechanisms account for visual hallucinations in sensory deprivation and blindness? It may be that sensory deprivation and visual loss somehow give rise to spontaneous discharges in the occipital lobes. This would be a phenomenon analagous to the cortex isole. One can produce spontaneous seizurelike discharges in cortex experimentally by physically isolating it.[22] In bilateral optic neuritis, electroencephalographic changes, including spike discharges, have been recorded from the occipital lobes.[23] Presumably the cortex is freed from inhibitory feedbacks and inputs by the lesion. It would appear from clinical experience, particularly the occurrence of hallucinations in blind half fields, that each hemisphere might independently behave as isolated cortex. There is also interhemispheric inhibition that at least is concerned with the areas corresponding to the visual field adjacent to the midline.[24] This probably is interrupted in certain of the lesions that cause occipital discharges. Further evidence indicating the relation of decreased sensory input to cortical activity concerns the ability to supress seizure discharges in some patients by specific sensory inputs. Most striking in this regard is the report of suppression of olfactory seizures in a patient with uncinate fits by the inhalation of substances having a particular odor.[25]

Visual hallucinations and drugs

There appear to be two mechanisms by which drugs precipitate visual hallucinations. In one, the drugs directly stimulate the visual areas of the brain, and in the other, withdrawal of drugs precipitates the hallucinations. Ethyl alcohol withdrawal typifies the second mechanism. Alcohol is primarily a depressant and does not appear to cause visual hallucinations. However, when the alcoholic stops drinking, hallucinations can occur. Similar sequences are seen in patients on high doses of meprobamate, chlordiazepoxide, glutethimide, and barbiturates.[26] According to Victor and Adams,[27] alcohol withdrawal symptoms begin within hours after cessation of drinking. Later the patient may have visual hallucinations. Initially these are present only when the eyes are closed, but later the patient continues to see the phantasms when the eyes are opened. At first the patient realizes they are not real, but as he progresses into the withdrawal state, losing insight because of confusion and agitation, his hallucinations seem real and may have a persecutory nature. At this point the patient may have frank delerium tremens with cardiovascular collapse and ensuing exhaustion. In some patients the hallucinations persist after recovery from delerium tremens. Not all sedatives and depressants cause hallucinations when they are withdrawn. The phenothiazines and diphenylhydantoin derivatives, both of which have sedative properties, are unlikely to cause visual hallucinations during or after treatment. Morphine, meperidine, and related drugs do not produce hallucinations while patients are taking them or upon withdrawal.

The drugs that produce hallucinations as a direct effect include parasympatholytic agents that are used topically in ophthalmology. Among these are scopolamine, atropine, and cyclopentolate. In the usual dose range and with topical application, central nervous system side effects are uncommon. But administration in higher dosages or swallowing of the eye drops may produce an organic psychosis, especially in children and the elderly. Visual hallucinations are virtually a constant finding, as are confusion, agitation, disturbances in memory, and a clouded sensorium. The patients are usually dry and have widely dilated pupils, tachycardia, and a cutaneous flush.

Cocaine and amphetamines also produce hallucinations. They are direct stimulators of the central nervous system. The abuser of these sympathomimetics regularly experiences an enhancement of mood and will continue to take the drug, despite the presence of toxic effects. After prolonged use of cocaine and amphetamines, a toxic psychosis may develop. Visual, auditory, and tactile hallucinations are very common. They occur in the face of a clear sensorium and with very little evidence of direct sympathomimetic effects. The clinical picture is difficult to distinguish from schizophrenia. Cessation of use of these drugs does not produce visual hallucinations or hyperactivity but tends to produce a depressed state, with fatigue and sleep.

Information about marijuana has only recently begun to become available. It is somewhat of a paradox pharmacologically in that it has some actions that mimic and enhance those of barbiturates and others that prolong the stimulant action of amphetamines. At "ordinary" doses, there is frequently a dreamy state with altered consciousness and disturbed perceptions, particularly involving time and distance. With very large doses, the patient may experience hallucinations. Withdrawal from marijuana produces minimal symptoms and no hallucinations.

LSD is the most potent of the hallucinogens. It is related to psilocybin and mescaline. The drug has a biologic half-life of about 3½ hours, and the LSD syndrome clears in about 12 hours.[28] Changes are usually perceived within minutes after administration. In the second or third hour visual symptoms become established. Micropsia and macropsia are often experienced, and occasionally, as noted above, paliopsia may also be present. Visual hallucinations of all kinds occur.[29, 30] The patient may or may not realize that what he sees are hallucinations. There are sometimes cross-overs from one sensory modality to another. The patient may hear colors or see sounds. The subject may perceive a change in the appearance of his body parts. With the eyes closed, there is a particular tendency for unformed visual hallucinations to occur. Van Rhijn has listed in detail the wide variety of content of the visual hallucinations in LSD intoxication.[30] There is no tendency towards stereotypy in the content of the hallucinations.

How does LSD produce hallucinations? It was once thought that its effect could be related to serotonin antagonism. This may be true, but some LSD derivatives that also antagonize serotonin do not produce visual hallucinations. If LSD interferes with serotonin, it appears to antagonize it as a competitive inhibitor. Recent work using organ-culture models consisting of serotonin-sensitive insect glands has demonstrated this effect.[31] LSD and related drugs directly stimulate the serotonin-sensitive cells. The effect continues even after the LSD is no longer bound. Another chemical hypothesis suggests that LSD interferes with synaptic transmission. A variety of electrophysiologic studies have also been reported. Purpura[32] found that LSD in doses up to 60 μg/kg facilitated cortical responses to photic stimulation in unanesthetized cats, but inhibition occurred with higher doses. The response of the cortex to stimulation of the lateral geniculate was facilitated with LSD. Apter and Pfeiffer[33] found that spontaneous retinal potentials occurred 10 minutes after 33 μg/kg of LSD were given to anesthetized cats. Simultaneous potentials were recorded from optic nerve and visual cortex. Sectioning the optic nerve eliminated the retinal discharges. Mescaline and LSD increased the time over which the ERG could be detected in the enucleated eye of the cat. Krill and associates[34] reported the effect of hallucinogenic agents on human retinal functions in normal subjects. Subjects receiving the agent at a dose sufficient to produce hallucinations had changes both in dark adaptation and the ERG. The ERG change was an increase in the scotopic b-wave amplitude. Many records showed an increase in the a-wave amplitude after larger doses of hallucinogens.

These data suggest several different mechanisms by which LSD could produce hallucinations. It could be that LSD inhibits serotonin-dependent cells in the reticular formation, resulting in the loss of input to occipital cortex. LSD could also deafferentate occipital cortex by impairing synaptic transmission. Finally, LSD could produce spontaneous potentials in the visual system.

Thorazine and other phenothiazines are potent antihallucinogens and will counteract the effects of LSD. How do phenothiazines work? They are known to have effects on all levels of the neuraxis.[35] The electroencephalogram shows changes when large doses are administered. There is a tendency to slowing, with low voltage, but this improves after a period of days or weeks. In animals the drug causes diminution in arousal and peripheral stimulation. Transmission across the corpus callosum is not affected by chlorpromazine, although chlorpromazine tends to normalize the depressant effect of amines and LSD on transcollosal responses. The phenothiazines also have important effects upon the basal ganglia. They decrease spontaneous firing of cells in the caudate nucleus and the globus pallidus, but they increase the firing rates in those nuclei after stimulation of the sciatic nerve. Thorazine enhances the response of the reticular formation to repetitive stimulation of the amygdala or globus pallidus paired with sciatic stimulation. Thorazine has depressant effects on the brain stem. Thorazine causes a decrease in the threshold for arousal produced by stimulation of the brain stem. It has a marked effect in blocking arousal produced by external stimuli. This is thought to indicate a selective effect of the drug on collateral pathways leading into the reticular formation. This contrasts to the mode of action of barbiturates, which act directly to depress the reticular formation. They produce a marked impairment of arousal regardless of the input. Some workers believe that Thorazine increases reticular activity, somehow producing a filtering effect that selects appropriate inputs.[36] There is also evidence that Thorazine impairs the uptake of catecholamines and 5 hydroxytryptamine by the brain. Which if any of these central nervous system effects of Thorazine is responsible for its anti-hallucinogenic properties is not known.

Visual hallucinations due to lesions of the midbrain and brain stem

Lhermitte[37] introduced the concept of midbrain hallucinations. He thought that lesions at the level of the peduncles were essential to their occurrence. It would seem that they can also occur in more caudal lesions. Pontine lesions were presumed to be the cause of hallucinations in a patient described by Garrel and associates.[38] They also described a case of midbrain origin. In both their cases the hallucinations were associated with insomnia. De Morsier[39] suggested that the hallucinations in patients with midbrain lesions may actually be due to associated thalamic lesions. The mechanism by which brain stem and midbrain hallucinations occur is unclear. Lhermitte believed it was somehow related to the induction of a dreamy state.[39] He stated that the usual combination of clinical findings is pathologic sleep, cerebellar signs, disorders of eye movement, and, sometimes, athetotic movements. The auditory hallucinations that infrequently occur are generally unformed and unrelated to the visions that the patient is experiencing. The patients tend to be sleepy but can be awakened, and they tend to have more hallucinations in the dark than in the light. The hallucinations are usually silent and mobile. They may be vivid pictures with bright colors that change like scenes in a motion picture. Some patients find them amusing, and authors have stated that peduncular hallucinations are rarely the cause of fear and anxiety. However, as Lhermitte has observed, peduncular hallucinations may produce fear and anxiety.

There is limited experimental data on the ability to elicit visual hallucinations by stimulation of the brain stem or midbrain. In 1970 Nashold[40] reported the results of stimulation of the midbrain in a 61-year-old man. The patient was being evaluated for phantom pain referred to his right arm, which had been lost due to an injury. Depth electrodes had been implanted in the left midbrain. Stimulation of an electrode estimated to lie beneath the surface of the superior colliculus and slightly dorsal to the Sylvian aqueduct produced phosphenes. The patient saw flashing lights that varied in intensity. The lights were of two varieties, "white or cold," arranged in straight or wavy lines. They were in his right visual field off the center and were superimposed on whatever he was looking at. In other patients, stimulation produced faulty spatial perception, and some commented on changes in the spatial relationship between real objects that they were observing (?visual allesthesia).

It would be profitable to consider dreams in considering the mechanisms by which brain stem lesions might produce hallucinations. Dreams fit the definition of hallucinations that I gave at the beginning of this chapter. Dement and associates[41] have observed that dreams represent the prototypical visual hallucinations. In recent years something has been learned of the neurophysiology and neurochemistry of dreams, and this information may be pertinent to the development of visual hallucinations after brain stem lesions. Apparently the best electroencephalographic correlate of dreams is not the rapid eye movement phase of sleep but rather discharges that have been called *PGO* (ponto-geniculo-occipital) *spikes.*[42] The data on which this conclusion is based were derived from observations on animals. The investigators assumed that the episodes of eye movement, sniffing, limb movement, vocalizing, and eye opening that occur during sleep in animals represented expressions of dream events. Since one cannot verify directly that animals dream, one must be cautious in applying the animal data to human dreams. PGO spike activity may be the basic ingredient in the production or energizing of vivid dream images. PGO spikes occur predominately during the REM phase of sleep but also occur to a lesser degree in nonREM sleep. PGO spikes can be potentiated by interrupting impulses ascending from the medial raphe nuclei of the pons. This can be achieved by surgical ablation of these nuclei, splitting the brain stem, or by pharmacologic means. These nuclei are rich in serotonin, and the administration of serotonin-blocking agents can potentiate PGO spikes. For example, reserpine is capable of inducing PGO spikes in the awake cat.[43] Other inhibitors of serotonin also appear capable of doing this. The administration of similar powerful serotonin antagonists in humans may produce florid hallucinations.[44] It should be recalled that LSD is both a powerful serotonin antagonist and a powerful inducer of hallucinations.

Visual hallucinations due to diseases of the cerebral hemispheres

Visual hallucinations are frequently associated with focal cerebral lesions. Some of these hallucinations are of ictal origin, and much of the pertinent neurophysiologic data currently available is from epileptic patients. The studies of Penfield and associates,[45-47] using focal brain stimulation, have provided an abundance of information. Penfield and Jasper[46] used two terms to designate the visual experiences associated with sensory seizures. By *visual seizures* they meant either photisms or diminution in vision. Visual hallucinations with more complex features were referred to as *psychical hallucinations.* Stimulation of the occipital lobes of their subjects never produced psychical hallucinations. In the experience of Penfield and co-workers, stimulation of the occipital lobes of conscious patients produced only photisms, shadows, and colors. It should be acknowledged that in man, the primary visual cortex is not readily accessible to stimulation. Most of the stimulations of the occipital lobe performed by Penfield and associates were actually in areas 18 and 19. The patients were quoted as describing the images from occipital stimulation as "flickering lights, dancing lights, colors, bright lights, stars, wheels, blue, green, and red colored discs, fawn and blue lights, colored whirling balls, radiating gray spots becoming pink and blue, a long white mark."[45] The investigators studied the effect of repeated stimulation by keeping the electrode in place and restimulating. Sometimes the subject would experience the same sensation, but at other times the subject would experience different sensations. Sometimes stimulation in the same place would produce the same image in a different location. Most of the images that were produced moved. They moved slowly or "danced, flickered or whirled in a given part of the visual field."[45] In instances in which the calcarine cortex itself was probably stimulated, the crude visual sensations were always in the contralateral field. Stimulation of prestriate and parastriate cortex produced visual impressions that might be located anywhere in the field of vision. In many patients with focal occipital seizures, and in the majority of experimentally induced seizures, the hallucinated images seemed to be located in front of the patient. Stimulation of the temporal lobe tended to produce psychical hallucinations. Penfield and associates believed that some of these were complex memories. They also reviewed cases of spontaneous focal seizures in which visual hallucinations occurred and found that the relation between the location of the lesion and the type of visual experience was the same as that found in the focal stimulation of those areas in conscious patients. When they occurred, unformed visual hallucinations tended to be mobile and bright. When formed hallucinations occurred, there were often distortions in the size of the figures, which were often brightly colored. In fact, formed black and white hallucinations are uncommon under any circumstances. Ictal and induced visual hallucinations are usually silent.

Formed hallucinations in cerebral disorders may occur in any part of the visual field and may be integrated with the environment. For example, small hallucinated figures may jump into the patient's hand or lap. One patient whom I interviewed claimed that he saw a truck drive up to the side of his hospital room and unload furniture through the window, which was closed. He was certain that it was a hallucinatory experience because he knew he was on the eighth floor of the hospital. Hallucinations of cerebral origin can be three-dimensional or two-dimensional. On rare occasions a visual hallucination may be associated with other sensory phenomena. Most notable is the association of hallucinated odors, generally unpleasant, with formed images in patients with uncinate fits. Hallucinations can assume or intrigue the patient, but some frighten the patient. Some of the hallucinations are quite believable to the patient, but others are clearly unreal. In some hallucinations, the patient may see himself or parts of himself.

Clinical and experimental evidence generally support the concept that formed hallucinations in cerebral disorders are typically associated with temporal and temporoparietal lesions. Photisms are more typical of posterior lesions. However, these generalizations break down too often for them to be employed as rules. Occipital lesions may produce formed hallucinations and temporal lesions may produce unformed hallucinations. Both types of hallucinations can coexist in a patient who has only one lesion. There is a tendency for stereotypy in a particular individual's visual hallucinations if they are of cortical origin. For example, ictal visual hallucinations are almost identical in a given patient from one episode to another. There is also a tendency for hallucinations to occur in hemianopic fields. A striking clinical observation has been the tremendous preponderance of right-sided lesions in association with visual hallucinations.[48]

There seem to be no features of visual hallucinations themselves that can help the physician determine the nature of the underlying pathologic condition. Migraine may be an exception. Visual hallucinations are a common feature of migraine. They are almost invariably unformed and characteristically expand and scintillate in a jagged fashion. This is thought to be correlated with the spread of cortical excitation and inhibition due to anoxia from vasospasm. I have often seen such hallucinations in patients with migraine. The only other situation in which I have seen it is in patients with lupus. Presumably, while the mechanism is vascular, it is peculiar to these diseases, since other vascular lesions tend not to produce the same phenomenon.

I have never seen a focal frontal lesion produce visual hallucinations unless it compressed or infiltrated visual pathways. However, unformed visual hallucinations were reported by one author in association with frontal lobe tumors.[49] Unfortunately, the tumors were not described in detail, and it is not known whether the patients had visual failure or compression of visual pathways.

SUMMARY

In the preceding section I have described positive visual phenomena that occur in normals and in patients with brain or ocular diseases or who use drugs. In essence, this has been a review of visual hallucinations. In Fig. 2-1 I have attempted to summarize mechanisms by which visual hallucinations might occur. While it would be satisfying to identify a single pathogenetic theme, the evidence suggests that there are multiple causes. Visual hallucinations can occur under a variety of circumstances, experimental and spontaneous, physiologic and pathologic. There is little or nothing inherent in the features of a given hallucination that will permit the physician to ascertain the nature of the responsible lesion. Generally, pure visual hallucinations in adult patients with a clear sensorium are not psychiatric in origin. If formed, the hallucinations are likely to be associated with a temporal lobe lesion; if unformed, they are likely to be occipital or ocular in origin. In a case of formed visual hallucinations due to focal brain disease, the chances are that the disease is in the right hemisphere. While these generali-

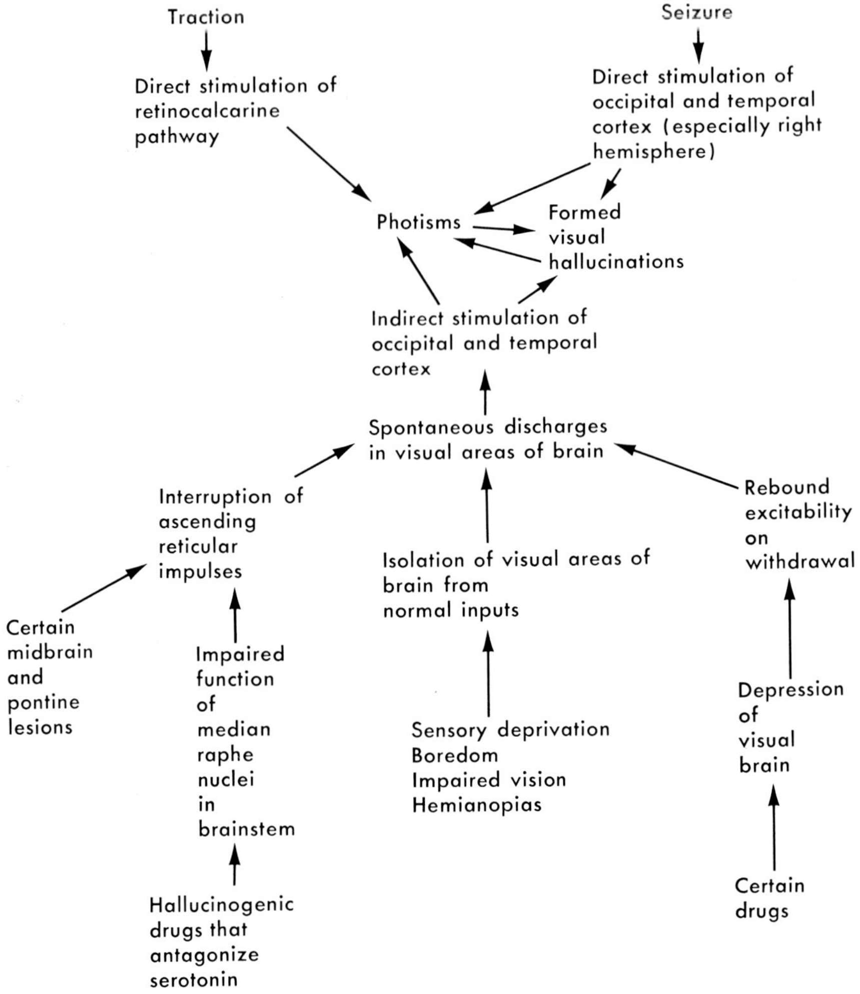

Fig. 2-1. Possible pathways for the development of visual hallucinations.

zations are largely true, exceptions are sufficiently common to make one reluctant to place absolute reliance upon them. On the other hand, one should not look upon visual hallucinations as worthless localizing symptoms. Just because a clinical phenomenon has many possible origins does not negate its importance. An analogy might be made to hypotension. It can occur physiologically or patholgically. It can be drug induced or drug reversed. It may indicate a serious disease in any one of a variety of organ systems. Since so many causes are capable of producing hypotension, it has poor localizing value. However, one certainly would not ignore hypotension in a patient and would at least explore the relevant possibilities and associations that would lead to the correct cause of the hypotension. The situation concerning visual hallucinations is similar. Hallucinations can be physiologic or pathologic, drug induced or drug reversed. They may reflect serious disease or be due to relatively inconsequential and readily reversible problems. Lesions in many loci may cause them, but their occurrence must alert the physician to search diligently for the appropriate cause.

REFERENCES

1. Critchley, M.: Types of visual perseveration: "Paliopsia" and "Illusory visual spread," Brain **74**:267-299, 1951.
2. Bender, M. B., Feldman, M., and Sobin, A. J.: Palinopsia, Brain **91**:321-338, 1968.
3. Kinsbourne, M., and Warrington, E. K.: A study of visual perseveration, J. Neurol. Neurosurg. Psychiatry **26**:468-475, 1963.
4. Esquirol, J. E. D.: Alienation mentale. In Adelon et al., editors: Dictionnaire des sciences medicales, vol. 2, Paris, 1817, Panckoucke.
5. Scheerer, R.: Die entoptische Sichtbarkeit der Blutbewegung im Auge und ihre klinische Bedeutung, Klin. Monatsbl. Augenheilkd. **73**:67-107, 1924.
6. Moore, R. F.: Subjective lightning streaks, Br. J. Ophthalmol. **19**:545-547, 1935.
7. Nebel, B. R.: The phosphene of quick eye motion, Arch. Ophthalmol. **58**:235-243, 1957.
8. Horowitz, M. J.: The imagery of visual hallucinations, J. Nerv. Ment. Dis. **138**: 513-523, 1964.
9. Oster, G.: Moire patterns and visual hallucinations, Psychedelic Rev. **7**:33-40, 1966.
10. Marti-Ibanex, R.: The gates to paradise, MD **9**:11-15, 1965.
11. Bender, L., and Vogel, B. F.: Imaginary companions of children, Am. J. Orthopsychiatry **11**:56-65, 1941.
12. Lhermitte, J. Les hallucinations. Clinique et physiopathologie, Paris, 1951, G. Doin and Co., pp. 47-55.
13. Bender, L.: Hallucinations in children. In A dynamic psychopathology of childhood, Springfield, Ill., 1954, Charles C Thomas, Publisher.
14. Lukiancwicz, N.: Hallucinations in nonpsychotic children, Psychiatr. Clin. (Basel) **2**:321-337, 1969.
15. Lukianowicz, N.: Imaginary sexual partner. Visual masturbatory fantasies, Arch. Gen. Psychiatry **3**:429-449, 1960.
16. Goodwin, D. W., Alderson, P., and Rosenthal, R.: Clinical significance of hallucinations in psychiatric disorders. A study of 116 hallucinatory patients, Arch. Gen. Psychiatry **24**:76-80, 1971.
17. Flynn, W. R.: Visual hallucinations in sensory deprivation. A review of the literature. A case report and a discussion of the mechanism, Psychiatr. Q. **36**: 55-65, 1962.
18. Tyler, H. R.: Cerebral disorders of vision. In Smith, J. L. editor: Neuro-ophthalmology, vol. 4, St. Louis, 1968, The C. V. Mosby Co., p. 266.
19. Lhermitte, J.: Les hallucinations. Clinique et physiopathologie, Paris, 1951, G. Doin and Co., pp. 52-53.
20. Fitzgerald, R. G.: Visual phenomenology in recently blinded adults, Am. J. Psychiatry **127**:1533-1539, 1971.
21. Lhermitte, J.: Les hallucinations. Clinique et physiopathologie, Paris, 1951, G. Doin and Co., p. 80.
22. Echlin, F. A., and Battista, A.: Epileptiform seizures from chronic isolated cortex, Arch. Neurol. **9**:64-71, 1963.
23. Chattha, A. S., and Lombrosco, C. T.: Electroencephalographic changes in childhood optic neuritis, Electroencephalogr. Clin. Neurophysiol. **33**:81-88, 1972.
24. Ehlers, N.: An extramacular inhibition phenomenon demonstration. The hemianopic border in normal subjects, Acta Neurol. Scand. **46**(suppl. 43):265-266, 1970.
25. Efron, R.: The effect of olfactory stimuli in arresting uncinate fits, Brain **79**:267-281, 1956.
26. Jaffe, J. H.: Drug addiction and drug abuse. In Goodman, L. S., and Gilman, A., editors: The pharmacological basis of therapeutics, ed. 4, New York, 1970, The Macmillan Company, pp. 276-313.
27. Victor, M., and Adams, R. D.: The

effect of alcohol on the nervous system, Res. Publ. Assoc. Res. Nerv. Ment. Dis. **32:**526-573, 1953.

28. Aghajanian, G. K., and Bing, O. H. L.: Persistence of lysergic acid diethylamide in the plasma of human subjects, Clin. Pharmacol. Ther. **5:**611-614, 1964.
29. Van Rhijn, C. H.: Variables in psycholytic treatment. Paper presented at the Second Conference On the Use of LSD in Psychotherapy. Cited in Malitz and Kanzler.[30]
30. Malitz, S., and Kanzler, M.: Effects of drugs on perception in man, Res. Publ. Assoc. Res. Nerv. Ment. Dis. **48:**35-53, 1970.
31. Berridge, M. J., and Prince, W. T.: Mode of action of hallucinogenic molecules, Nature (New Biol.) **243:**283-284, 1973.
32. Purpura, D. P.: Electrophysiological analysis of psychotogenic drug action. I. Effect of LSD on specific afferent systems in the cat, Arch. Neurol. **75:**122-131, 1956.
33. Apter, J. T., and Pfeiffer, C. C.: Change in spontaneous and evoked potentials on the electroretinogram induced by drugs: strychnine, atropine, LSD-25, mescaline, Am. J. Ophthalmol. **45:**718, 1958.
34. Krill, A. E., Wieland, A. M., and Ostfeld, A. M.: The effect of two hallucinogenic agents on human retinal function, Arch. Ophthalmol. **64:**724-733, 1960.
35. Jarvik, M. E.: Drugs used in the treatment of psychiatric disorders. In Goodman, L. S., and Gilman, A., editors: The pharmacological basis of therapeutics, ed. 4, New York, 1970, The Macmillan Company, pp. 151-203.
36. Killam, K. F., and Killam, E. K.: Drug action on pathways involving the reticular formation. In Jasper, H. H., Proctor, L. D., Kinghton, S. S., Noshay, W. C., and Costello, R. T., editors: Reticular formation of the brain, Boston, 1958, Little, Brown and Company, pp. 111-222.
37. Lhermitte, J.: Syndrome de la calotte du pedoncule cerebral. Les troubles psycho-sensorials dans les lesions du mesocephale, Rev. Neurol. (Paris) **29:**1359-1365, 1922.
38. Garrel, S., Fau, R., Perret, J., and Chatelain, R.: Disturbances of sleep in two brain-stem vascular syndromes, one with anatomoclinical confirmation, Electroencephalogr. Clin. Neurophysiol. **23:**290, 1967.
39. De Morsier, G.: Les hallucinations etude oto-neuro-ophtalmologique, Rev. Otoneuro-ophtalmol. **16:**241-352, 1938.
40. Nashold, B. S., Jr.: Phosphenes resulting from stimulation of the midbrain in man, Arch. Ophthalmol. **84:**433-435, 1970.
41. Dement, W., Halper, C., Pivik, T., Ferguson, J., Cohen, H., Henriksen, S., McGarr, K., Gonda, W., Hoyt, G., Ryan L., Mitchell, G., Barchas, J., and Zarcone, V.: Hallucinations and dreaming, Res. Publ. Assoc. Res. Nerv. Ment. Dis. **48:**335-359, 1970.
42. Jouvet, M., Michel, F., and Courjon, J.: Sur un stade d'activite electrique cerebrale rapide au cours du sommeil psychologique, C. R. Soc. Biol. (Paris) **153:**1024-1028, 1959.
43. Delorme, F., Jeannerod, M., and Jouvet, M.: Effects remarquables de la reserpine sur l'activite EEG phasique ponto-geniculo-occipitale, C. R. Soc. Biol. (Paris) **159:**900-903, 1965.
44. Engelman, K., Lovenberg, W., and Sjoerdsma, A.: Inhibition of serotonin synthesis by parachlorophenylalanine in patients with the carcinoid syndrome, N. Engl. J. Med. **277:**1103-1108, 1967.
45. Penfield, N., and Rasmussen, T.: The cerebral cortex of man. A clinical study of localization of function, New York, 1968, Hafner Publishing Co., Inc.
46. Penfield, W., and Jasper, H.: Epilepsy and the functional anatomy of the human brain, Boston, 1954, Little, Brown and Company.
47. Penfield, W., and Perot, P.: The brain record of auditory and visual experience. A final summary and discussion, Brain **86:**595-696, 1963.
48. Teuber, H. L., Battersby, W. S., and Bender, M. B.: Visual field defects after penetrating missile wounds of the brain, Cambridge, Mass., 1960, Harvard University Press, pp. 104-105.
49. Tarachow, W.: The clinical value of hallucinations in localizing brain tumors, Am. J. Psychiatry **94:**1434-1442, 1941.

Chapter 3

Microscopic anatomy of the optic nerve

Douglas R. Anderson

INTRODUCTION

Optic nerve microanatomy was reviewed at a previous symposium,[1] but since that volume has not been widely available, a slightly revised reprinting of that chapter is presented here as a companion to the new subsequent chapter on mechanisms of optic nerve disease. The original sources of anatomic and physiologic information are not cited here, but the scholarly can find them in the bibliography of recent optic nerve studies[2-6] and three articles on glial cells.[7-9]

The optic nerve is made up of two compartments: the *neuroectodermal compartment,* the nervous tissue proper, and the *mesodermal compartment,* whose function is to support and nourish the neural tissue. These two compartments differ in structure and function and are best considered separately. The mesodermal compartment will be considered first, after which the neuroectodermal compartment will be investigated in much more detail.

MESODERMAL COMPARTMENT

The mesodermal compartment is a collagenous connective tissue that contains blood vessels. Apart from the blood vessels, the main cellular elements are fibroblasts and meningothelial cells. Within the mesodermal compartment are some nonmyelinated nerve fibers, namely the peripheral nervous system fibers that accompany the central retinal vessels. These are not part of the central nervous system visual fibers and are hence not considered part of the neuroectodermal compartment in this discussion.

Supported in part by U.S. Public Health Service Research Grant Number EY-00031 from the National Eye Institute, National Institutes of Health, Bethesda, Maryland.

Intraorbital portion of the optic nerve

The intraorbital portion of the optic nerve is completely invested by connective tissue in the form of meninges (Fig. 3-1). The dura mater is a dense connective tissue with very compact collagen and few vessels. The inner surface of the dura mater is lined by a layer of meningothelial cells that ultrastructurally are quite similar to fibroblasts, except that they lie at the surface of the collagenous tissue rather than within the collagen. These cells form a mesothelium that lines the potential subdural space between the dura mater and the arachnoid mater.

The arachnoid mater consists primarily of several layers of meningothelial cells. These cells are held together by desmosomes and contain cyto-

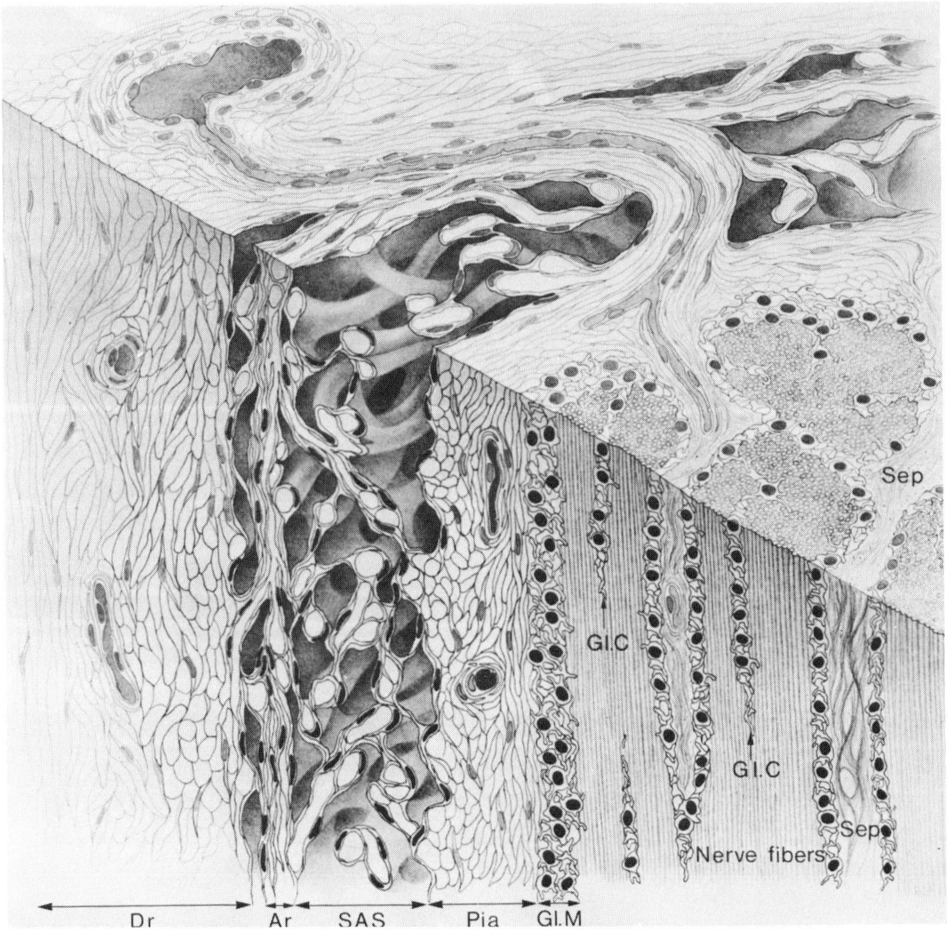

Fig. 3-1. Schematic drawing of vaginal sheaths of the human optic nerve, showing relationships of dura mater *(Dr)*, arachnoid mater *(Ar)*, subarachnoid space *(SAS)*, pia mater *(Pia)*, peripheral glial mantle of Fuchs *(Gl. M)*, pial septa *(Sep)*, and glial columns *(Gl. C)*. (From Anderson, D. R.: Arch. Ophthalmol. **82:**659, 1969.)

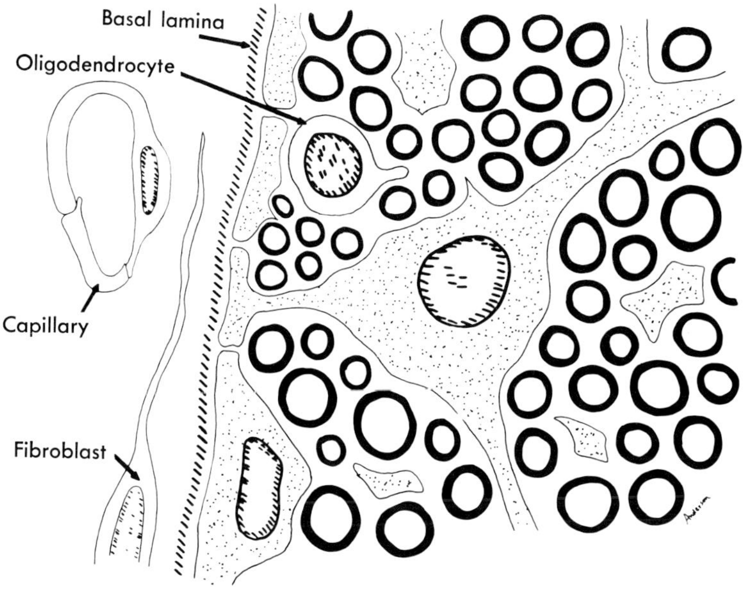

Fig. 3-4. Diagram of the boundary between mesodermal neuroectodermal compartments in the intraorbital portion of optic nerve. The boundary is marked by the basal lamina (basement membrane). Astroglial cells and foot plates (stippled) make a complete lining at the boundary, separating completely the oligodendrocytes and myelinated nerve fibers (black rings) from the mesodermal compartment, which contains a fibroblast and capillary. Note also that within the neuroectodermal compartment the various elements are separated by a thin extracellular space, and that there is a narrow extracellular space separating the astroglial cells and foot plates from one another at the mesodermal-neuroectodermal interface.

The astrocyte processes extend from the perinuclear cytoplasm (perikaryon) and insinuate themselves among the other neuroectodermal components, such as the myelinated axons and oligondendrocytes in the case of the intraorbital portion of the optic nerve. The shape of the external surface of the astrocytes conforms to the outer shape of the other neuroectodermal elements, so that the processes tend to fill in all the available space within the central nervous system.

At least some of the astrocyte processes end in the form of a foot plate that, in most of the central nervous system, makes contact with blood vessels. In the case of the optic nerve, the foot plates make contact with the pial septa (Fig. 3-4), which contains the blood vessels. These astrocyte processes along with a few astrocyte cell bodies make a complete lining not only along all blood vessels and each pial septum, but also wherever the neuroectodermal compartment makes contact with connective tissue. A basement membrane marks the boundary.

This universal relationship can be seen well in all parts of the optic nerve:

in the orbital portion of the optic nerve, where the astroglia form a lining along each pial septum; beneath the pia mater, where it is called the peripheral glial mantle of Fuchs, and around the central connective tissue core. This universal relationship is particularly well illustrated in the optic nerve head (Plates 1 and 2). Here it can be noted that not only does the glial tissue fill in the space between the collagenous sheets of the lamina cribrosa, but the edge of each perforation in the collagen sheet is lined with astroglia that thus separate the collagen of the connective tissue sheet from the nerve fibers passing through the perforation. An astroglial layer is also present along the inner surface of the scleral canal, where the astroglial tissue is known as the border tissue of Jacoby. Astroglia also form a lining layer over the surface of the disc, where the layer is known as the internal limiting membrane of Elschnig. This internal limiting membrane over the disc is quite analagous to the internal limiting membrane of the retina, which is made up of foot plates of Muller cells, which are modified astrocytes in the retina.

Thus the astrocytes form a complete lining layer that separates neuroectodermal components from mesodermal connective tissue. No other element of the neuroectodermal compartment ever makes direct contact with the mesoderm.

Several functions have been proposed for astrocytes, although it has been difficult to establish these functions with certainty. Astrocytes are usually considered the "connective tissue" of the central nervous system, providing support for the other elements and, by means of their long tenuous processes, holding them together in the proper relationships to allow neural function. This function of astrocytes is seemingly well illustrated in the optic nerve head. Here the arrangement of the astrocytes seems particularly well suited to support the optic nerve fibers as they make a 90° bend. Also, in this region the tonofilaments are particularly prominent in the astrocyte processes, and desmosomes seem to be more numerous.

Because of the relationship between astrocytes and blood vessels, it was previously thought that astrocytes were important to the nutrition of other elements in the central nervous system. In the early days of electron microscopy, when it was thought that the extracellular space of the central nervous system did not exist, it was thought that nutrients might pass from the capillaries into the foot plate cytoplasm, through which they would diffuse to reach axons that are remote from the capillaries. In this way astrocyte cytoplasm was envisioned to serve the same function that extracellular space serves in other parts of the body. This concept now turns out to be incorrect, and it is unsupported by recent physiologic data.

More careful inspection of electron micrographs has shown that there is a thin fluid-filled space between the various neuroectodermal elements (neuropil). Tracer studies and physiologic evidence have now shown that various substances can diffuse through this space and that the space is the ionic environment of the nerve fibers. It is thus a true extracellular space, and this space, not the astrocyte cytoplasm, serves the usual functions of extracellular spaces.

It has also been proposed from indirect evidence that astrocytes might act as a metabolic reservoir. In this capacity they would store substances that could be used to nourish the neural elements in times of acute but transient inadequacy of blood flow or in times of unusually great nervous activity that requires more than the usual nutrition. This concept is illustrated by the presence of glycogen in astrocytes that is rapidly consumed in periods of anoxia. While it may be a function of astrocytes, providing emergency nourishment other than glycogen has not been demonstrated.

Another important function attributed to astrocytes is the regulation of ions and water in the extracellular space between the cells. This function is quite hypothetical, and it is clear from physiologic data that the composition of extracellular fluid depends in part if not entirely on the composition of plasma, modified by hemodynamic factors and the blood vessel wall, just as it does elsewhere in the body. It has also been proposed that astrocytes serve to prevent the spread of impulses from one neurite to another by isolating synapses and preventing the spread of transmitter substance through the extracellular space. This hypothetical function does not apply to the optic nerve, where there are no synapses.

The astrocytes, then, are thought to contribute generally to the support and nurture of the other neuroectodermal components, but the details of how they perform this function are not completely worked out.

Oligodendrocytes and myelin

There are several kinds of oligodendrocytes with slightly different anatomic features, differing relationships to other neural structures, and biochemical differences. The oligodendrocytes are grouped together morphologically because in contrast they are smaller and have fewer processes than astrocytes. The kind of oligodendrocyte found in the optic nerve is the interfascicular oligondendrocyte, which is typically found in rows in the white matter tracts of myelinated nerve fibers.

By electron microscopy, oligodendrocytes have a small dense nucleus in comparison with astrocytes (Fig. 3-5). Surrounding the nucleus is a thin rim of cytoplasm that contains many ribosomes and no glycogen. Only occasionally does the plane of section happen to pass through one of the processes. Microtubules are seen regularly extending throughout the length of the oligodendrocyte process, and these microtubules extend into the perinuclear cytoplasm (Fig. 3-6). The microtubules serve as an identifying feature of oligodendrocyte processes, since the astrocyte processes contain filaments rather than microtubules.

The different types of oligodendrocytes presumably have different func-

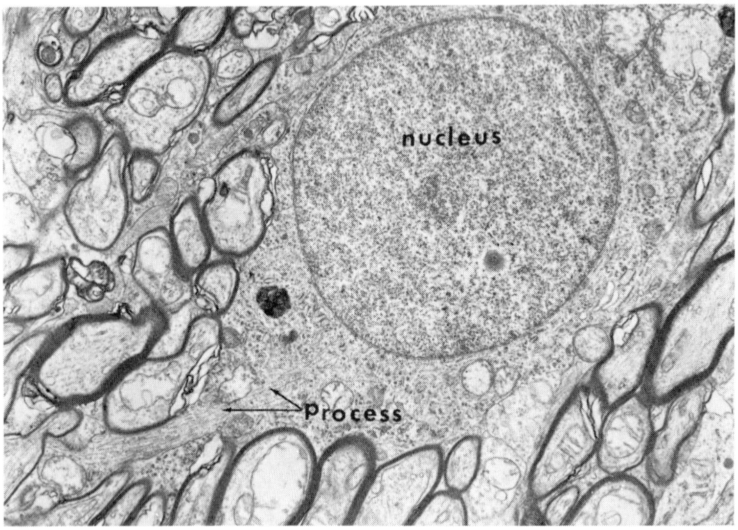

Fig. 3-5. Monkey optic nerve oligodendrocyte. The nucleus is surrounded by a narrow rim of cytoplasm from which cytoplasmic process emerges. (×20,000; from Anderson, D. R., and Hoyt, W. F.: Arch. Ophthalmol. **82**:506, 1969.)

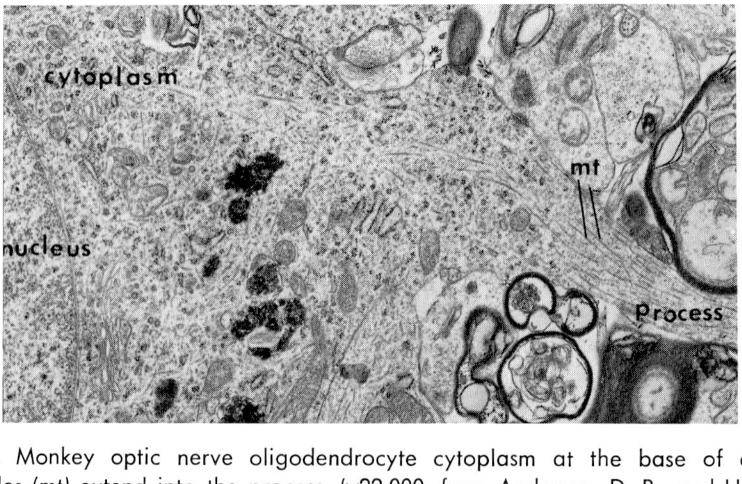

Fig. 3-6. Monkey optic nerve oligodendrocyte cytoplasm at the base of a process. Microtubules *(mt)* extend into the process. (×22,000; from Anderson, D. R., and Hoyt, W. F.: Arch. Ophthalmol. **82**:506, 1969.)

tions. For most of the varieties of oligodendrocytes, the function has not been thoroughly established. It is well established, however, that the interfascicular oligodendrocyte, as found in the optic nerve, is concerned with myelination. The oligodendrocytes are obviously needed to manufacture myelin, which consists of multiple layers of oligodendrocyte plasma membrane. In addition, oligodendrocytes, with their rich supply of enzymes and ribosomes and their high metabolic rate, are assumed to be necessary for the maintenance of myelin after it is formed.

Since the earliest microscopic studies, several lines of evidence have pointed to the oligodendrocyte as the source of myelin. Oligodendrocytes appear in the embryo at the time that myelination first begins. Secondly, wherever myelin is found in the central nervous system, oligodendrocytes appear conspicuously in rows within the white matter fiber tracts. This is particularly well illustrated in the case of the optic nerve, since oligodendrocytes are present in the orbital portion, which is myelinated, but are absent in the optic nerve head, where the nerve fibers are unmyelinated. Also, in silver-stained preparations oligodendrocytes are occasionally seen to send a process toward a nerve fiber and end at its surface as if attached to it.

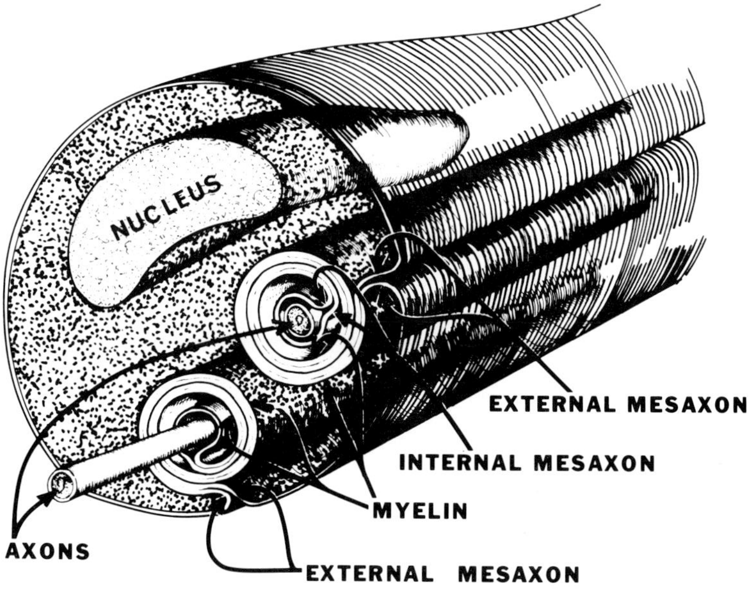

Fig. 3-7. Diagram of myelinated nerve in the peripheral nervous system. The myelin and the nerve fiber are enclosed within the Schwann cell cytoplasm. If analogy is made to the unmyelinated nerve fibers, it appears that myelin is formed by a spiral of mesaxon around the nerve fiber (Fig. 3-8). Between the outside of the Schwann cell and the myelin sheath is a mesaxon called an external mesaxon. There is also an internal mesaxon, which extends between the nerve fiber and the innermost layer of the myelin sheath.

Despite these observations, there was previously some doubt about whether the oligodendrocyte was responsible for myelination in the central nervous system. The doubts arose because oligodendrocytes were not seen in the peripheral nerves that are myelinated. In peripheral nerves, it was supposed that the Schwann cell was responsible for myelination, but doubt about this also arose because Schwann cells were not present in the central nervous system, even in the myelinated nerve tracts.

Uncertainties about the source of myelin were resolved with the advent of electron microscopy. With this technique it was clearly demonstrated that in the *peripheral* nervous system Schwann cells were responsible for the formation of myelin. The electron micrographs not only demonstrated the cell of origin for myelin but also provided the unexpected observation that in the peripheral nervous system myelin is formed by multiple wrapping of the plasma membrane of Schwann cells. The manner in which myelin is derived from the plasma membrane of Schwann cells is shown in Fig. 3-7. Compare this with the relationship of unmyelinated fibers to Schwann cells (Fig. 3-8).

In the central nervous system, myelin was found to consist of spiral

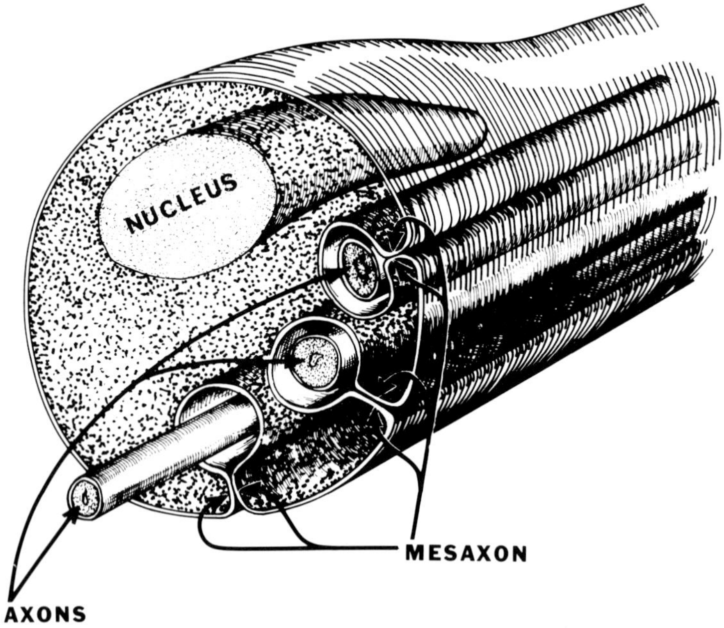

Fig. 3-8. Diagram of an unmyelinated nerve fiber in the peripheral nervous system. The nerve fibers (axons) are enclosed within the cytoplasm of a Schwann cell. A trough is present that represents the invagination of the nerve fiber from the surface of the Schwann cell. The opposed walls of the trough have been called a mesaxon, in analogy to the mesentery.

wrappings of plasma membrane just as in the peripheral nervous system. It was expected from the evidence cited above that the oligodendrocytes were the cell of origin for the myelin. In addition, it is now recognized that the cytoplasm trapped within the myelin or in the cytoplasmic loops at the node of Ranvier contain microtubules, which are typical of oligodendrocyte cytoplasm. It proved difficult, however, to demonstrate a direct connection between the myelin sheath and the plasma membrane of an oligodendrocyte.

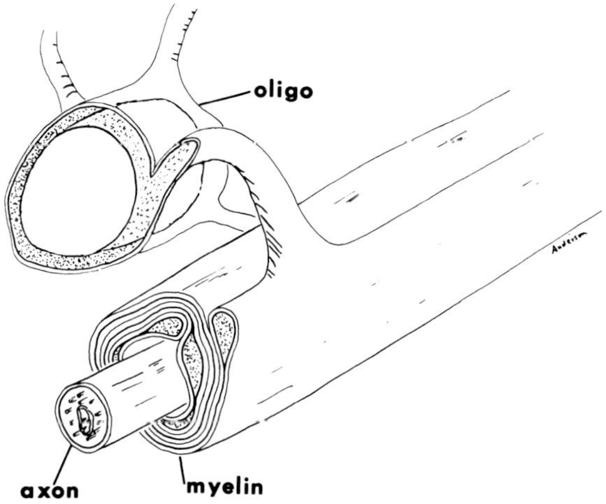

Fig. 3-9. Diagram of CNS myelin. In the central nervous system the myelin sheath is derived from the oligodendrocyte plasma membrane, but unlike in the peripheral nervous system, the myelinated nerve fiber is not enclosed within the cell cytoplasm. Therefore, there is no external mesaxon but rather a tag of cytoplasm on the external surface of the myelin representing the extension of oligodendrocyte cytoplasm. An internal mesaxon can be seen wherever oligodendrocyte cytoplasm has been trapped within the myelin sheath.

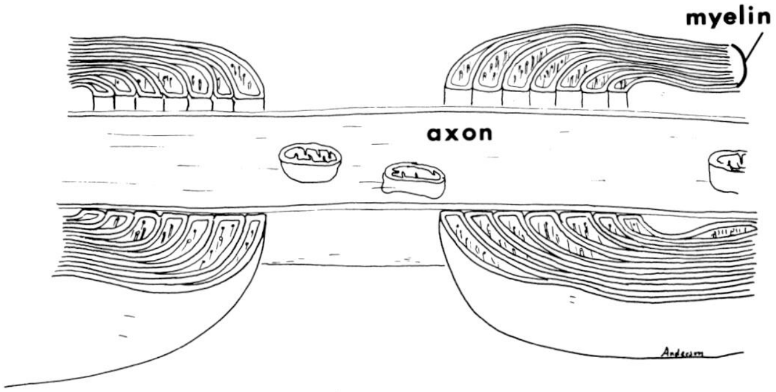

Fig. 3-10. Diagram of the node of Ranvier in the central nervous system. The myelin lamellae split as they approach the node to form loops that contain oligodendrocyte cytoplasm.

Later, such connections with oligodendrocytes were demonstrated in embryonic tissue and in remyelination after a disease process. Now it has been demonstrated also in adult tissue, but even after knowing that such connections exist, many hours of diligent search may fail to show a place where such connections are included within the plane of section. The current concept of myelin formation from oligodendrocytes is shown in Fig. 3-9.

Ranvier was the first to note interruptions in the myelin sheath in the peripheral nervous system, called nodes of Ranvier. Similar structures also occur in the central nervous system and are also called nodes of Ranvier, despite the fact that Ranvier himself believed that such nodes did not occur in the central nervous system but only in the peripheral nervous system. These interruptions occur where one myelin-producing cell ends its myelin contribution and another cell takes over. The myelin layers end in the form of loops, as shown in Fig. 3-10, and there is a short piece of naked axon at the node.

It is interesting that Ranvier thought that the nodes were attachment points that prevented the myelin sheaths from slipping down the nerve fiber in response to gravity. This idea no longer seems reasonable in light of current knowledge. It is not really necessary to postulate that nodes of Ranvier have a function, since they could merely be the result of anatomic necessity when several cells contribute sections of myelin sheaths along the lengths of the nerve.

It appears, however, that the nodes of Ranvier do serve a function. Although unmyelinated nerve fibers are depolarized along their entire length as the nerve impulse is propagated, myelinated nerve fibers are depolarized only at the nodes of Ranvier. Thus the nerve fiber where it is wrapped by myelin is not depolarized and the impulse is transmitted by sequential depolarization of adjacent nodes (saltatory conduction). There are two important results of saltatory conduction: first, conduction of impulse is much more rapid, and second, the metabolic energy is conserved because active repolarization needs to be done only at the nodes, not in between.

Microglia

Microglia are classically conceived as mesodermally derived cells residing in the central nervous system tissue that in times of disease become phagocytic and participate in repair. There is now some evidence that inflammatory cells can enter the central nervous system from the blood stream when disease arises. Because of this, there is some question whether microglia in the classical sense—mesodermal cells that lie dormant in the central nervous system until there is disease—exist; possibly, the small, densely nucleated cells thought to be microglia microscopically are in fact another type of oligodendrocyte that is embryologically of neuroectodermal origin.

Nerve fibers

The visual fibers within the optic nerve are axons that extend from ganglion cells of the retina to the lateral geniculate body. There may also be some axons whose impulse travels toward the eye instead of away from it (centrifugal fibers). However, it is not known with certainty whether such centrifugal fibers exist, and, assuming they exist, their number, origin, destination, and functions are unknown. There are no anatomic criteria for identifying these centrifugal fibers or differentiating them from visual nerve fibers.

The nerve fibers of the optic nerves vary in size from less than a micrometer to several micrometers in diameter. Fibers of the same size sometimes seem to be grouped together, but when the entire nerve is counted it is seen that the diameters of the nerve fibers form a continuous spectrum rather than being of several discreet sizes. The ultrastructure of the axons is relatively simple. There are microtubules and a few filaments that run lengthwise through the axon. The chief metabolic organelle is the mitochondrion. These are particularly numerous in the unmyelinated fibers of the optic nerve head. The myelinated fibers are depolarized and repolarized only at the nodes of Ranvier and thus require less metabolic energy than the unmyelinated nerve fibers. Corresponding to this, mitochondria are less common in the myelinated portion of the fibers and tend to be aggregated near the nodes of Ranvier.

CLINICAL IMPLICATIONS

Although this chapter has been concerned with pure anatomy for its own sake, it seems appropriate to cite a few examples of how knowledge of anatomy may help in understanding the nature of disease processes.

Consider for example the strict dependence of myelin upon oligodendrocytes and the implications of this relationship in demyelinating diseases. In certain experimental demyelinating conditions, recovery with remyelinization of the nerve fibers can occur. It appears from these experiments that remyelinization can occur if, as the disease process subsides, (1) the axons are intact or can regenerate and (2) oligodendrocytes have not been destroyed.

In multiple sclerosis, electron microscopy of the lesion reveals that axons as well as astrocytes remain. However, oligodendrocytes are absent, and there is no remyelinization. These findings suggest that multiple sclerosis may be a disease of oligodendrocytes rather than a disease of myelin itself, and such considerations will obviously be pertinent as we come to know more about this disease.

Another currently interesting question is the role of astrocytes in the pathogenesis of glaucoma disc cupping. In *nonglaucomatous* optic atrophy the nerve fibers are lost from the optic nerve head, but astroglia remain, accounting for a relatively flat disc. This circumstance can be recognized in histopathologic sections, even though the architecture is distorted as the tissues collapse to fill in the spaces left by the degenerated nerve fibers.

In contrast, in total glaucomatous cupping there is absence of both nerve fiber and astroglia. The histopathology of nonglaucomatous optic atrophy suggests clearly that astrocytes are not lost secondary to nerve fiber loss. Therefore, the absence of glia in glaucoma immediately suggests that the site of glaucomatous damage is at the optic disc, since if the nerve fibers were damaged primarily in the retina there would not be a secondary loss of astrocytes at the optic nerve head.

If astrocyte loss in glaucoma is not secondary to nerve fiber damage, only two alternatives remain: (1) astrocytes and nerve fibers are each independently destroyed by a common insult resulting from glaucoma or (2) astrocytes are the primary target of glaucoma and nerve fibers are lost secondarily when the supportive and nutritive function of the glia are lacking. The second alternative is given some support by the observation that cupping (? loss of glia) often proceeds to a marked degree before a visual field defect (loss of nerve fibers) can be detected. Also suggestive is the clinical impression that partially cupped discs are more susceptible to damage from moderately elevated intraocular pressure than are uncupped discs. If this sequence (glia first, then nerve fibers) is correct, the loss of nerve fibers might be blamed on the loss of the support and nutritive function of the astrocytes.

REFERENCES

1. Anderson, D. R.: Microscopic anatomy of the optic nerve. In Smith, J. L.: Neuro-ophthalmology, vol. 5, Hallandale, Florida, 1969, Huffman Publishing Co., pp. 49-68.
2. Anderson, D. R., and Hoyt, W. F.: Ultrastructure of intraorbital portion of human and monkey optic nerve, Arch. Ophthalmol. **82:**506, 1969.
3. Anderson, D. R.: Ultrastructure of meningeal sheaths: Normal human and monkey optic nerve, Arch. Ophthalmol. **82:** 659, 1969.
4. Anderson, D. R.: Ultrastructure of human and monkey lamina cribrosa and optic nerve head, Arch. Ophthalmol. **82:**800, 1969.
5. Anderson, D. R.: Ultrastructure of the optic nerve head, Arch. Ophthalmol. **83:** 63, 1970.
6. Anderson, D. R.: Vascular supply to the optic nerve of primates, Am. J. Ophthalmol. **70:**341, 1970.
7. Kuffler, S. W.: The physiology of neuroglial cells. Ergeb. Physiol. **57:**1, 1966.
8. Bunge, R. P.: Glial cells and the central myelin sheath, Physiol. Rev. **48:**197, 1968.
9. Blunt, M. J., Baldwin, F., Wendell-Smith, C. P.: Gliogenesis and myelination in kitten optic nerve, Z. Zellforsch. Mikrosk. Anat. **124:**293, 1972.

Chapter 4

Mechanisms of optic nerve disease

Douglas R. Anderson

AUTOREGULATION

The retina and optic nerve are part of the central nervous system, and their vessels have typical characteristics of central nervous system vessels. Anatomically the endothelial cells of the vessels lack fenestrations and are united by tight junctions.[1, 2] Physiologically, vessel walls form a blood-brain barrier. Fluorescein, for example, does not leak from normal vessels in the retina or optic nerve. In the late phases of fluorescein angiography the dye appears in the optic nerve head, but this is due to diffusion from the adjacent choroid, which lacks a blood-brain barrier. Vessels in the nerve tissue itself do not leak fluorescein.[3]

An important characteristic of central nervous system vessels is *autoregulation* of blood flow.[4] This general term covers several physiologic mechanisms that serve to maintain a fixed rate of blood flow. Reduced to basics, flow rate is determined by (1) difference in arterial and venous pressure and (2) the total resistance along the pathway. If arterial pressure rises, flow would be expected to increase were it not for autoregulatory mechanisms that increase resistance in the vascular pathway. An example of this is the contraction of retinal arteries in response to high blood pressure. Similarly, if arterial pressure falls, the vessels dilate to reduce resistance and maintain flow.

One way autoregulation is apparently accomplished is *myogenic auto-*

Supported in part by PHS Research Grant EY-00031 awarded by the National Institutes of Health, Bethesda, Maryland.

regulation, a mechanism by which the vessels themselves detect, or are sensitive to, hydrostatic pressure and adjust their muscular tone accordingly. Another mechanism is *metabolic autoregulation,* by which rate of flow is moderated by metabolic needs. This mechanism depends upon the fact that the level of nutrients (for example, oxygen) and metabolic products (for example, carbon dioxide) results from a balance between metabolic rate and the rate of perfusion of an area by blood. Hence an increase in local carbon dioxide level ordinarily represents either an increased metabolism or an impaired blood flow. Either way, the mechanism of metabolic autoregulation corrects the problem by causing the vessels to dilate, thus promoting blood flow and restoration of normal tissue levels of carbon dioxide. Conversely, a decrease in carbon dioxide level results in an increased vascular tone and slowing of blood flow. Included in metabolic autoregulation is the vascular response to carbon dioxide, oxygen level, pH, and perhaps other factors. The phenomenon of metabolic autoregulation is witnessed clinically when oxygen is administered to newborn infants and a high arterial oxygen level causes retinal vascular constriction. The result is reduced flow, which may suffice to supply oxygen but be inadequate to supply the other metabolic needs or to take away metabolic products, and this may result in vascular proliferation in an effort to overcome the deficiencies. One is trying to make use of metabolic autoregulatory mechanisms when one uses carbon dioxide to dilate central nervous system vessels therapeutically, hoping to increase the delivery of oxygen and other nutrients by increasing blood flow. As a third clinical example, a considerable portion of the carotid artery must be occluded before the volume of flow to the brain is reduced, and I imagine that part of the explanation is that flow is maintained by autoregulatory mechanisms that reduce resistance in the vascular bed distal to the partial occlusion.

One must be careful when trying to extrapolate from basic considerations to clinical realities. For instance, consider the use of carbon dioxide in an effort to increase blood flow, as just mentioned. Is it possible that in an ischemic area, carbon dioxide levels are already high and the vessels in the ischemic region are already dilated to a maximum? Can we be sure that the administered carbon dioxide will affect the ischemic area any further than the local level of carbon dioxide has already done? Might it even be that such therapy would steal from the ischemic area by dilating all the cerebral vessels instead of just the ischemic ones?

One must also keep in mind that the autoregulatory mechanisms occur in normal vessels. As pointed out by Doctor Scheinberg at this symposium last year, in an ischemic area the vessels themselves may not be properly functional and may not have their usual normal autoregulatory responses. Hence they may not be capable of responding to carbon dioxide. Other disease states may also cause inadequacy in the normal regulatory capacity. For example, normal vessels constrict when blood pressure rises, and if the blood pressure is brought into the normal range the vessels redilate. However, after longstanding hypertension the vessels become sclerotic and may not be capable of redilating when the blood pressure is normalized; in physiologic terms, the vessels have lost their ability to autoregulate. When the blood pressure is brought into the normal range in such instances, the area supplied by these nondilatable vessels may become ischemic. Although scientific data is lacking, we can wonder whether such failure of autoregulatory mechanism has something to do with ischemic papillitis in patients with high blood pressure or perhaps helps to explain accelerated glaucomatous damage to the disc when high blood pressure is treated.

What then are the details of autoregulation in the optic nerve as presently known? First, the autoregulatory capacity of the anterior visual pathway has been well demonstrated in the retina[5-9] and might be presumed to be present in the majority of the optic nerve as in the rest of the central nervous system. However, the regulatory capacity in the optic nerve head (optic disc) is questionable. Doubt first arose because choroidal blood flow, unlike that of the retina, was found to be highly dependent on intraocular pressure.[7, 10-14] This occurs because when intraocular pressure rises, so does pressure in the veins that drain intraocular structures. This results in a reduced difference between arterial and venous pressure. Flow in the choroid was found to decrease with this reduced perfusion pressure, which is to say that autoregulatory compensation is not sufficient to maintain the usual blood flow, even though there is some capacity for regulatory response in the choroid.[7, 14-18] Since the optic nerve head receives arterial branches from the same source as the choroid, namely, from the posterior ciliary arteries, the question arises whether there is a similar deficiency of autoregulation in the optic nerve head. If one knew that the main autoregulatory capacity resided in the larger arterial branches that supply both the disc and choroid, one could assume that the disc circulation behaves like the choroidal circulation; but it isn't known how much of the regulatory capacity resides in the smaller arterial branches supplying only the disc. Therefore, to understand disc circulation one must study the vascular physiology of the disc itself rather than the more easily studied choroidal circulation. Efforts to accurately assess blood flow and its regulation in the optic nerve head have not been conclusive, with some studies seeming to demonstrate autoregulation at least at the disc surface,[19-21] and other studies failing to demonstrate autoregulation.[13] Nonetheless, one can't help wondering whether a lack of autoregulatory capacity would make the disc particularly susceptible to ischemia when there is diffuse vascular disease affecting vessels supplying the optic nerve head, as for example in hypertensive arteriolar sclerosis or giant cell arteritis.

ANASTOMOSES

When the carotid artery is partially occluded, intact autoregulatory mechanisms cause the vascular bed to dilate so that total resistance along the pathway remains stable and a normal volume of blood flow is maintained. However, autoregulation is only part of the explanation for the maintenance of flow in the cerebral hemispheres even when there is a significant partial occlusion in the carotid artery. As the vessels beyond the obstruction dilate, the reduced resistance in the distal vascular pathway causes the dilated vascular bed to begin to borrow from adjacent areas by means of the important arterial anastomoses, especially as the obstruction becomes total and the dilated vascular bed is markedly dilated. However, the adjacent areas from which the blood is stolen do not suffer if they reduce their resistance by autoregulatory mechanisms, and in the end an adequate flow is maintained via one carotid to both vascular territories. Trouble develops when the summated effects of occlusion in anastomotic arteries exceed the capacity of the more distal vascular beds to dilate.

With this background we can turn our attention to the anterior visual pathways. The retina does not have arterial anastomoses. A branch artery occlusion will result in an infarction of a wedge of retina supplied by the occluded artery. The rest of the anterior visual pathway is more fortunate. The vessels of the pia mater are called a *plexus,* which indicates their rich anastomoses. Arterial anastomoses also occur around the optic nerve head by virtue of the arterial circle of Zinn-Haller, and there are retrograde branches from the peripapillary choroid into the pia mater of the optic nerve behind the globe.[22-26] Are these anastomoses sufficient to help prevent disaster when arteries are diseased? There is evidence that blood flow in the disc is segmental, which is to say that there are segments of the disc that each normally receive flow from individual feeding arterioles.[27] When a feeding arteriole is occluded, fluorescein may be slow in appearing in its usual territory, that is, linear flow is slow.* Yet in the laboratory, the disc somehow survives rather well after major interference with arterial supply, suggesting that an adequate volume of flow is maintained by means of a favorable combination of anastomoses and autoregulation. Experimental occlusion of the posterior ciliary arteries usually results only in a minute or partial infarction of the optic nerve head in the majority of monkeys, and the majority of nerve fibers are saved.[28, 29] If these results apply to human conditions, it would seem that major ischemia of the optic nerve head can result only from simultaneous involvement of multiple arteries in addition to the posterior

*When a vascular bed is dilated, it has a greater intravascular volume. Thus linear flow is slower in a dilated vascular bed than in a constricted vascular bed, even though the volumes of flow through the beds per unit time are the same. Angiography reflects linear flow rate, and valid conclusions about the volume of flow cannot be reached unless one also estimates the changes in intravascular volume.

ciliary arteries, a diffuse disease of the microvascular bed, or conceivably an interference with venous drainage. There is a tendency for the disc to be involved in vascular disease, but it is difficult to determine whether this results from a relative deficiency of anastomoses, a relative deficiency in autoregulation compared to neighboring central nervous system structures, or a predilection for these particular vessels to be involved in vascular diseases such as hypertension or giant cell arteritis. In any event, when segmental optic nerve infarction occurs (for example, to produce an altitudinal defect in the visual field), one must assume that there is multiple artery involvement that exceeds whatever ability the vessels have to dilate by autoregulation and that they can no longer steal by means of arterial anastomoses from adjacent vascular beds, which may be having their own troubles because their arterial feeder vessels may also be compromised. Segmental infarction can be accounted for by partially embarrassed flow in a vessel that is adequate for the needs of its territory despite attempted steal from adjacent beds while the amount stolen is not adequate for the neighboring territory whose artery is completely cut off.

GLAUCOMA

Glaucoma is of interest in a discussion of ischemic optic nerve disease because the present working hypothesis is that glaucomatous optic nerve damage is an ischemic condition of the optic nerve that results when intraocular pressure interferes with blood flow in the optic disc.[23, 30-34] One of the puzzling things about the vascular theory of glaucomatous cupping is that in some individuals the discs are relatively resistant to damage from intraocular pressure, whereas in other individuals the discs are sensitive to slight increases in intraocular pressure. One explanation is that the decrease in flow resulting from an elevation of intraocular pressure may be compounded by the presence of concurrent vascular disease that would make the disc more susceptible to the effect of intraocular pressure, and indeed, a history of cardiovascular or hematologic disease is frequent in patients who develop glaucomatous cupping with only slight elevations of intraocular pressure.[35] At the bottom of the spectrum are patients who develop glaucomatous cupping with intraocular pressure in the normal range. This is thought to occur because of an exceptionally bad vascular disease, but this brings into question the distinction between this type of low tension glaucoma and ischemic optic neuropathy.[36, 37] If low tension glaucoma and ischemic optic neuropathy present differently clinically, and I think at least some of the cases are clearly in one category or the other, what is the difference in the nature of the vascular disease that accounts for the progressive loss of glia and nerve tissue a bit at a time by one patient, while another develops ischemic papillitis in one or several major episodes?

One possible solution to the riddle would arise by invoking nonvascular factors in glaucomatous damage. A possibility that seems intriguing to me[38] is that the abundant glial cells, which support blood vessels and nerve fibers in the optic nerve head, may be weaker in some individuals than in others. Particularly weak glia may gradually give way spontaneously, causing gradual damage to axons and the appearance of glaucomatous excavations, without either elevation of intraocular pressure or vascular disease. Slightly stronger glia may be mechanically damaged with slight elevation of intraocular pressure, allowing collapse of the capillaries they support and infarction of the adjacent bundles of nerve fibers. In strong discs, the glia may not collapse under the influence of hydrostatic pressure, and if autoregulation is efficient, the intraocular pressure may not influence blood flow or result in ischemia of the disc. Though purely speculative, this hypothesis offers an alternative to the purely vascular theory and could explain some of the puzzling clinical features in glaucoma.

Another hypothesis to explain glaucomatous cupping of recent interest is that intraocular pressure mechanically interferes with axoplasmic transport along the optic nerve, resulting in neuronal death. Axoplasmic transport is a biological phenomenon in which materials synthesized in a ganglion cell (protein and so on) are actively transported along nerve fibers.[39, 40] Such a mechanism is needed since structural protein needed at the axon terminal can only be manufactured in the endoplasmic reticulum near the cell nucleus. This process is of interest in glaucoma because external pressure on the axon, such as by a ligature, is known to interfere with axoplasmic transport. Moreover, it has now been shown that elevated intraocular pressure causes an obstruction to flow in the axons where they exit from the globe through the *lamina cribrosa scleralis,*[41] and there is currently considerable speculation about the meaning of this observation. One must be careful about interpreting these experiments. Axoplasmic transport is an active transport depending on local metabolism at every point along the axon. Axoplasmic transport is interrupted wherever a segment of axon (for example, the segment in the optic nerve head) is ischemic. Thus, interruption of axoplasmic transport at the disc may reflect local ischemia or local mechanical compression or both.

PAPILLEDEMA

The pathophysiologic alterations in the optic disc that account for the production of papilledema have been an intriguing and elusive mystery. It is clear that elevation of intracranial pressure, which is transmitted into the vaginal sheaths of the optic nerve, compresses and causes elevation of pressure in the central retinal vein.[42] Because of the reduced difference in arterial and venous pressure, a decrease in blood flow might result except where there is adequate autoregulatory compensation. We have already seen that in the retina there is autoregulation, and one might expect that retinal blood flow would not be altered. With fluorescein angiography the blood flow does seem to be slowed, but presumably this is only slowing of linear velocity along the vessel due to an increased total intravascular volume, and the volume of flow per unit time is maintained. In the disc we are not certain about the presence or absence of autoregulation, and one might postulate that the disc, which is drained by the central retinal vein, could develop ischemia. The clinical appearance of papilledema could conceivably be the result of swelling caused by local malnutrition combined with a plethora of engorged vessels. By now it may seem that I am trying to attribute every abnormal condition of the optic disc to ischemia, but hopefully it is clear, especially with regard to papilledema, that there are practically no facts available and one can speculate practically however one wishes. What other mechanisms might be considered?

It has also been suggested that elevated intracranial pressure would obstruct axoplasmic transport and that intraaxonal swelling in papilledema could represent material that was prevented from flowing down the axon. Undoubtedly, reports that investigate the influence of intracranial pressure on axoplasmic transport will soon appear in the literature.

Many other factors could be considered. Papilledema could really be the result of several factors rather than a single one. Consider, for example, that there is frequently protein in cerebral spinal fluid when there is an elevated intracranial pressure associated with papilledema. At one time I designed a series of experiments in which I hoped to show that papilledema resulted when proteinaceous fluid was forced by high intracranial pressure into the vaginal sheath and from there into the extracellular space of the optic disc. These experiments failed and I bring them up here only to show that in discussing papilledema one can produce at least three widely variant theories (ischemia, axoplasmic transport, extracellular protein) to explain the production of papilledema. Perhaps the correct theory has not yet been conceived.

EPILOGUE

The preceding discussion, designed to be a display of the scientific evidence for current concepts and theories, is also a display of the current state of our ignorance. But understanding where our ignorance lies may help us recognize which blocks of data we need to build our future House of Knowledge.

REFERENCES

1. Anderson, D. R.: Ultrastructure of human and monkey lamina cribrosa and optic nerve head, Arch. Ophthalmol. **82:** 800-814, 1969.
2. Cohen, A. I.: Is there a potential defect in the blood-retinal barrier at the choroidal level of the optic nerve canal? Invest. Ophthalmol. **12:**513-519, 1973.
3. Grayson, M. C., and Laties, A. M.: Ocular localization of sodium fluorescein:

Effects of administration in rabbit and monkey, Arch. Ophthalmol. **85:**600, 1971.
4. Betz, E.: Cerebral blood flow: Its measurement and regulation, Physiol. Rev. **52:**595, 1972.
5. Frayser, R., and Hickam, J. B.: Retinal vascular response to breathing increased carbon dioxide and oxygen concentrations, Invest. Ophthalmol. **3:**427-431, 1964.
6. Alm, A., and Bill, A.: The oxygen supply to the retina. I. Effects of changes in intraocular pressure and arterial blood pressures, and in arterial Po_2 and Pco_2 on the oxygen tension in the vitreous body of the cat, Acta Physiol. Scand. **84:**261, 1972.
7. Alm, A., and Bill, A.: The oxygen supply to the retina. II. Effects of high intraocular pressure and of increased arterial carbon dioxide tension on uveal and retinal blood flow in cats, Acta Physiol. Scand. **84:**306-319, 1972.
8. Tsacopoulos, M., and David, N. J.: The effect of arterial Pco_2 on relative retinal blood flow in monkeys, Invest. Ophthalmol. **12:**335-347, 1973.
9. Tsacopoulos, M., Baker, R., Johnson, M., Strauss, J., and David, N. J.: The effect of arterial Pco_2 on inner retinal oxygen availability in monkeys, Invest. Ophthalmol. **12:**449-455, 1973.
10. Bill, A.: Intraocular pressure and blood flow through the uvea, Arch. Ophthalmol. **67:**336-348, 1967.
11. Bill, A.: Uveal circulation; a review of methods and results. In Leydhecker, W., editor: Glaucoma: Tutzing Symposium XX International Congress of Ophthalmology, Basel, 1967, S. Karger Ag.
12. Friedman, E.: Choroidal blood flow, Arch. Ophthalmol. **83:**95-99, 1970.
13. Alm, A., and Bill, A.: Ocular and optic nerve blood flow at normal and increased intraocular pressures in monkeys *(Macaca irus):* A study with radioactively labelled microspheres including flow determinations in brain and other tissues, Exp. Eye Res. **15:**15-29, 1973.
14. Alm, A., and Bill, A.: Blood flow and oxygen extraction in the cat uvea at normal and high intraocular pressures, Acta Physiol. Scand. **80:**19-28, 1970.
15. Chandra, S. R., and Friedman, E.: Choroidal blood flow, Arch. Ophthalmol. **87:**67-69, 1971.
16. Perkins, E. S.: Sympathetic innervation of the blood supply to the optic nerve. In Cant, J. S., editor: The optic nerve, St. Louis, 1972, The C. V. Mosby Co., pp. 40-47.
17. Friedman, E., and Chandra, S. R.: Choroidal blood flow. III. Effects of oxygen and carbon dioxide, Arch. Ophthalmol. **87:**70-71, 1972.
18. Best, M.: Autoregulation of ocular blood flow, Arch. Ophthalmol. **89:**143, 1973.
19. Ernest, J. T., and Potts, A. M.: Pathophysiology of the distal portion of the optic nerve. IV. Local temperature as a measure of blood flow, Am. J. Ophthalmol. **72:**435-444, 1971.
20. Ernest, J. T.: In vivo measurement of optic disc oxygen tension, Invest. Ophthalmol. **12:**927-933, 1973.
21. Ernest, J. T.: Autoregulation of optic disc oxygen tension, Invest. Ophthalmol. **13:**101-106, 1974.
22. Hayreh, S. S.: Blood supply and vascular disorders of the optic nerve, Anal. Inst. Barraquer **4:**7-109, 1963.
23. Ernest, J. T., and Potts, A. M.: Pathophysiology of the distal portion of the optic nerve. II. Vascular relationships, Am. J. Ophthalmol. **66:**380-387, 1968.
24. Anderson, D. R.: Vascular supply to the optic nerve of primates, Am. J. Ophthalmol. **70:**341-351, 1970.
25. Henkind, P., and Levitzky, M.: Angioarchitecture of the optic nerve. I. The papilla, Am. J. Ophthalmol. **68:**979-986, 1969.
26. Francois, J., and Neetens, A.: Vascularization of the optic pathway. I. Lamina cribrosa and optic nerve, Br. J. Ophthalmol. **38:**472-488, 1954.
27. Hayreh, S. S.: Pathogenesis of visual field defects: Role of the ciliary circulation, Br. J. Ophthalmol. **54:**289, 1970.
28. Hayreh, S. S., and Baines, J. A. B.: Occlusion of the posterior ciliary artery. III. Effects on the optic nerve head, Br. J. Ophthalmol. **56:**754-764, 1972.
29. Anderson, D. R., and Davis, E. B.: Retina and optic nerve after posterior ciliary artery occlusion, Arch. Ophthalmol. **92:**422, 1974.
30. Hayreh, S. S.: Optic disc changes in

glaucoma, Br. J. Ophthalmol. **56:**175-185, 1972.
31. Duane, T. D., Jaeger, E. A.: Glaucoma and ocular circulation: Theories of field loss, Survey Ophthalmol. **15:**364-369, 1971.
32. Begg, I. S., Drance, S. M., and Sweeney, V. P.: Ischemic optic neuropathy in chronic simple glaucoma, Br. J. Ophthalmol. **55:**73-90, 1971.
33. Francois, J., and Neetens, A.: Increased intraocular pressure and optic nerve atrophy, Brussels, 1966, Editions Arscia S. A.; the Hague, 1966, Dr. W. Junk, Publishers.
34. Phelps, C. D.: The pathogenesis of optic nerve damage in glaucoma: a review of the vascular hypothesis. In Blodi, F. C., editor: Current concepts in ophthalmology, vol. 3, St. Louis, 1972, The C. V. Mosby Co., pp. 142-161.
35. Drance, S. M.: Some factors in the production of low tension glaucoma, Br. J. Ophthalmol. **56:**229-242, 1972.
36. Drance, S. M.: Shock-induced optic neuropathy: A cause of non-progressive glaucoma, N. Engl. J. Med. **288:**392, 1973.
37. Hayreh, S. S.: Pathogenesis of cupping of the optic disc, Br. J. Ophthalmol. **58:** 863, 1974.
38. Anderson, D. R.: Pathogenesis of glaucomatous cupping: A new hypothesis. In New Orleans Academy of Ophthalmology: Symposium on glaucoma St. Louis, The C. V. Mosby Co., 1975.
39. Obstbaum, S. A., and Podos, S. M.: Axoplasmic transport, Invest. Ophthalmol. **13:**81, 1974.
40. Ochs, S.: Fast transport of materials in mammalian nerve fibers, Science **176:** 252, 1972.
41. Anderson, D. R., and Hendrickson, A.: Effect of intraocular pressure on rapid axoplasmic transport in monkey optic nerve, Invest. Ophthalmol. **13:**771-783, 1974.
42. Rios-Montenegro, E. N., Anderson, D. R., David, N. J.: Intracranial pressure and ocular hemodynamics, Arch. Ophthalmol. **89:**52-58, 1973.

Chapter 5

The neuroradiology of the optic chiasm and adjacent structures as demonstrated by polytomoencephalography

John C. Johnson
Martin Lubow

Advances in medical science continue to shower us with new toys and tools. For the experienced clinician, each technique has its demonstrated attributes and limitations. If priorities were assigned in the study of patients with retrobulbar visual problems, certainly the highest priority would be given to the clinical history. At most institutions, the ophthalmoscopic examination would be the next most important procedure.

Disease processes affecting the optic chiasm and related structures are often difficult to evaluate by the more routine clinical and radiographic methods such as radionuclide brain scanning and arteriography. Some patients have impressive subjective complaints but minimal or no findings by routine radiographic and neurologic examinations. For us the two most rewarding methods, following conventional clinical and radiographic studies, have been the visual field examination and polytomoencephalography.

Tomography in the investigation of diseases of the brain and its adjacent osseous structures is by no means new. Vallebona[11] first applied autotomography in the calvarium. Autotomography was later used by Ziedses des Plantes[2] and Schechter and De Gutierrez-Mahoney[3] to study the cerebral ventricles and cisternal spaces. Bourdon[4] and Valentino[5] utilized linear tomography during encephalography. More recently, DiChiro[6] brought the combination of pneumoencephalography and linear tomography to a high degree of sophistication.

Since the development of the polytome apparatus, fractional pneumoencephalography seems to have had a rebirth in popularity. A number of authors[7-10] have utilized the polytome in conjunction with pneumoencephalography. Other workers[11-19] have specifically used tomoencephalography in the region of the optic chiasm. We were impressed with the need for a reliable and reproducible method for demonstrating radiographically the optic chiasm and adjacent structures. We began evolving our present methodology approximately 2½ years ago. Since then we have examined 80 patients, ranging from the pediatric to the elderly age groups. We have not encountered any significant complications.

Most of these patients were referred for radiographic investigation of the sellar-suprasellar region because of visual loss or pituitary disturbances of various types. Several have full neurodiagnostic investigation, including conventional pneumoencephalography, interpreted as normal on repeated hospitalizations.

The patient is routinely premedicated with atropine and a sedative. Because many of our patients eventually prove to have pituitary or hypothalamic lesions, they are also premedicated with corticosteroids in an attempt to avoid any difficulties resulting from clinically unrecognized hypopituitarism. We have not found the routine administration of pressor agents necessary. General anesthesia is rarely necessary except in children below the age of 10. In many children, we have found intravenous fentanyl citrate to be very useful.

An intravenous saline drip is maintained during the procedure for safety and convenience. We are presently evaluating the use of intravenous mannitol just prior to the procedure in selected patients in an attempt to decrease brain volume and increase the capacity of the suprasellar or optochiasmatic cistern. Urea may be used for the same purpose.

Prior to lumbar puncture, preliminary polytomographic sections in anteroposterior (AP) and, occasionally, lateral projections should be exposed for localization and assessment of radiographic technique. We have relied primarily on tomograms in the brow-up, anteroposterior projection although we agree with other investigators that lateral views are sometimes helpful. In general, however, the frontal view tomograms have been underemphasized in the demonstration of the optochiasmatic cistern.[16] If a primary tumor of the optic pathways is suspected, oblique views may also be helpful. The radiographic magnification factor is approximately 1.3.

After lumbar puncture with the patient in the sitting position, 12 cc of air are slowly injected with the patient seated and the neck in the routine semiflexed position to facilitate ventricular filling. If a chair is not being used, the shoulders are supported from behind and the patient is instructed to lean back slightly and extend the neck moderately. With the patient in this position, there is a tendency for the air to ascend anterior to the spinal cord and brain stem and collect in the suprasellar area. This injection also requires 12 cc of air. Injection of air with the patient in this position is a critical part of the examination, since in our experience, the routine position for ventricular filling cannot be relied upon to consistently fill the optochiasmatic cistern. Interestingly, when the air is injected slowly into the ventricular system, very little if any headache is encountered. However, the patient always experiences headache when the neck is extended and the basal cisterns are filled. After injection of the total of 24 cc of air as described above, the lumbar needle is withdrawn and the patient quickly assumes the brow-up, supine position on the radiographic table. The patient is then pulled to the top of the table and the neck is extended so that the head is allowed to drop below the level of the table for a few seconds before being returned to the standard brow-up position. Positioning the head in this semihanging position momentarily is important because it ensures filling of the anterior recesses of the third ventricle, as well as the sella turcica if it is empty.[19]

Filming in the brow-up, AP position is then carried out. Multiple sections are exposed over a depth of 2.5 or 3 cm centered on the midportion of the sella. This interval will include the entire optochiasmatic cistern with some allowance anteriorly and posteriorly for slight variations in positioning. The distance between sections should be no greater than 2 mm, and sections at 1-mm intervals are sometimes obtained. The films must be processed and viewed immediately since the air may remain in the desired areas only

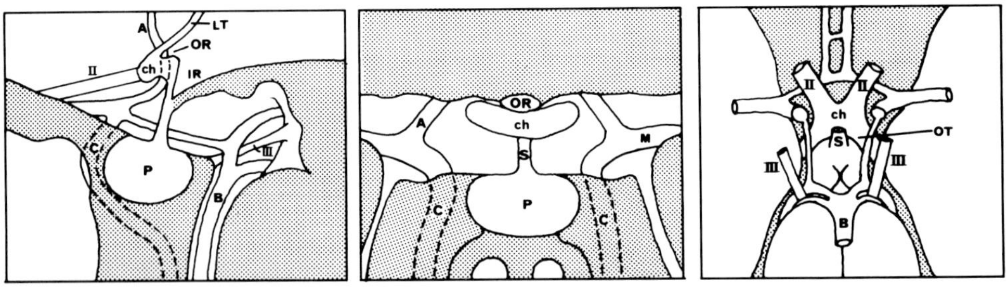

Fig. 5-1. *A,* Anterior cerebral artery; *OR,* optic recess of the third ventricle; *ch,* optic chiasm; *II,* optic nerves; *C,* carotid artery; *P,* pituitary gland; *B,* basilar artery; *III,* third nerve; *S,* pituitary stalk; *IR,* infundibular recess of the third ventricle; *OT,* optic tract; *LT,* lamina terminalis. *Lateral view,* Posterior portion of optic chiasm is bounded superiorly by optic recess of third ventricle. Farther anteriorly, superior aspect of chiasm is bounded by suprachiasmatic cistern. Infundibular recess of third ventricle projects down toward pituitary stalk. *Frontal view,* At this level, chiasm is shown bounded superiorly by optic recess of third ventricle. Pituitary stalk courses from chiasm superiorly down to diaphragma sellae. *Base view,* Pituitary stalk emanates from hypothalamus in posterior chiasmatic notch. Anterior chiasmatic notch lies between optic nerves just anterior to chiasm. (From Johnson, J. C., Lubow, M., and Stears, J.: Radiology **114:**629, 1975.)

fleetingly. If anatomic demonstration is not considered adequate on the first film series, a second series can be performed immediately since sometimes the air may be distributed more favorably by that time. Although the optic chiasm is consistently well demonstrated by this method (Figs. 5-1 to 5-3), visualization of the intracranial segments of the optic nerves in the straight AP position is less predictable (Figs. 5-4 and 5-5). If the optic nerves posterior to the optic canal are of specific interest, following the AP film series the patient's head is immediately turned into the 40-degree oblique projection to visualize the optic canal. Sections are then taken at 1- or 2-mm intervals starting at the cranial end of the optic canal and extending posteriorly toward the chiasm. It is assumed that the intracranial portion of the optic nerve has about the same orientation as the long axis of the optic

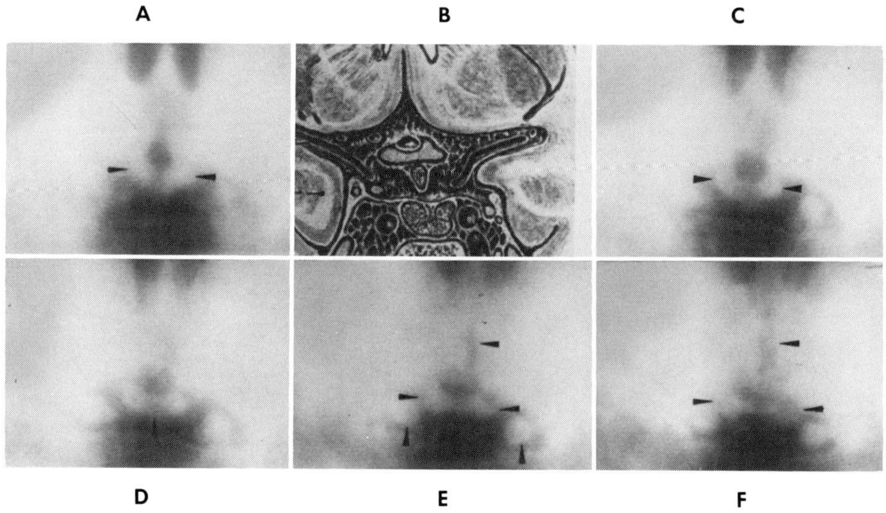

Fig. 5-2. Brow-up, AP polytomographic sections from pneumoencephalogram are arranged with most posterior section in **A** proceeding anteriorly to **F. A,** Approximately at level of dorsum, two optic tracts (arrows) can be seen separated in midline by infundibular recess of third ventricle. **B,** Drawing from coronal section of anatomic specimen taken through level of chiasm. Chiasm is bounded superiorly in its midportion by optic recess of third ventricle. Cut end of pituitary stalk is seen below chiasm. **C,** Anteroposterior polytomographic sections from pneumoencephalogram at approximately same level as in anatomic specimen in **B.** Optic chiasm in this area tends to be U-shaped and is bounded superiorly by optic recess of third ventricle. **D,** Two millimeters anterior to **C,** optic chiasm (arrow) is just beginning to assume figure-eight, or dumbbell, configuration. **E,** Two millimeters anterior to **D,** chiasm (two central arrows) has definite dumbbell configuration at level just posterior to anterior chiasmatic notch. Upper arrow points to interhemispheric fissure while two lower arrows show carotid siphons. **F,** Additional 2 mm forward, two optic nerves (two inferior arrows) are seen. Superior arrow points to interhemispheric fissure. (From Johnson, J. C., Lubow, M., and Stears, J.: Radiology **114:**629, 1975.)

canal. A second lumbar puncture is occasionally necessary after the second film series if filling of the ventricular system or optochiasmatic cistern is not considered adequate.

The optic chiasm is well seen in most patients in whom it has not been affected by some pathologic process, and it is the central structure within the optochiasmatic cistern. According to Fischgold and associates,[13] the height of the optochiasmatic cistern averages about 13 mm. Tumors arising from the hypothalamus, such as gliomas and craniopharyngiomas, encroach upon the optochiasmatic cistern from above (case 4). Tumors of the pituitary gland narrow the cistern from below (cases 1 and 2). Tumors arising from the optic chiasm itself, such as gliomas and meningiomas, fill the cistern beginning first in its central portion and then extending into the periphery of the cistern (cases 3 and 7).

In the region of the posterior chiasmatic notch, the diverging optic tracts can be seen to be separated by the infundibular recess of the third ventricle (Figs. 5-2, *A*, 5-3, *A*, and 5-5, *F*). Usually only the undersurfaces of the optic tracts can be seen since the optic apparatus in this area tends

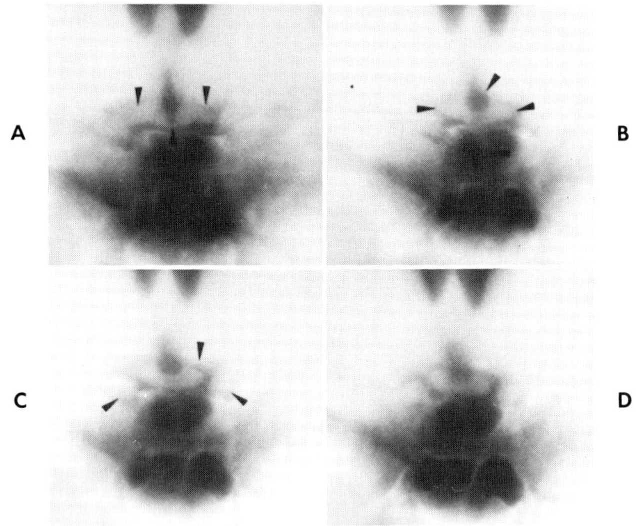

Fig. 5-3. A, Brow-up, AP polytomographic cut from pneumoencephalogram at level of dorsum, showing relatively long and narrow infundibular recess of third ventricle (inferior arrow) separating optic tracts lateral to it (superior arrows). **B,** Few millimeters farther anterior, more bulbous configuration of optic recess of third ventricle (superior arrow) comes into focus. Horizontal opposing arrows mark chiasm at this level. Inferior arrow points to pituitary stalk coursing inferiorly from posterior chiasmatic notch down into partially empty sella. **C,** Lateral inferior arrows mark round outlines of carotid siphons at this level. Chiasm is also well seen (superior arrow). **D,** Two millimeters farther anterior, chiasm is beginning to assume dumbbell shape. (From Johnson, J. C., Lubow, M., and Stears, J.: Radiology **114:**629, 1975.)

to be closely applied to the hypothalamus. Just anterior to the infundibular recess, the posterior portion of the chiasm, bounded superiorly by the optic recess of the third ventricle, tends to be U-shaped (Figs. 5-2, *B* and *C*, 5-3, *B*, and 5-6, *B*). Near the anterior chiasmatic notch, just behind the nerve-chiasm junction, the chiasm is usually dumbbell shaped. While this pattern seems to be the most common, there is considerable variation in the shape of the chiasm (Fig. 5-7). It is sometimes more nearly oval. However, to our knowledge we have not seen a normal patient in whom the chiasm was thicker in the midline than laterally. Even if the chiasm is minimally thicker in the midline, we consider this to be abnormal, usually representing a glioma. This impression is reinforced by minimal effacement of the optic recess of the third ventricle (case 9).

In patients with an empty sella, the entire chiasm tends to be U- or V-shaped (Fig. 5-7, *C*). Sometimes the chiasm may appear to lie com-

A B C

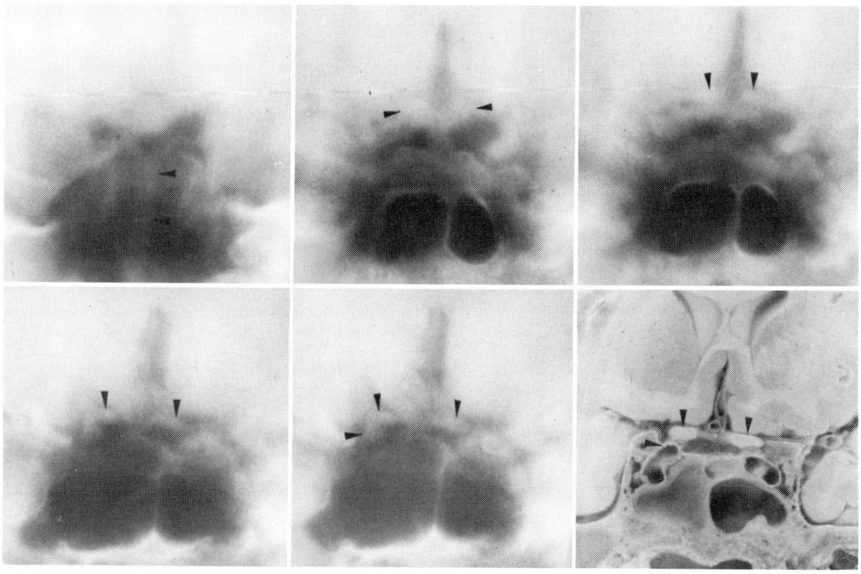

D E F

Fig. 5-4. Normal intracranial optic apparatus. **A,** Cut taken posteriorly at level of prepontine and interpeduncular cisterns. Arrows point to basilar artery. **B,** More anteriorly, arrows illustrate optic chiasm of normal size and shape. Pituitary stalk courses inferiorly from posterior chiasmatic notch to diaphragma sellae. **C,** Arrows point to anterior cerebral arteries immediately superior to chiasm. **D,** More anteriorly, optic nerves (arrows) begin to come into focus. **E,** Still farther anteriorly, optic nerves (vertical arrows) are well illustrated in frontal polytomographic cut. Horizontal arrow points to carotid siphon. **F,** Photograph of anatomic specimen cut in coronal plane at level of optic nerves for comparison with **E.** Arrows are arranged similarly to those in **E,** and illustrate exactly same anatomic structures.

pletely within the sella when it is developmentally empty secondary to an incompetent sellar diaphragm. While the optic apparatus may have an unusual appearance in the developmentally empty sella syndrome, in our experience this situation has not been associated with visual deficit.

In our normal series, the transverse diameter or width of the chiasm ranged from 14 to 20 mm, most normal chiasms measuring about 17 or 18

A B C D E F

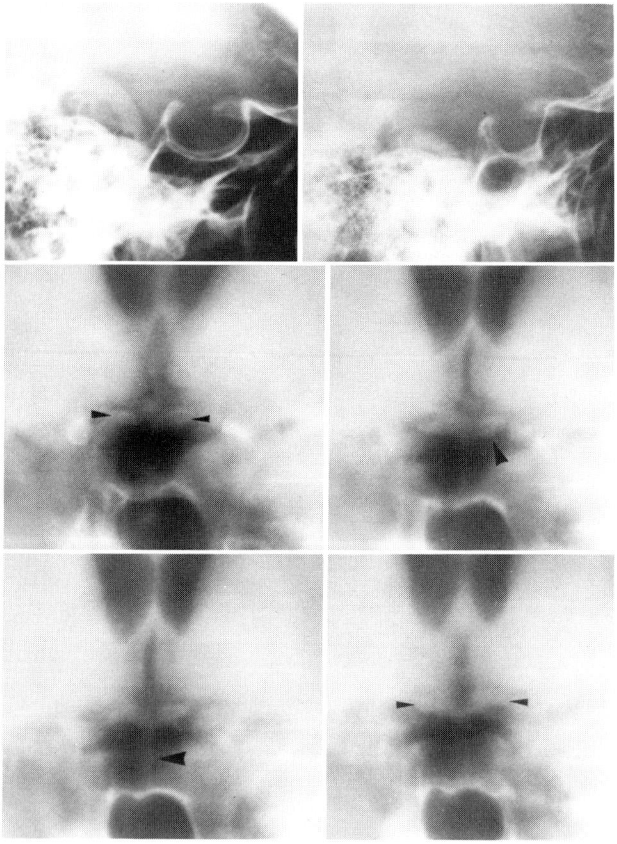

Fig. 5-5. A, Enlarged sella of acromegalic male. **B,** Within a year after transphenoidal hypophysectomy, sellar size had returned to normal. Note surgical defect in sellar floor. **C** to **F,** Brow-up, AP polytomographic cuts of the pneumonencephalogram proceeding from anterior to posterior. In spite of previous transphenoid hypophysectomy, polytomoencephalography was performed due to continued acral growth and persistent elevation of growth hormone levels. **C,** Note visualization of optic nerves (arrows) with anterior communicating artery projecting just above nerves in anterior chiasmatic notch. Note mound of soft tissue in left side of largely empty sella. This apparently was source of patient's continued growth hormone secretions. **D,** A few millimeters posterior to **C,** optic chiasm (arrow) is well seen. Note its oval shape in this patient. **E,** Still farther posterior, chiasm is again well seen and pituitary stalk (arrow) is well outlined. **F,** Posteriorly at level of dorsum, optic tracts are well seen separated by infundibular recess of third ventricle in midline.

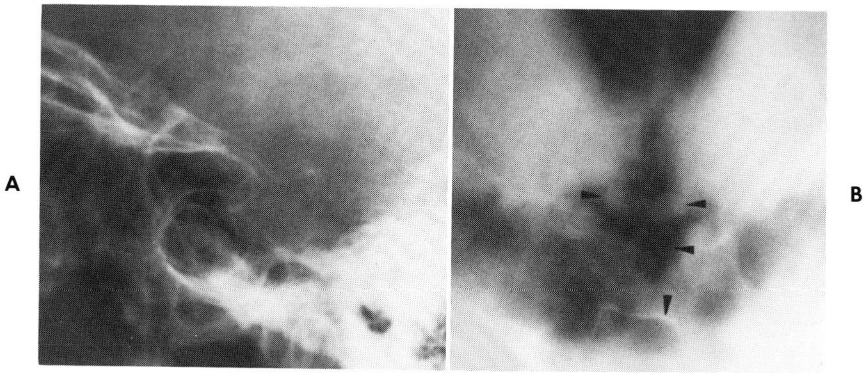

Fig. 5-6. Another example of normal optic chiasm as well as variation of the diaphragma sellae. **A,** Enlarged sella in middle-aged woman. **B,** Upper two arrows show optic chiasm of normal size and configuration. Middle arrow indicates large defect in left side of diaphragma sellae admitting air into sella. Note that floor of sella is deepest (inferior arrow) on side of defect in diaphragma.

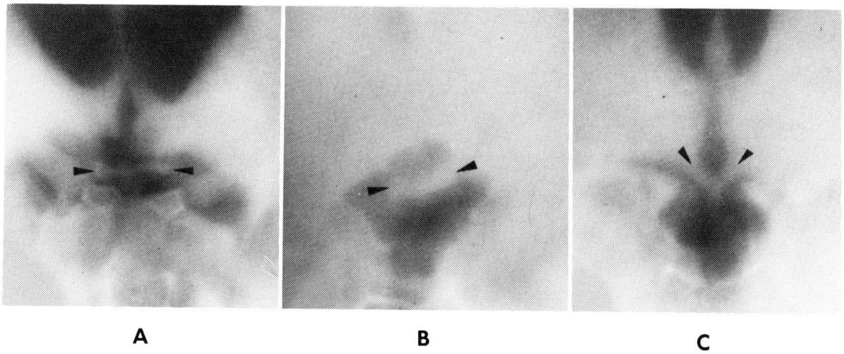

Fig. 5-7. A, Unusually thin optic chiasm in elderly woman who underwent pneumoencephalography because of enlarged sella and acromegaly. Chiasm was found to be only 3.5 mm thick, well below average. Patient's vision was normal. **B,** Tilted chiasm in child with neurofibromatosis who underwent pneumoencephalography to investigate possible intracranial extension of clinically obvious, left orbital mass. Sphenoid ridge was elevated on left secondary to orbital enlargement. Optic chiasm was found to be of normal size and shape (arrows) but was tilted because of osseous abnormality. Plexiform neuroma was found in left orbit. **C,** Partially empty sella in middle-aged woman who underwent pneumoencephalography because of sellar enlargement. Right inferior arrow marks level of anterior clinoid, expected point of attachment of diaphragma. Chiasm (upper arrows) sags down into sella somewhat and together with pituitary stalk assumes Y-configuration. In developmentally empty sella, chiasm often assumes unusual configurations, but vision is rarely if ever affected. (From Johnson, J. C., Lubow, M., and Stears, J.: Radiology **114:**629, 1975.)

mm in the central portion of the chiasm. If sections are taken at intervals greater than 2 mm, it may not be possible to reliably measure the chiasm. Since the vertical height or thickness of the chiasm is a smaller measurement, it is inherently less reliable. In our series, the chiasm varied from 4 to 7 mm in thickness. Taking into account the magnification produced by the radiographic apparatus, these dimensions approximately agree with the average 4 mm by 12 mm chiasm observed anatomically.[20] In addition to the measurements, Caille and Piton[11] and Fischgold and associates[13] indicate that symmetry of the chiasm in the frontal tomograms is an important point of evaluation. We have relied heavily on this. We have utilized lateral sections only occasionally (cases 4 and 8), but Fischgold and co-workers[13] have provided normal measurements in the lateral view for the distance between the chiasm and the tuberculum.

The oblique view is used in selected patients in an attempt to evaluate the size and shape of the optic nerve as it runs between the cranial end of the optic canal and the chiasm. The optic nerves are less consistently well demonstrated on our studies than the chiasm. This may be because even the several minutes required to perform the AP film sequence may be long enough for the cistern to empty of air and refill with fluid. We also think that it is more difficult to demonstrate the optic nerves in patients with a so-called prefixed chiasm, that is, short optic nerves. It seems easier to obtain a good image of the optic nerve when the optic chiasm is situated relatively posteriorly. In this situation, the intracranial segments of the optic nerves are longer and more likely to be completely enveloped by air. The patient's age and the shape of the skull may also influence how well the optic nerves can be demonstrated radiographically. In children, the optic apparatus tends to be more vertically oriented, and the interpeduncular and optochiasmatic cisterns tend to be deeper. The more capacious suprasellar cisternal spaces in children would seem to allow better demonstration of the optic apparatus, but this is not neceessarily the case. In younger patients, the optic chiasm is located more anteriorly, near the so-called chiasmatic sulcus of the sphenoid bone just anterior to the sella.[11] In adults, the chiasm is not closely related to the chiasmatic sulcus and is located more posteriorly and superiorly. This means that the optic nerves tend to be longer in adults than in children, which probably accounts for the findings in adults that suprasellar extension of pituitary tumors tend to spread and elevate the optic nerve while displacing the chiasm posteriorly. The length of the optic nerves may also be related to the shape of the skull; the chiasm tends to be more rostral in the brachycephalic skull and more posteriorly located in the dolichocephalic skull.[19] In spite of these variations, we have had a number of cases in which the oblique views provided valuable information, showing optic nerve enlargement that could not be appreciated in the AP sections (case 6). We believe it is of importance to define accurately the extent of optic gliomas within the anterior optic pathways since some evidence suggests a better prognosis when the tumor is limited to the nerve.[18]

Because it is a small structure, the optic nerve in the oblique view is rather difficult to measure accurately on the films. It normally has an oval configuration averaging about 3½ mm vertically by 6 mm horizontally (Figs. 5-8 to 5-11).

The diaphragma sellae is another structure that is consistently demonstrated well by polytomoencephalography (Figs. 5-12 and 5-13). Rarely, visualization is hindered by arachnoid adhesions. In our experience, the diaphragma is most commonly slightly concave superiorly; that is, it sags

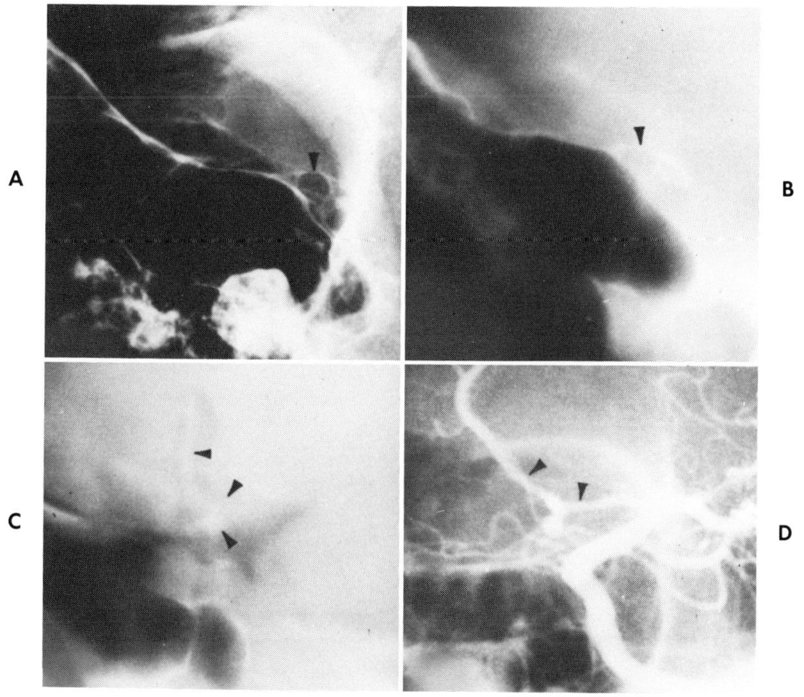

Fig. 5-8. A, Oblique view of the left orbit. Head has been rotated 40° opposite side being examined. This is routine position for radiographing optic canal (arrow). **B,** Same patient as in **A.** Polytomographic section has been taken through level of midportion of optic canal (arrow) in same 40° oblique projection. **C,** Polytomographic cut from pneumoencephalogram in same patient at level of about 0.5 cm posterior to **B,** also in 40° oblique position. Lower arrow illustrates optic nerve (seen on end). Assumption has been made that long axis of intracranial portion of optic nerve follows about same axis as optic canal. Note that, as expected, optic nerve in this position is oval shape with long axis of oval being oriented horizontally. Upper two arrows point to anterior cerebral artery as it courses superior to optic nerve. **D,** Oblique view of left carotid arteriogram in patient with berry aneurysm. Compare to arterial anatomy in **C.** Arrows indicate approximately same segment of anterior cerebral artery as in **C.**

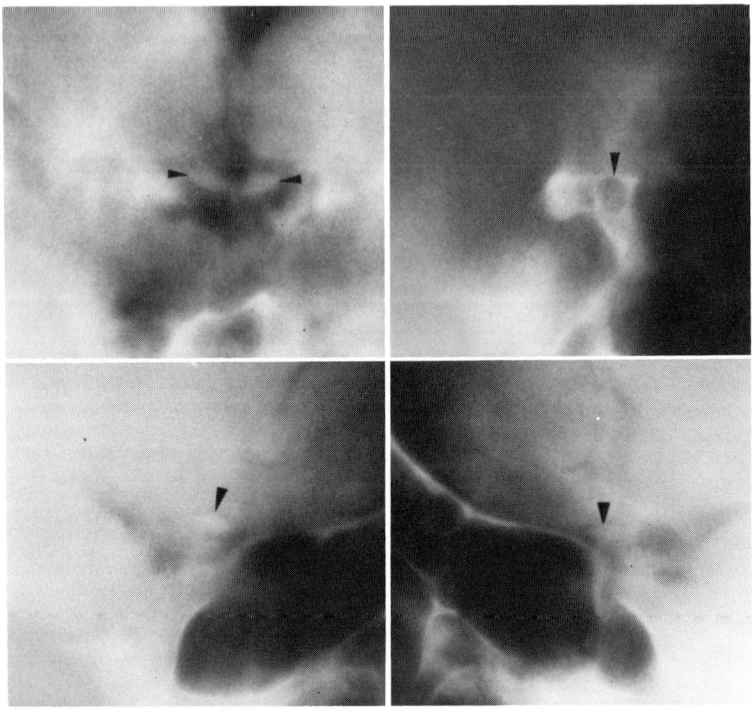

A B C D

Fig. 5-9. A, Brow-up, AP polytomographic section through midportion of sella in patient with enlarged, asymmetric, partially empty sella. Optic chiasm (arrows) is well visualized and looks normal. **B,** If optic nerves are to be investigated in oblique projections, preliminary cut to localize optic canal must be taken prior to injection of air. **C** and **D,** Right and left optic nerves (arrows), respectively, are well visualized. Again noted is typical oval shape.

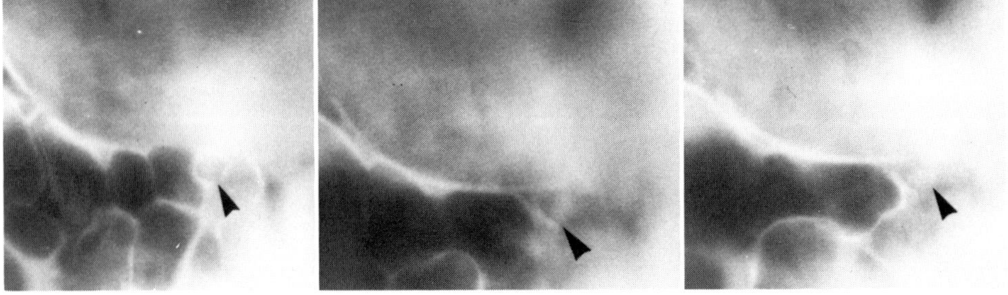

A B C

Fig. 5-10. Three successively more posterior, oblique polytomographic cuts of left optic nerve during pneumoencephalography. **A,** Arrow indicates left optic canal. **B,** At cranial end of optic canal, optic nerve (arrow) can be faintly seen. **C,** A few millimeters more posterior, oval-shaped optic nerve can be clearly seen.

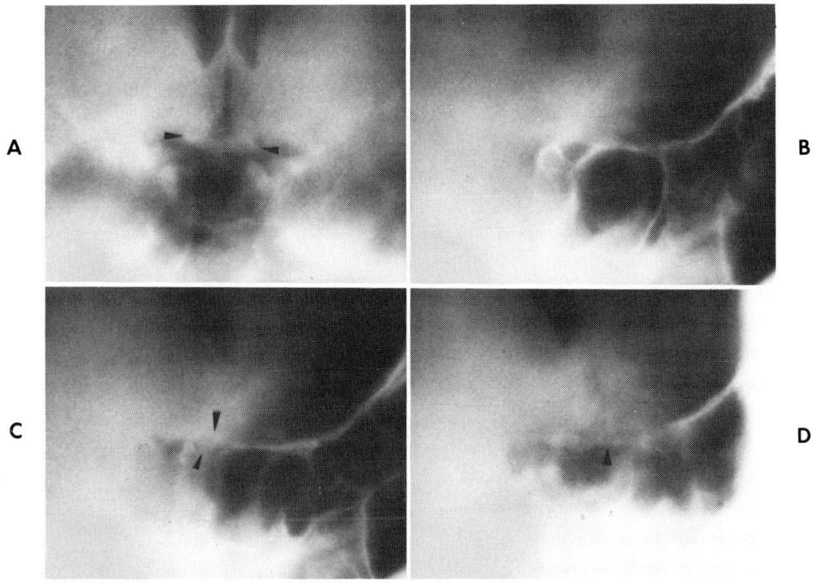

Fig. 5-11. A, Arrows indicate rather thin but normal optic chiasm. Note bulbous optic recess of third ventricle above chiasm. **B,** Polytomographic section performed in oblique projection through right optic canal. **C,** Section in oblique projection as in **B,** posterior to optic canal. Right optic nerve (upper arrow) is noted. Small round density just below nerve (lower arrow) probably represents ophthalmic artery. **D,** Section taken in same position as in **B** and **C** but several millimeters more posterior. Left optic nerve (arrow) can be seen "from side" coursing from optic chiasm on left toward left orbit on right.

slightly downward into the sella. It may also be perfectly flat (Fig. 5-12). On the basis of our experience to date, we presently think that even minimal upward convexity of the diaphragma indicates early suprasellar extension of an intrasellar tumor. However, a firm statement on this point must await more experience in this area. Analysis of the shape and position of the diaphragma sellae on the tomograms is a critical part of the examination since suprasellar extension of pituitary tumors cannot be consistently predicted from the shape of the sella on plain films (cases 1 and 2). Furthermore, the visual fields may be normal in the presence of considerable suprasellar extension.[21]

Many anatomic structures in the suprasellar area can be demonstrated by polytomoencephalography. These include the internal carotid, basilar, posterior cerebral, superior cerebellar, and anterior cerebral arteries (Figs. 5-2, *E,* 5-4, *C,* 5-12, *A,* and 5-14). The pituitary stalk (Figs. 5-4, *B,* and 5-5, *E*) and the anterior recesses of the third ventricle (Figs. 5-2, *B* and *C,* and 5-3, *B*) as well as the adjacent bony structures are also well seen. Certainly, not all of these structures will be seen on every study. However, the optic chiasm, the diaphragma sellae, and the anterior recesses of the third ventricle are uniformly well demonstrated if the examination has been properly performed and should be searched for routinely on each study. If the key structures are not well defined, a space-occupying lesion must be strongly suspected. Conversely, if no anatomic abnormality is found on a technically good study, the possibility of a surgically remedial or space occupying lesion becomes remote. In this situation, some other reason for visual difficulty becomes more likely, such as degenerative, toxic, or vascular causes.[13]

We have found optochiasmatic arachnoiditis to be very difficult to diagnose preoperatively. Fischgold and co-workers[13] state that optochiasmatic arachnoiditis typically allows good air filling of the suprasellar area but that the optochiasmatic cistern and its contents are irregular in appearance and compartmentalized by the adhesions. However, we have observed cases (case 11) in which the arachnoid adhesions acted as a mass enlarging the image of the chiasm and also affecting the anterior recesses of the third ventricle.

In our series, the confirmed pathologic diagnoses include pituitary tumors, craniopharyngioma, germinoma, metastases, optochiasmatic arachnoiditis, empty sella syndromes, and optic pathway gliomas. Our experience in the optic glioma patients continues to add to the controversy regarding the natural history and management of this disease.[22] The remarkable clinical and radiographic findings as well as response to medical therapy in our optic glioma series will be the subject of a separate report.

A 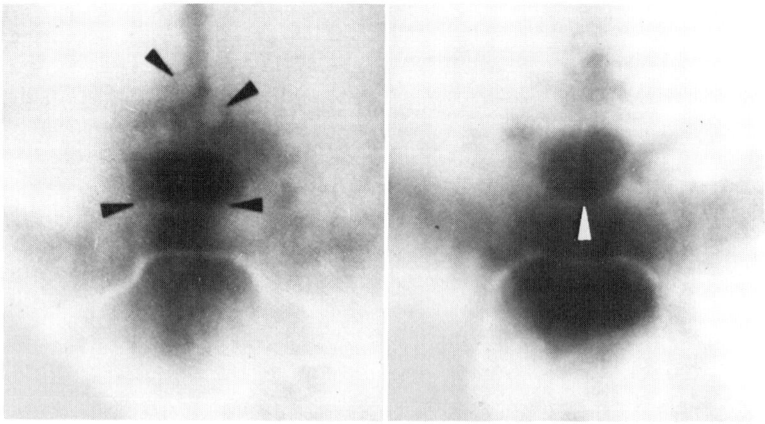 B

Fig. 5-12. A, AP polytomographic section through midportion of sella. Diaphragma (two lower arrows) is perfectly flat, or horizontal. Two upper arrows point to anterior cerebral arteries entering interhemispheric fissure. **B,** AP section. Arrow points to diaphragma sellae that is concave upward or sags downward into sella slightly. These two configurations are both considered normal.

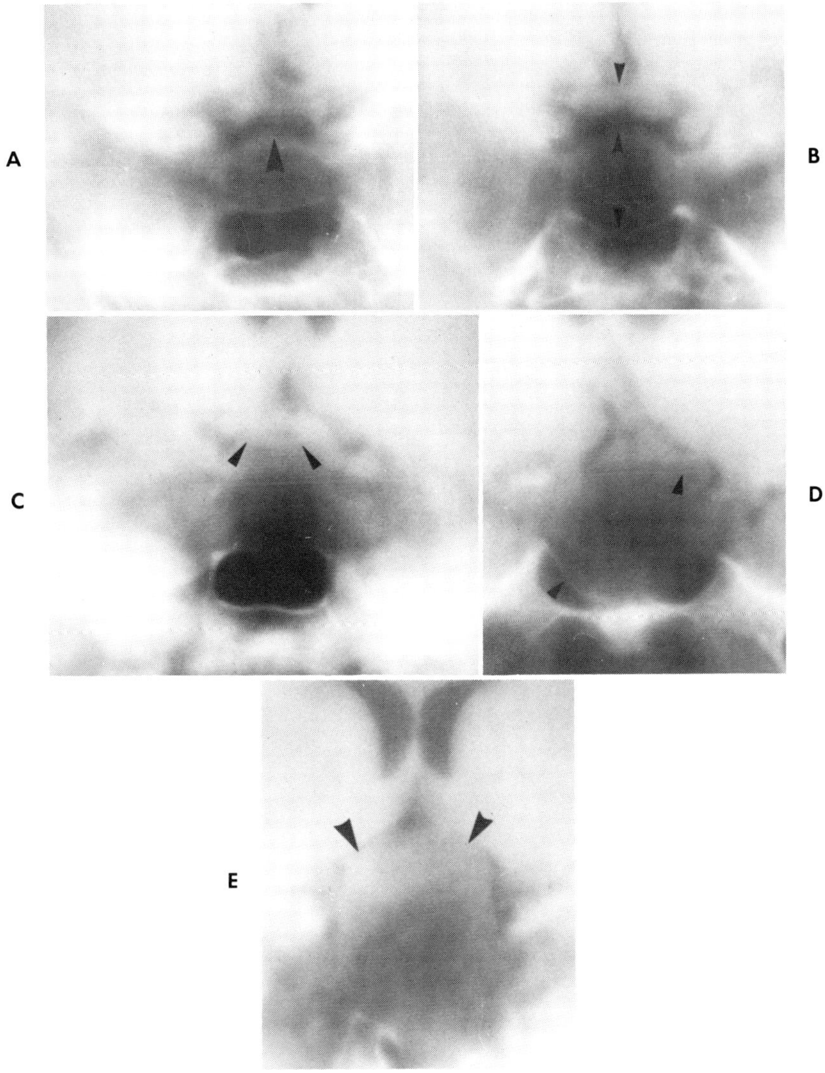

Fig. 5-13. Five brow-up, AP polytomographic sections from pneumoencephalograms on five different patients, all with pituitary tumors. **A,** Diaphragma sellae (arrow) shows minimal but definite upward convexity. Cisternal space between diaphragma and undersurface of optic chiasm is well preserved. **B,** Diaphragma sellae (middle arrow) bulges upward somewhat more than in **A,** but cisternal space between diaphragma and chiasm (marked on its superior aspect with an arrow) is still patent. **C,** Still more suprasellar extension of chromophobe adenoma. Undersurface of chiasm (arrows) can still be seen but suprasellar cistern has been completely obliterated. **D,** Even more distortion of the chiasm. Chiasm (arrow) appears draped over surface of tumor. Depressed sellar floor (inferior arrow) can be seen on right. **E,** Massive suprasellar extension of chromophobe adenoma. Marked upward bulging of diaphragma sellae (arrows) has completely obliterated details of optic apparatus.

A B C

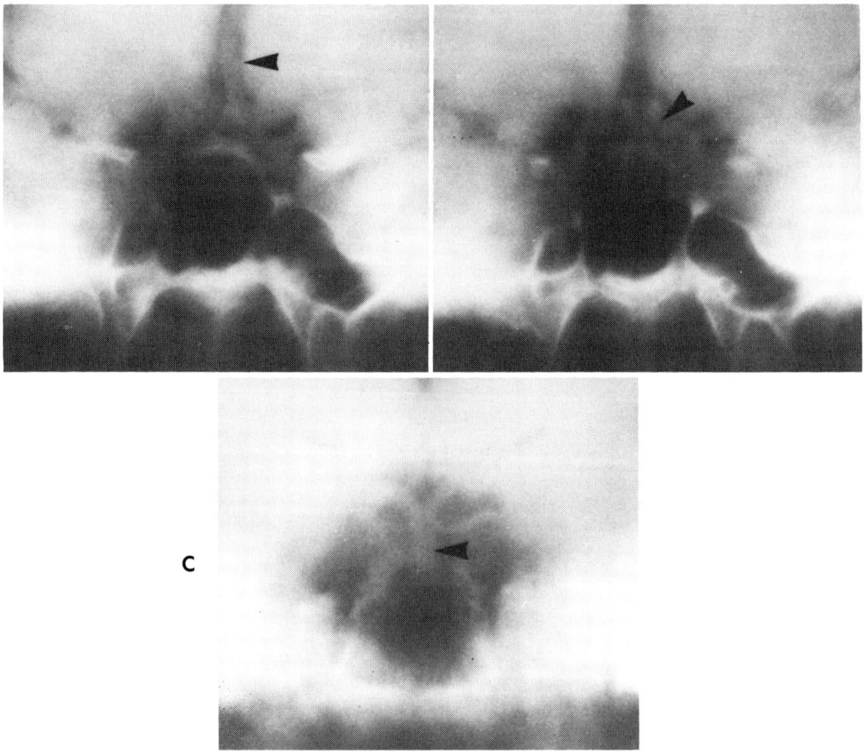

Fig. 5-14. A, AP polytomographic cut from pneumoencephalogram taken through level of planum sphenoidale. Arrow points to anterior cerebral arteries coursing superiorly in interhemispheric fissure. **B,** A little farther posterior, two anterior cerebrals can be seen side by side (arrow) forming anterior communicating artery. **C,** Cut at level of prepontine and interpeduncular cistern. Arrow points to basilar artery. Superior to arrow, posterior cerebral and superior cerebellar arteries can be seen branching off.

SUMMARY AND CONCLUSIONS

We have found this specific method of fractional pneumoencephalography combined with polytomography to be uniformly rewarding in the workup of patients with chiasmal syndromes manifested by localizing visual field abnormalities despite otherwise normal general neurologic and physical examinations.

The chiasmatic area lends itself well to radiographic analysis by polytomoencephalography. The detailed anatomic demonstration obtained is not presently available by any other diagnostic modality. In many of our patients, plain films of the skull, brain scan, and cerebral angiography were normal or equivocal while the polytomoencephalogram showed convincing anatomic abnormalities. If necessary, the examination can be repeated and compared to the earlier study. This feature will provide additional insight in the future concerning the natural history of optic gliomas.

As with any relatively new method, we are concerned about the tendency to overuse and overestimate this technique. However, the information has proven to be highly reliable, and at our institution, polytomoencephalography has become the final specific diagnostic test in this area short of craniotomy.

Table 3. Summary of case reports*

Patient	Diagnosis	*Visual fields*	*Plain films*	*Brain scan*	*Angio-gram*	*Orbito-gram*	*Pneumo-encepha-logram*
1. I. H.	Pituitary adenoma	+	±	–	+	NA†	+
2. G. E.	Pituitary adenoma	+	±	–	–	NA	+
3. M. W.	Meningioma	+	–	+	+	NA	+
4. D. M.	Germinoma	+	–	NA	–	NA	+
5. W. P.	Optic glioma	+	+	NA	NA	+	+
6. D. S.	Optic glioma	+	+	NA	NA	+	+
7. J. G.	Optic glioma	+	+	–	NA	+	+
8. G. J.	Optic glioma	+	±	–	–	NA	+
9. T. B.	Optic glioma	+	–	–	NA	–	+
10. M. P.	Metastatic carcinoma	+	–	–	–	NA	+
11. J. L.	Arachnoiditis	+	–	–	–	NA	+

*Note that the pneumoencephalogram and the visual fields are abnormal in all patients.
†NA, not available.

CASE REPORTS

Case 1. I. H., a 43-year-old laborer, was seen in January 1973 complaining of a decrease in vision OD for six months. This followed an unusual sudden decrease in vision OS 14 months earlier for which he was hospitalized in February and again in August 1972. Both hospital workups included angiography and PEG, and all studies were negative on both occasions, failing to clarify his unexplained visual loss.

His past history was noncontributory. He was in good general health.

Visual acuity was 20/25 OD, 20/200 OS. Color visions were abnormal. He could see 9/18 OD and 1/18 OS. Visual fields were abnormal OU with prominent bitemporal hemianopias to white and red targets.

Brain scan and cerebral angiography were considered normal. Plain films of the skull were initially thought to be normal, but in retrospect, a subtle double floor anteriorly was noted. PEG was grossly abnormal.

Frontal craniotomy demonstrated an atypical tumor on the tuberculum sellae and around the anterior portion of the chiasm, biopsy of which showed a pituitary chromophobe adenoma.

A

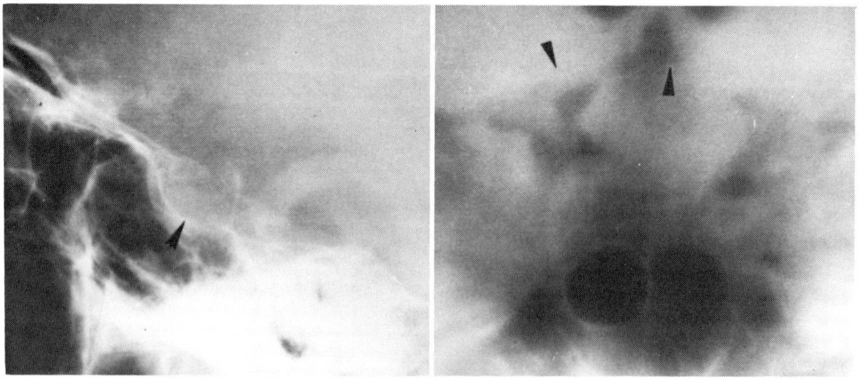

B

A, Lateral plain film of skull shows sella of normal size with well-mineralized floor (arrow). Subtle double floor can be seen anterior to arrow. **B,** AP view from polytomoencephalogram through midportion of sella shows large suprasellar mass seeming to rise up out of sella markedly effacing third ventricle (arrow up). Right anterior cerebral artery (arrow down) is elevated.

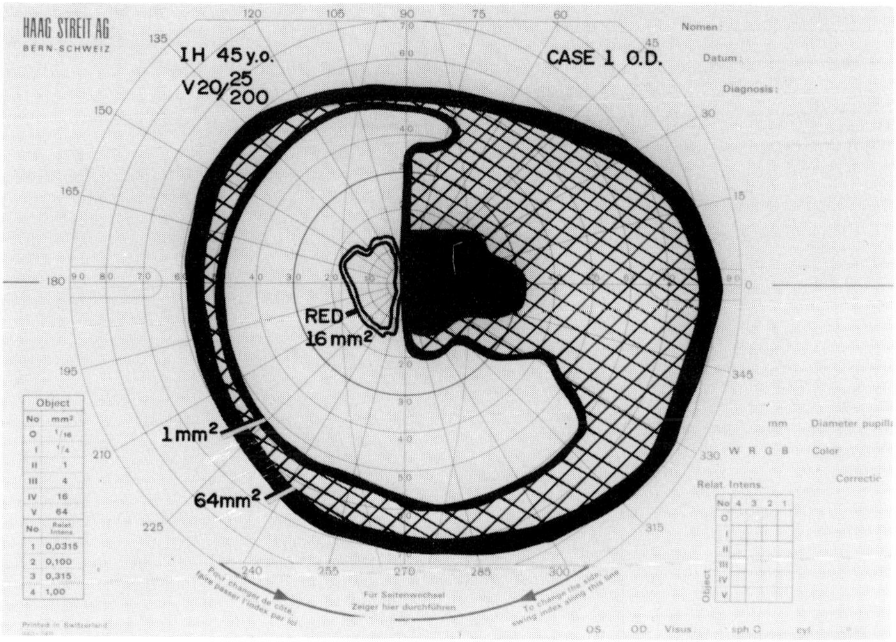
HAAG STREIT AG
BERN-SCHWEIZ
IH 45y.o.
V20/25/200
CASE 1 O.D.
RED
16 mm²
1mm²
64mm²

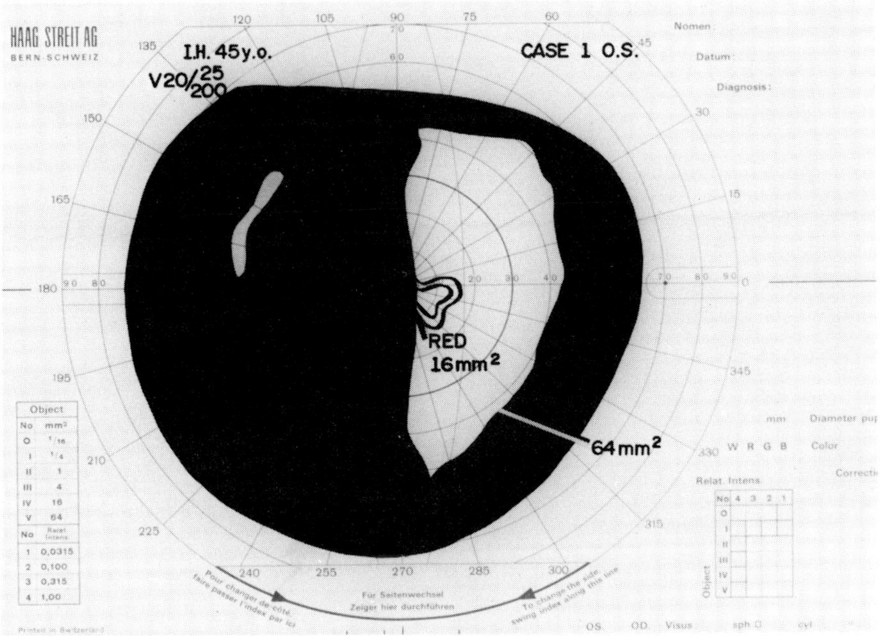
HAAG STREIT AG
BERN-SCHWEIZ
I.H. 45y.o.
V20/25/200
CASE 1 O.S.
RED
16mm²
64mm²

Case 2. G. E., a 50-year-old white housewife, was seen in October 1973 complaining of decreased vision OD for four months, attributed to a recurrent macular cyst. She had a history of transient decreased vision due to macular edema OU in 1971.

Her general health was good. Menopause at age 48 years was presumed to be normal.

Visual acuity was 20/70 OD, 20/40 OS. The visual fields were abnormal with bitemporal hemianopia to red targets and an enlarged blind spot and superior temporal constriction to white targes in OD only. The opic discs appeared normal.

Brain scan and angiogram were normal. Plain films of the skull were equivocal. The sella was of normal size but a double floor was noted.

Frontal craniotomy revealed chromophobe adenoma with suprasellar extension in the anterior chiasmatic notch. The tumor was partially necrotic.

A

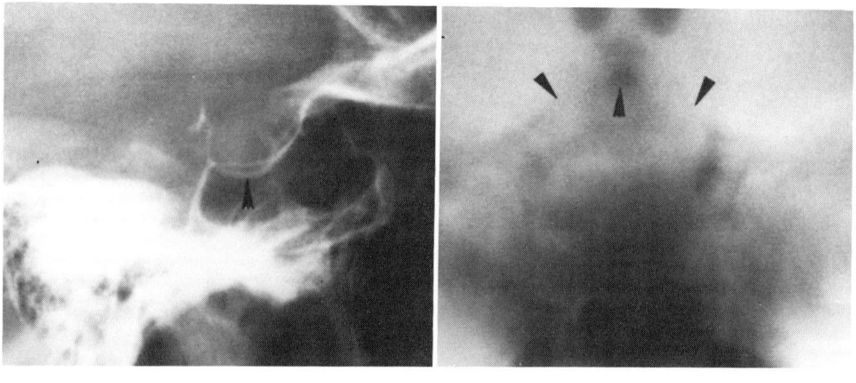

B

A, Lateral plain film shows normal-sized sella. Double floor is present. This can be normal variant. **B,** AP section from polytomoencephalogram shows large suprasellar mass (lateral arrows) markedly elevating third ventricle (central arrow).

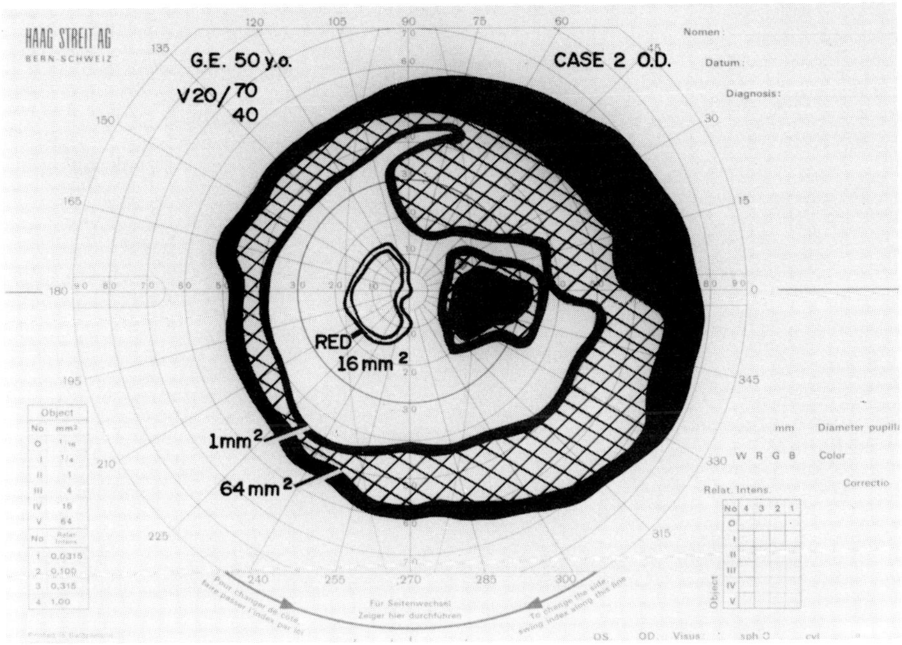
HAAG STREIT AG
BERN SCHWEIZ
G.E. 50 y.o.
CASE 2 O.D.
V20/70 40
RED
16 mm 2
1mm 2
64 mm 2
Nomen
Datum
Diagnosis
Diameter pupill
Color
Relat. Intens.
Für Seitenwechsel
Zeiger hier durchführen

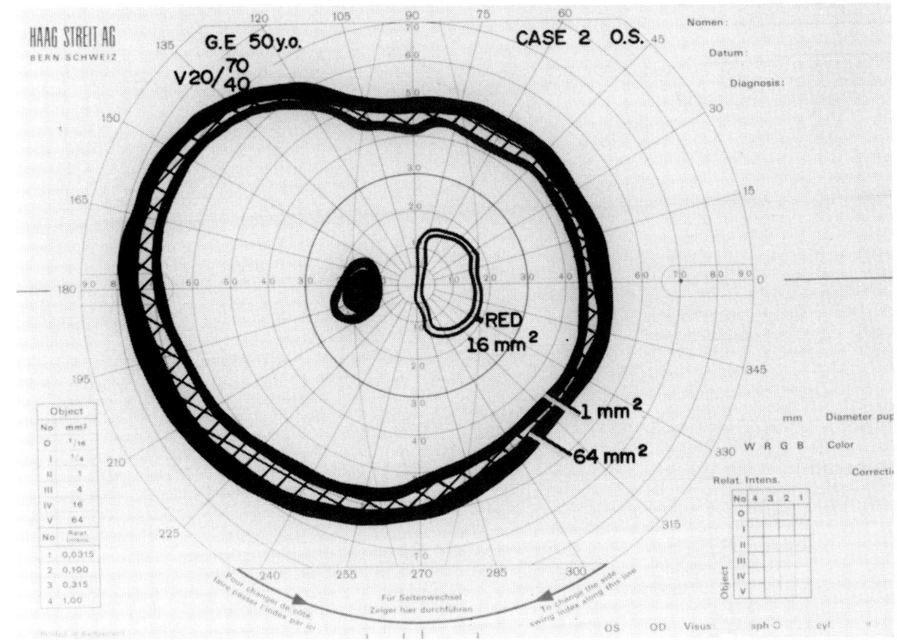
HAAG STREIT AG
BERN SCHWEIZ
G.E 50 y.o.
CASE 2 O.S.
V20/70 40
RED
16 mm 2
1 mm 2
64 mm 2
Nomen
Datum
Diagnosis
Color
Relat. Intens.
Für Seitenwechsel
Zeiger hier durchführen

Case 3. M. W., a 50-year-old white female harness maker, was seen in August 1973 complaining of gradual painless loss of vision OS for six months. This problem had been evaluated and attributed to chronic optic neuritis. Steroid treatment for six months was unsuccessful.

Visual acuity was 20/25 OD, 20/70 OS. Color visions were 18/18 OD, 0/18 OS. Visual fields were abnormal with nonspecific contraction and enlarged blind spot OS to white targets and bitemporal heminaopias to red targets. There was mild pallor of her left optic disc.

Routine plain films and brain scan were normal. Cerebral angiography suggested a suprasellar mass. PEG showed an apparently intrachiasmatic tumor.

At craniotomy, a meningioma enveloping the optic apparatus was found. It probably arose from the left side of the tuberculum.

A

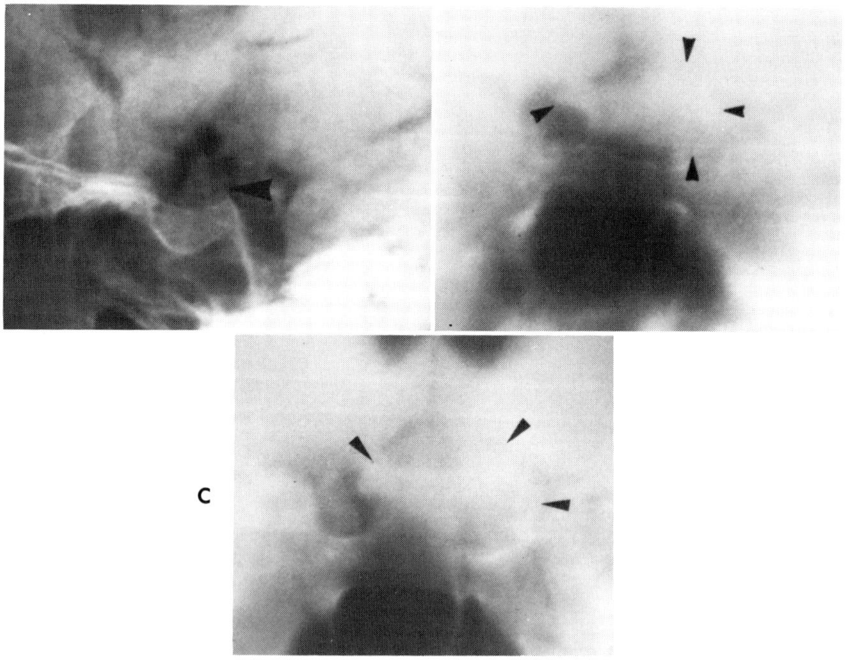

B

C

Intrachiasmatic meningioma. **A,** Lateral view from pneumoencephalogram shows sella of normal size and mineralization. Arrow points to tumor. **B,** Polytomoencephalography showed lesion to be intrachiasmatic. Chiasm at this level measures 15 by 31 mm. **C,** Patient's vision continued to worsen. Approximately one year later repeat polytomoencephalography showed increase in size of tumor.

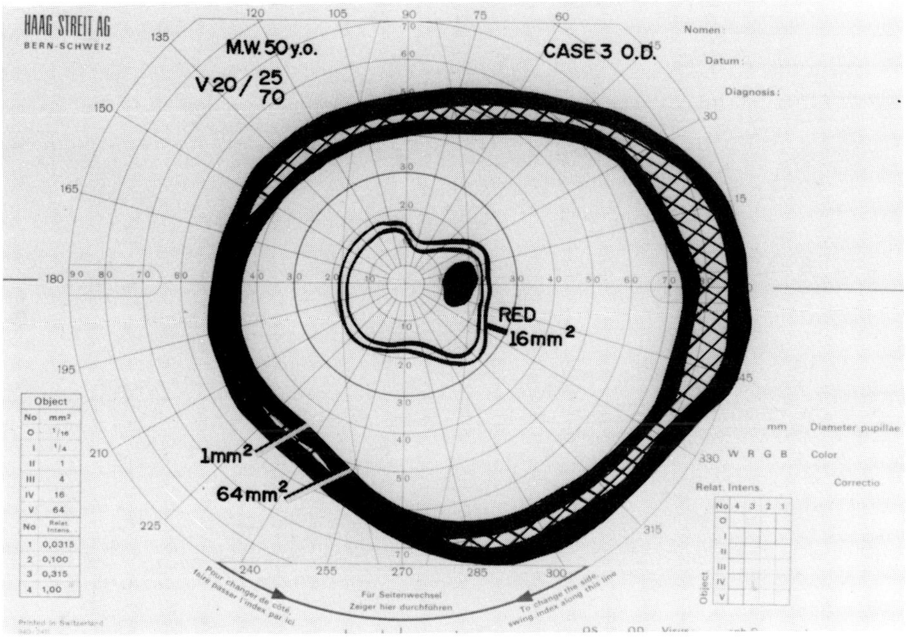
HAAG STREIT AG
BERN-SCHWEIZ
M.W. 50 y.o.
CASE 3 O.D.
V20/25/70
RED
16mm²
1mm²
64mm²
Nomen:
Datum:
Diagnosis:
Object
Für Seitenwechsel
Zeiger hier durchführen

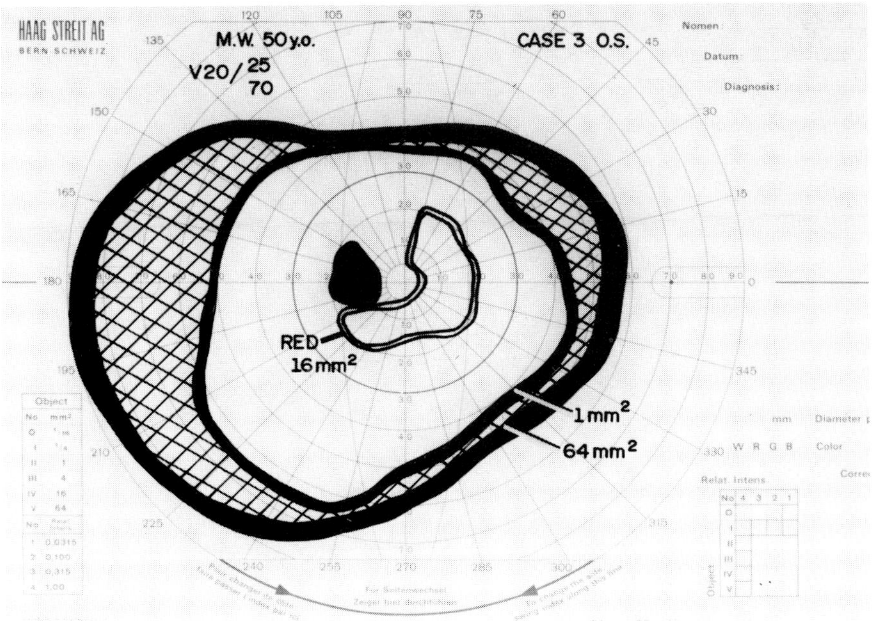
HAAG STREIT AG
BERN-SCHWEIZ
M.W. 50 y.o.
CASE 3 O.S.
V20/25/70
RED
16mm²
1mm²
64 mm²
Nomen:
Datum:
Diagnosis:
Object
Für Seitenwechsel
Zeiger hier durchführen

Case 4. D. M., a 21-year-old white male clerk, was seen July 1973 complaining of decreasing vision OU for three months. There was an interesting past history of polyuria for three years and an unusual high-pitched voice for which he was evaluated without benefit when 14 years old.

Visual acuities were 20/200 OD, counts fingers OS. Color visions were 6/18 OD and 0/18 OS. Visual fields were abnormal OU with prominent bitemporal scotomatous heminanopias. There was optic atrophy OU.

Routine skull films and angiogram were normal. The PEG was abnormal as was a positive contrast ventriculogram.

Right frontal craniotomy revealed a suprasellar germinoma, apparently arising from the hypothalamus and invading the chiasm.

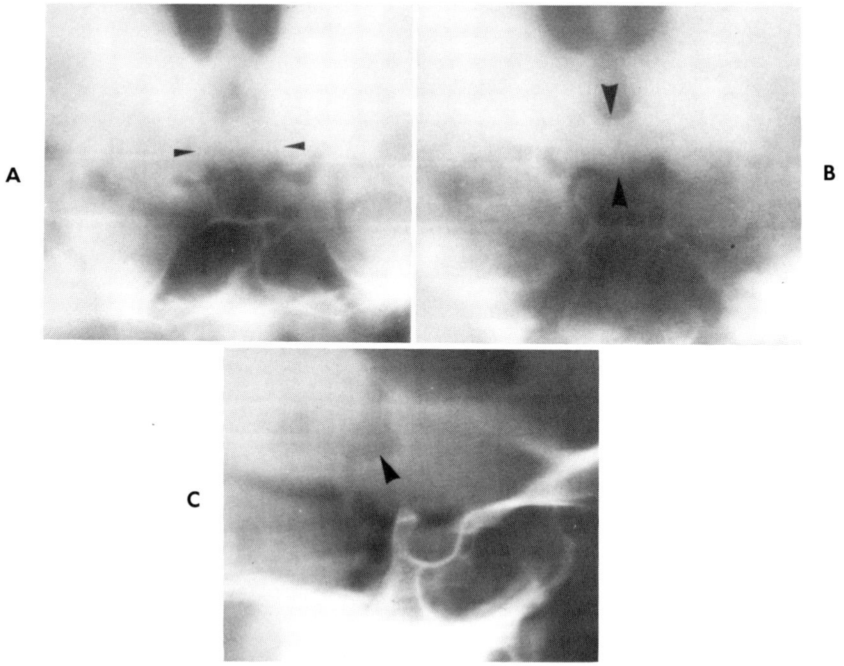

A, Brow-up, AP polytomographic section at level of midportion of sella shows markedly enlarged optic chiasm (arrows). Optic recess of third ventricle, normally well visualized at this level, cannot be identified. **B,** Farther posterior, at the level of dorsum, infundibular recess of third ventricle (upper arrow), normally long and narrow, is effaced and displaced superiorly. Tumor has grown inferiorly and now touches dorsum (inferior arrow). **C,** Lateral cut confirms nonfilling of anterior recesses of third ventricle as result of hypothalamic-chiasmatic mass.

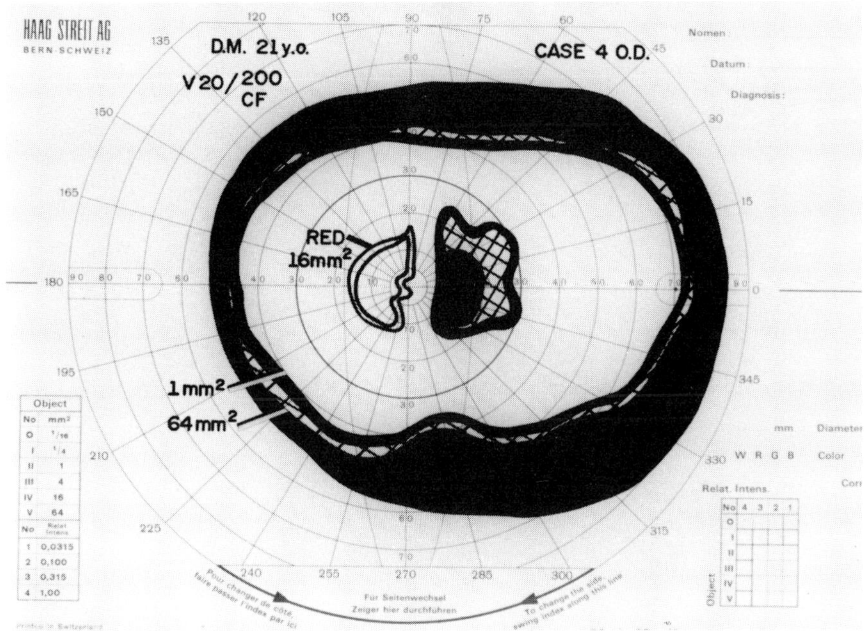
HAAG STREIT AG
BERN-SCHWEIZ
D.M. 21y.o.
CASE 4 O.D.
V20/200
CF
RED
16mm²
1mm²
64mm²

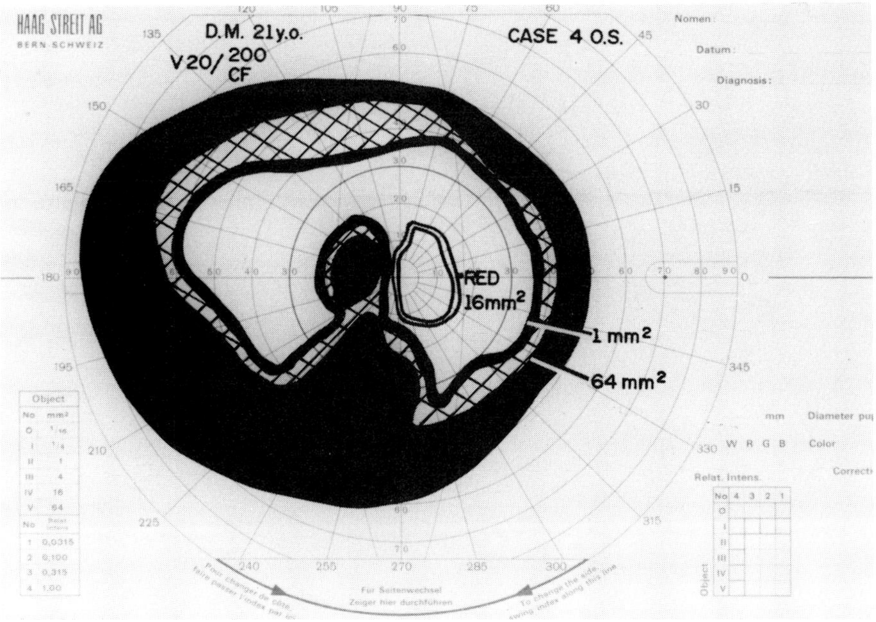
HAAG STREIT AG
BERN-SCHWEIZ
D.M. 21y.o.
CASE 4 O.S.
V20/200
CF
RED
16mm²
1 mm²
64 mm²

Case 5. W. P., a 5-year-old white boy, was seen because of proptosis OD for one month and poor vision OD with a lazy eye for one year. There was a family history of skin nodules in his father and his paternal grandfather.

Visual acuity in the proptotic right eye was no light perception with optic disc edema. Visual acuity in OS was 20/20 wtih normal disc and visual field. Iris surface nodules were noted OU.

Plain films demonstrated an enlarged right optic canal. Positive contrast orbitogram was abnormal, showing a tumor of the right optic nerve. PEG was abnormal, showing enlargement of the chiasm and the left hypothalamic area.

Craniotomy was not performed. The presumed diagnosis was neurofibromatosis with optic gliomas involving the right optic nerve, chiasm, and the left hypothalamic area.

A B C D

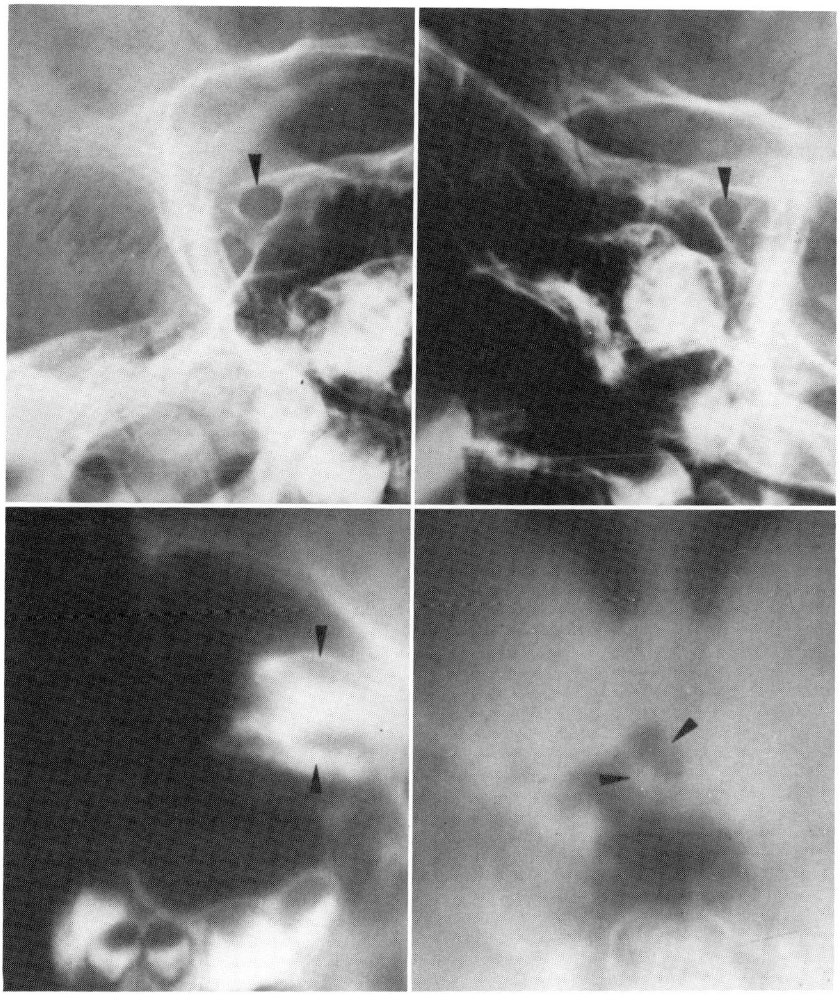

A and **B,** Optic canals (arrows) are asymmetric, right being considerably larger than left **C,** Lateral polytomographic section from positive contrast orbitogram shows marked enlargement of right optic nerve (arrows). **D,** AP polytomographic cut from pneumoencephalogram at level of midportion of sella shows right side of optic chiasm (horizontal arrow) to be of normal size and shape. It is separated from hypothalamus. Left side of chiasm appears enlarged and is continuous with hypothalamus. Optic recess of third ventricle (oblique arrow) is minimally but definitely deformed and displaced. Findings are indicative of tumor involving left side of chiasm and left side of hypothalamus as well as right optic nerve.

Case 6. D. S., a 12-year-old schoolgirl, was seen in May 1974, referred for "congenital" optic atrophy OD. Her past medical history indicated muscle surgery in 1970 for right exotropia found at age 7 years with poor vision and optic atrophy OD.

Visual acuity was hand movements OD, 20/20 OS. There was an afferent pupillary defect and optic atrophy OD. Visual field OD showed only a small nasal remnant; visual field OS showed only nasal constriction. Skin café au lait spots and iris surface nodules were noted OU.

A positive contrast orbitogram demonstrated a tumor of the right optic nerve and a diffuse enlargement of the left optic nerve. PEG showed bilateral enlargement of the prechiasmal intracranial optic nerves and obliteration of the perichiasmal spaces.

Craniotomy was not performed. The presumed diagnosis was neurofibromatosis with optic gliomas involving right and left optic nerves and the chiasm.

A B C D E F

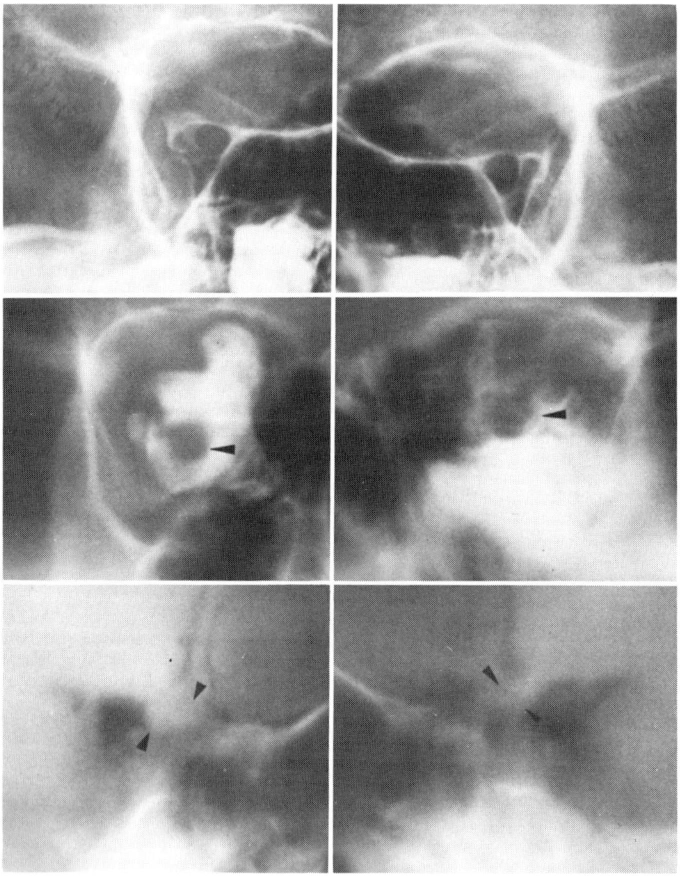

A and **B,** Optic canals were both of borderline size. **C** and **D,** AP polytomographic cuts of right and left positive contrast orbitography show bilateral enlargement of orbital segments of optic nerves (arrows). **E,** Oblique view of the right optic nerve shows it to be markedly enlarged (arrows). In this view, right optic nerve measures 5 by 11 mm, average normal measuring about 3.5 by 6 mm. **F,** Left optic nerve (arrows) is not as well visualized but is also enlarged. AP cuts also showed that optic chiasm was enlarged.

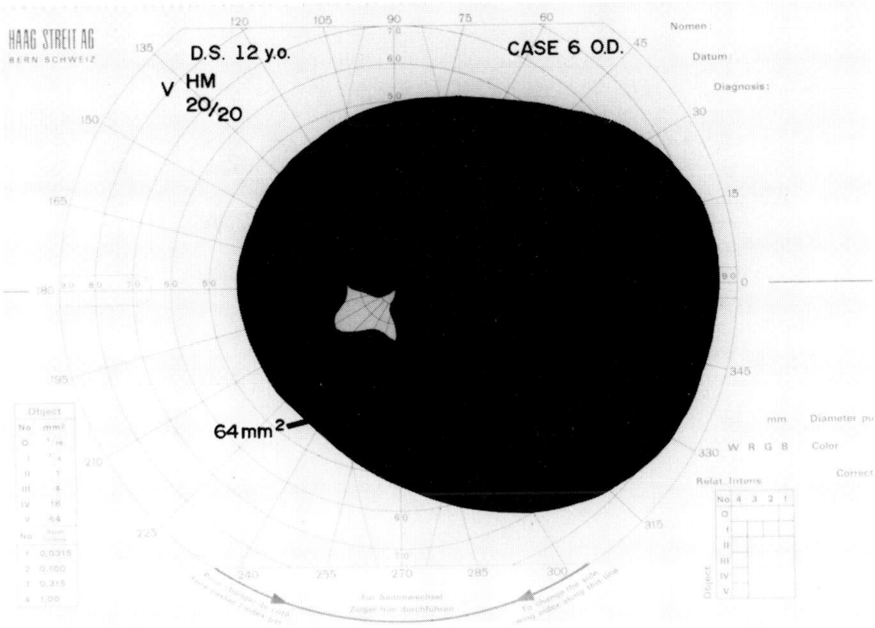
HAAG STREIT AG
BERN SCHWEIZ
D.S. 12 y.o.
CASE 6 O.D.
V HM
20/20
64mm²
Nomen:
Datum:
Diagnosis:

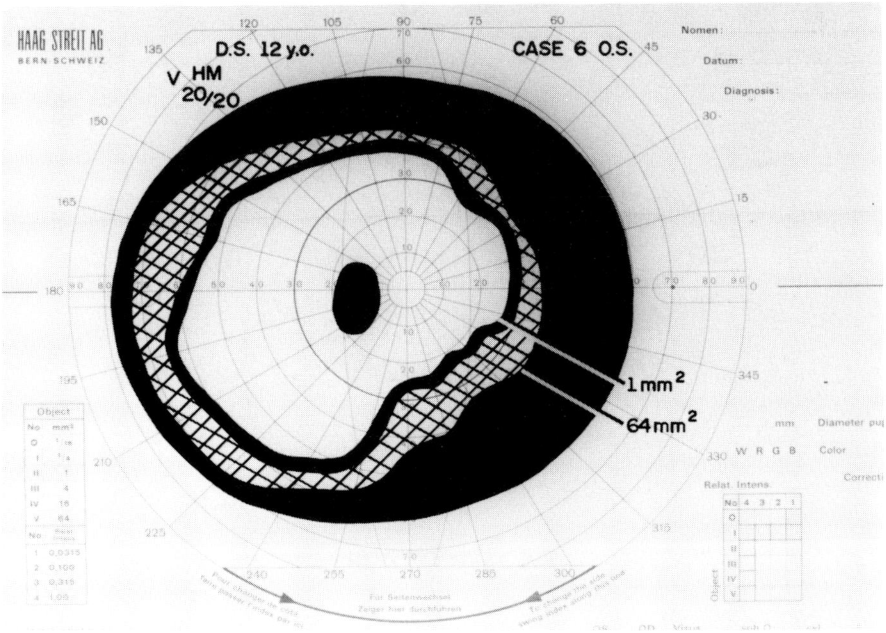
HAAG STREIT AG
BERN SCHWEIZ
D.S. 12 y.o.
CASE 6 O.S.
V HM
20/20
1mm²
64mm²
Nomen:
Datum:
Diagnosis:

Case 7. J. G., a 22-year-old housewife, was admitted on September 11, 1973, with a referral diagnosis of severe optic neuritis (papillitis) OD. Her history indicated pain and blurred vision OD on September 1, with progression to count fingers OD by September 7. By September 10 vision was no light perception OD with optic disc edema.

When she was admitted her visual acuity was no light perception OD, 20/20 OS. She had 3 mm of proptosis OD, with lid edema and pain on elevation. There was optic disc edema OD. The left eye was normal.

Routine skull films showed a normal sella, but optic canal views showed the right optic canal to be minimally but definitely enlarged. Brain scan was normal. Positive contrast orbitogram was abnormal with an enlarged right optic nerve. PEG showed marked asymmetry of the optic chiasm.

The proptosis and central scotoma of OD improved markedly after three days of treatment. Steroid therapy was stopped after seven days.

Follow-up examination one month later revealed visual acuity 20/20 OU. There was an afferent pupillary defect OD. The right optic disc appeared pale normal; the left optic disc was normal. No craniotomy was performed. The presumed diagnosis was optic glioma of the right optic nerve and chiasm.

A

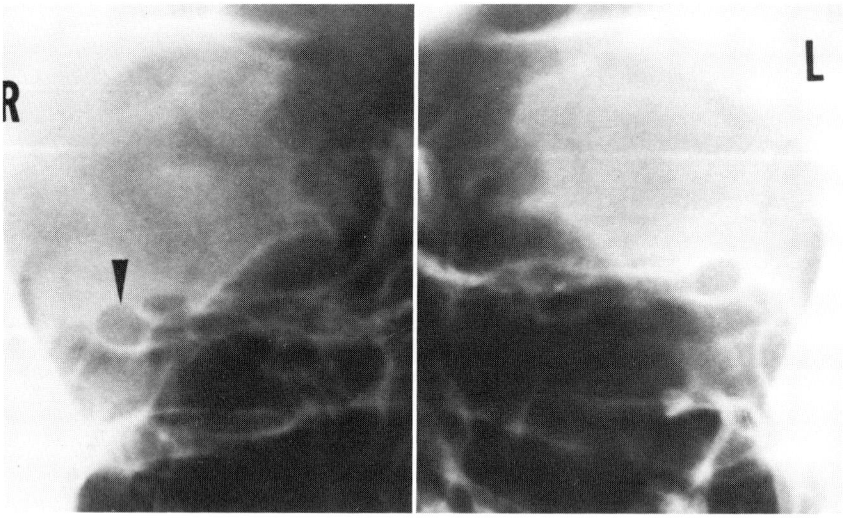

B

A, Right optic canal is enlarged (arrow). **B,** Left optic canal is normal.

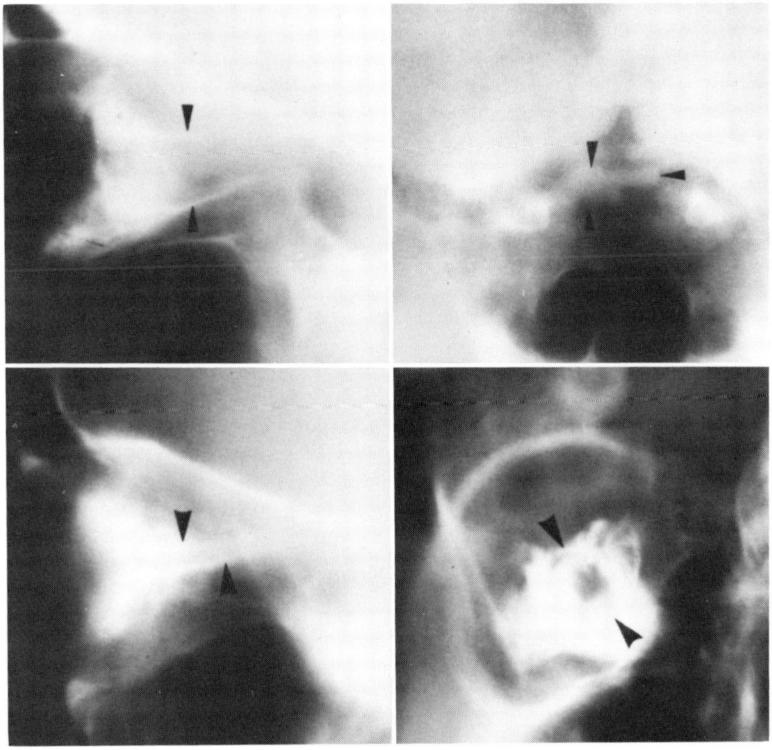

A, Lateral polytomographic cut of positive contrast orbitogram OD shows markedly enlarged optic nerve (arrows). **B,** AP polytomographic section from pneumoencephalogram shows that right side of optic chiasm (vertical opposing arrows) is at least twice as thick as left (horizontal arrow). **C,** Positive contrast orbitogram on different patient, showing normal-sized optic nerve (arrows), for comparison with **A**. **D,** AP view of positive contrast orbitogram, again showing enlargement of right optic nerve. (From Johnson, J. C., Lubow, M., and Stears, J.: Radiology **114:**629, 1975.)

Case 7—cont'd

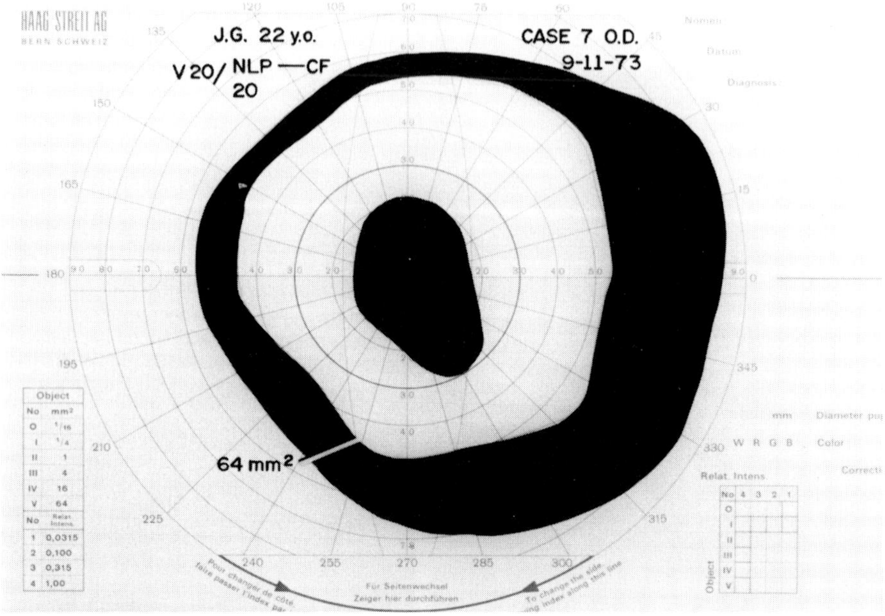
HAAG STREIT AG
BERN SCHWEIZ
J.G. 22 y.o.
V 20/20 NLP —CF
CASE 7 O.D.
9-11-73
64 mm²

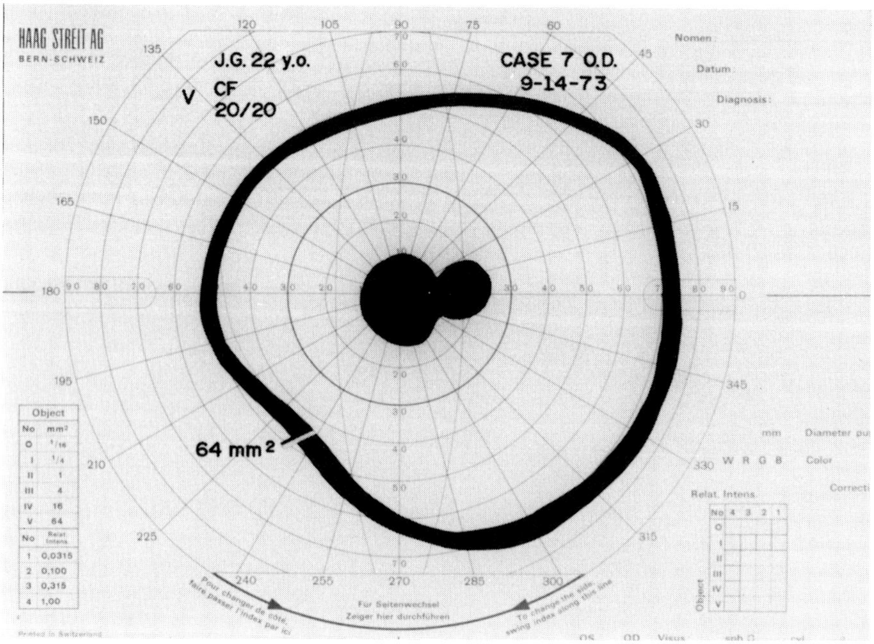
HAAG STREIT AG
BERN-SCHWEIZ
J.G. 22 y.o.
V CF
20/20
CASE 7 O.D.
9-14-73
64 mm²

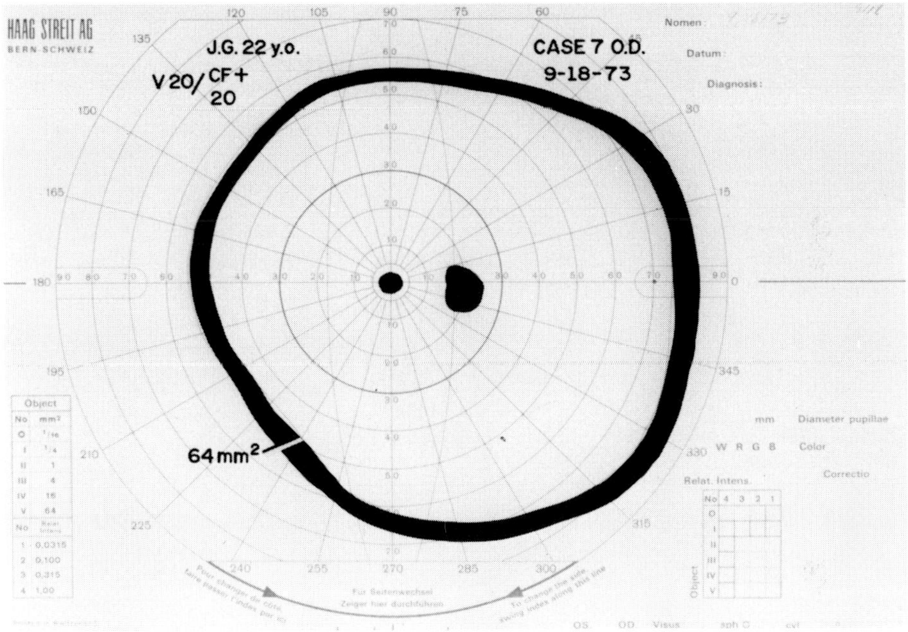
HAAG STREIT AG
BERN-SCHWEIZ
J.G. 22 y.o.
V 20/CF+ 20
CASE 7 O.D.
9-18-73
64 mm²
Nomen
Datum
Diagnosis
Object
Diameter pupillae
Color
Correctio
Relat. Intens.

Case 8. G. J., a 17-year-old schoolboy, was first seen in 1971 complaining of poor vision found on a school examination six months earlier. Visual acuity then was 20/40 OD and 20/25 OS, with an unusual form of hereditary dyslexia. He returned in 1973 because of progressive visual loss with visual acuity 20/400 OD, 20/200 OS. Visual fields were now abnormal, with bilateral cecocentral scotomas not present in 1971.

Plain skull films were normal, with a prominent chiasmatic sulcus. Brain scan was normal. PEG was abnormal, with a suprasellar mass and asymmetry of the optic chiasm. Cerebral arteriogram was abnormal, indicating suprasellar mass.

Craniotomy revealed a grossly enlarged right optic nerve indicative of an optic glioma. No biopsy was performed. The final diagnosis was optic glioma of the right optic nerve, chiasm, and hypothalamus plus hereditary dyslexia. No change in the visual acuities or visual fields were found at the follow-up examination two years later.

A

B

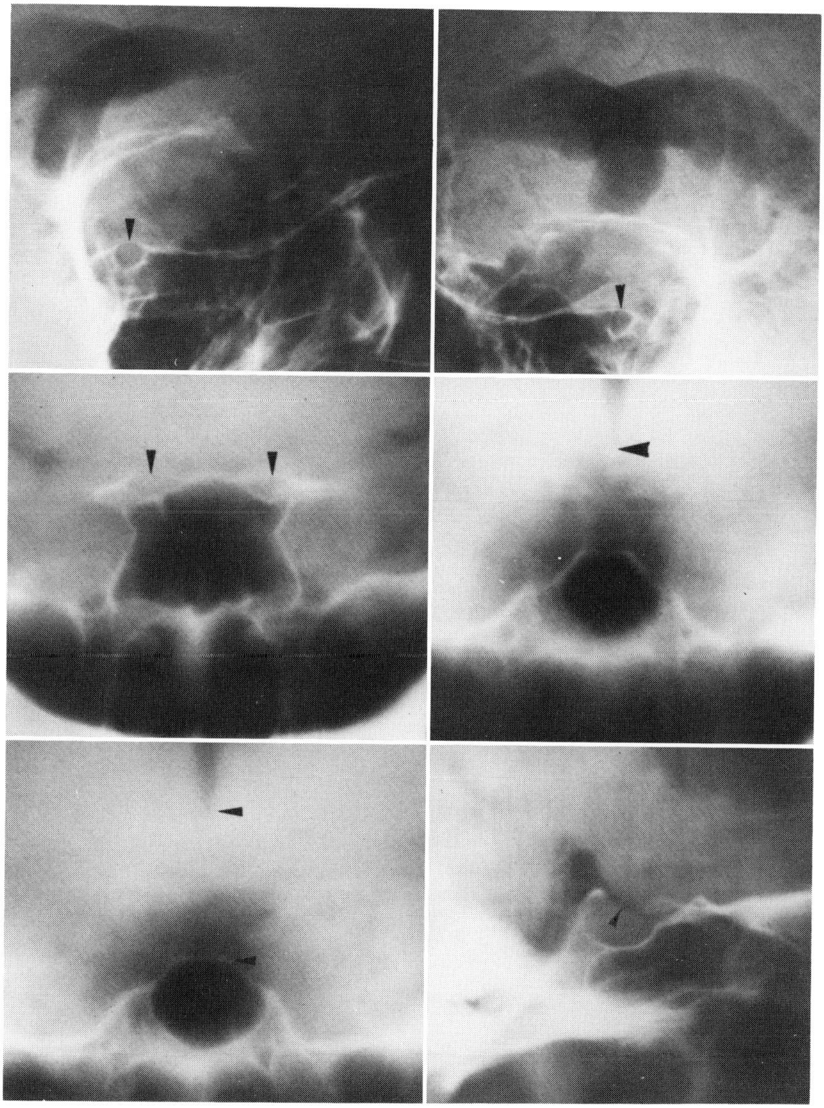

C

D

E

F

A and **B**, Plain films show normal-size optic canals (arrows), but right optic canal in **A** is slightly larger and its superior wall bulges upward slightly compared to superior wall on left. **C**, AP polytomographic cut taken during pneumoencephalogram shows that roof of cranial end of right optic canal is partially destroyed. **D**, AP polytomographic cut at level of posterior portion of sella shows that anterior recesses of third ventricle do not fill. Inferiormost extent of third ventricle (arrow) is more than a centimeter above dorsum. **E**, Section a few millimeters anterior to **D** in midportion of sella, usual level of optic recess of third ventricle. Anteriormost portion of third ventricle (upper arrow) is situated markedly superior to its expected location. Floor of sella (inferior arrow) looks normal. **F**, Lateral tomographic section shows that chiasmatic-hypothalamic mass touches diaphragma sellae. Note also that chiasmatic sulcus just anterior to sella is quite prominent.

Case 8—cont'd

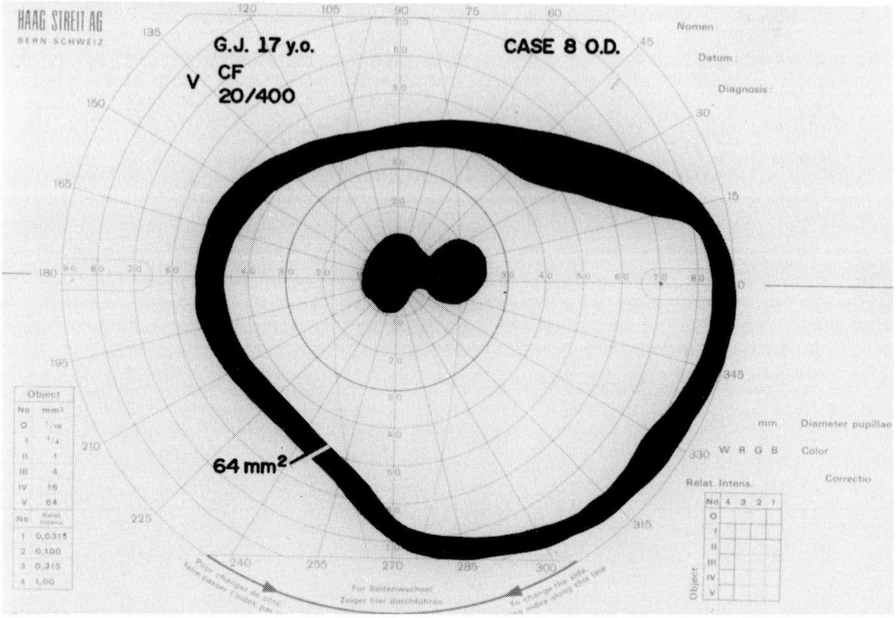
HAAG STREIT AG
BERN SCHWEIZ
G.J. 17 y.o.
CASE 8 O.D.
V CF
20/400
64 mm²
Nomen
Datum
Diagnosis
Object
Relat. Intens.

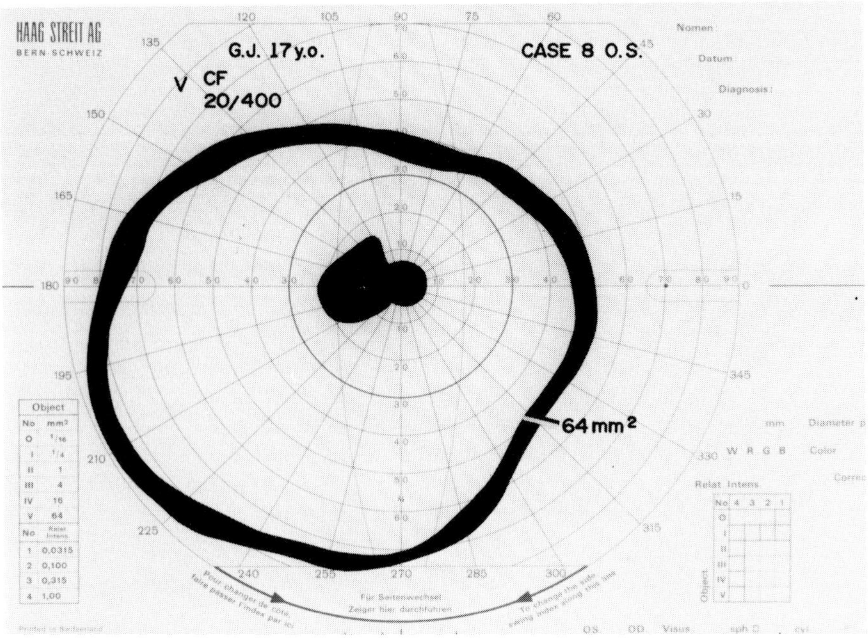
HAAG STREIT AG
BERN SCHWEIZ
G.J. 17 y.o.
CASE 8 O.S.
V CF
20/400
64 mm²
Nomen
Datum
Diagnosis
Object
Relat. Intens.

Case 9. T. B., a 15-year-old schoolgirl, was seen in December 1974 complaining of progressive right orbital pain, photophobia, and blurred vision for approximately two weeks. Visual acuity was known to have been normal several weeks earlier on an examination at Childrens Hospital.

Past history and family history were noncontributory.

Visual acuity was 20/60 OD, 20/20 OS. Visual field OD was contracted with an enlarged blind spot. The visual field OS was normal. There were scattered iris surface nodules OU.

Plain skull films, brain scan, and angiogram were normal. PEG was abnormal, showing an enlarged chiasm. Positive contrast orbitogram was unsatisfacory for interpretation.

Because of the increase in her symptoms, the enlarged chiasm, and the presence of iris nodules, medical decompression was started and the symptoms cleared. The visual acuity and visual field improved to normal OD. No craniotomy was performed. The presumed diagnosis was optic glioma of the right optic nerve and chiasm associated with neurofibromatosis.

A

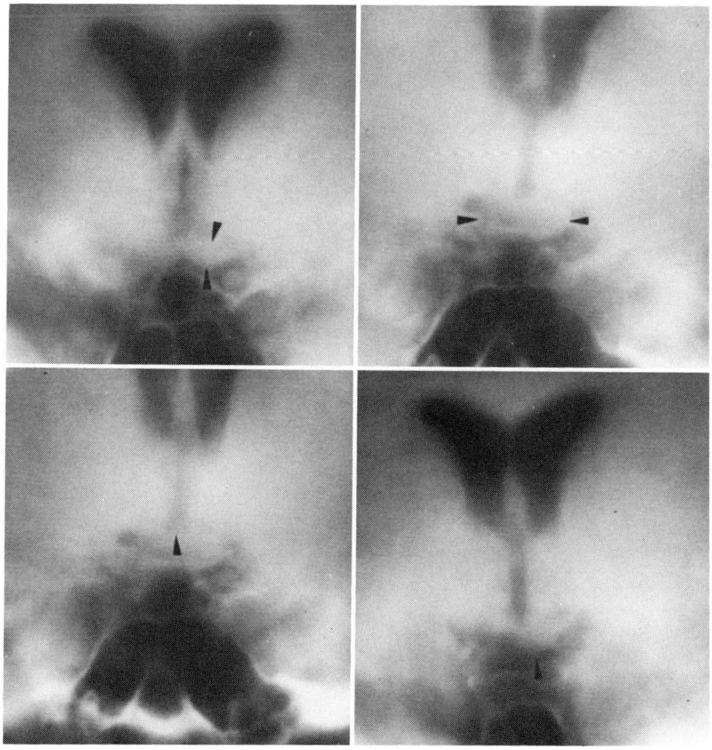

B

C

D

A, Section taken anterior to chiasm. Arrows point to moderately enlarged left optic nerve. Right optic nerve is not surrounded by air and therefore is not demonstrated, which suggests that right optic nerve is even more enlarged than left. **B,** Entire optic chiasm (arrows) is enlarged. It measures 22 by 10 mm, the average optic chiasm measuring about 18 by 5 mm. **C,** Section showing effacement and flattening of normally smoothly rounded optic recess of third ventricle. **D,** Still farther posterior, at the level of dorsum, infundibular recess of third ventricle comes into focus. Left optic tract (arrow) is enlarged.

Case 9—cont'd

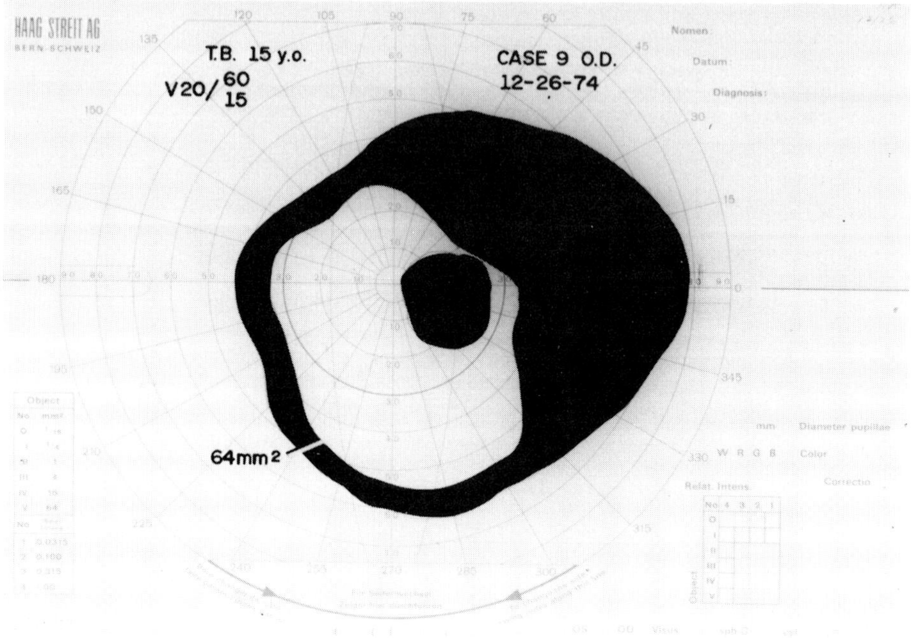
HAAG STREIT AG
BERN SCHWEIZ
T.B. 15 y.o.
V20/60/15
CASE 9 O.D.
12-26-74
64mm²

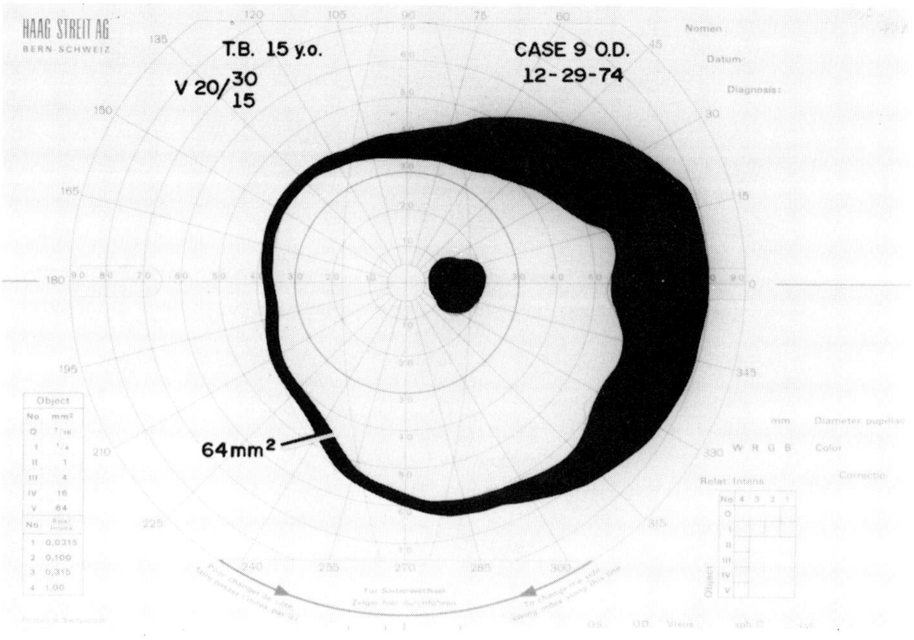
HAAG STREIT AG
BERN SCHWEIZ
T.B. 15 y.o.
V 20/30/15
CASE 9 O.D.
12-29-74
64mm²

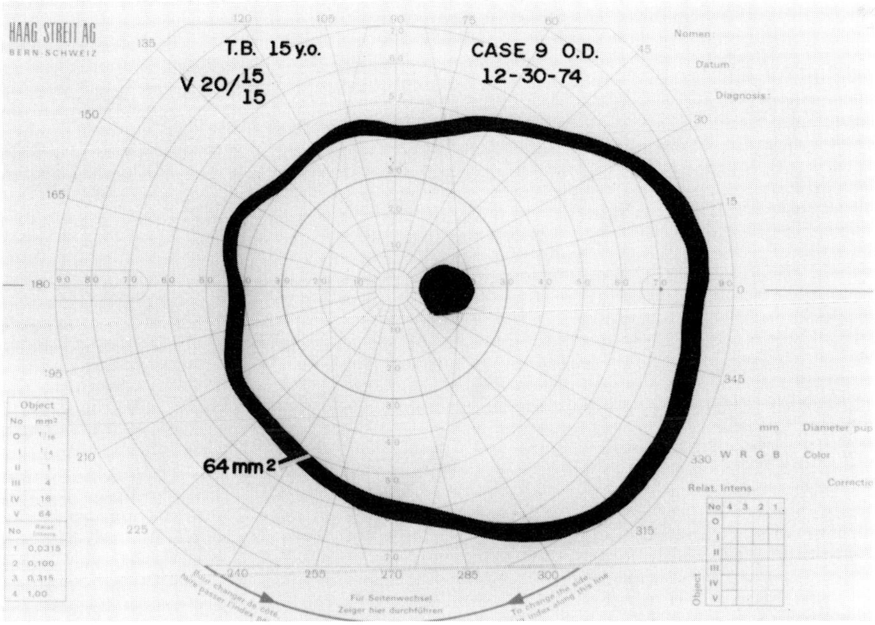
HAAG STREIT AG
BERN-SCHWEIZ
T.B. 15 y.o.
V 20/15 15
CASE 9 O.D.
12-30-74
64 mm²

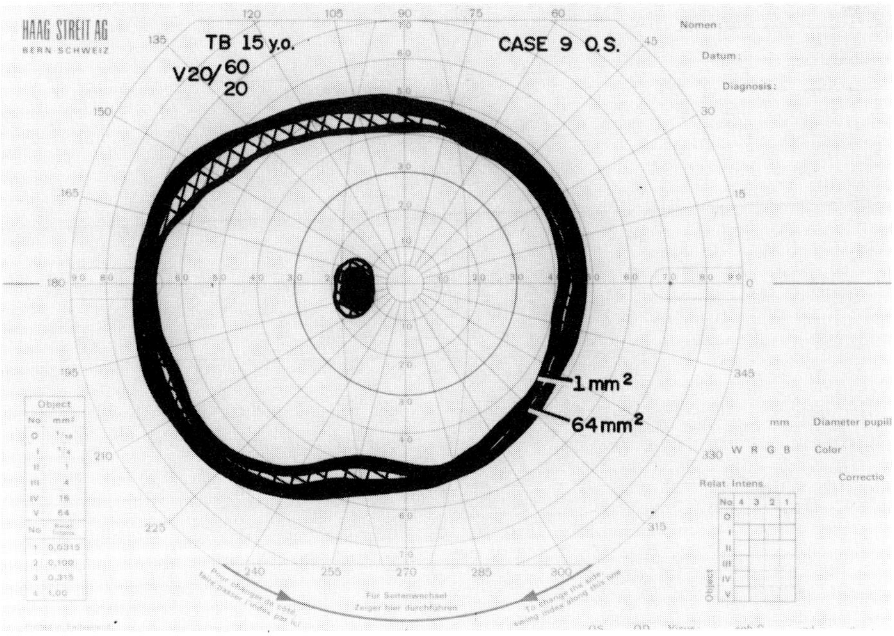
HAAG STREIT AG
BERN SCHWEIZ
TB 15 y.o.
V20/60 20
CASE 9 O.S.
1 mm²
64 mm²

Case 10. M. P., a 70-year-old white female clerk, was seen in April 1974 complaining of unexplained decreased vision OU for two months despite hospital workup elsewhere that showed no abnormality.

She considered her general health good except for the decreased vision, despite a past history of mastectomy for adenocarcinoma (1969).

Visual acuity was 20/70 OD, 20/40 OS. Visual fields showed bitemporal hemianopia to white and red targets. The optic discs were normal.

Plain skull films, brain scan, and angiogram were normal. PEG was abnormal, demonstrating a suprasellar mass continuous with the diaphragma anteriorly.

Craniotomy revealed an encapsulated tumor resembling a chromophobe adenoma, which on histologic study revealed metastatic adenocarcinoma compatible with breast origin.

A

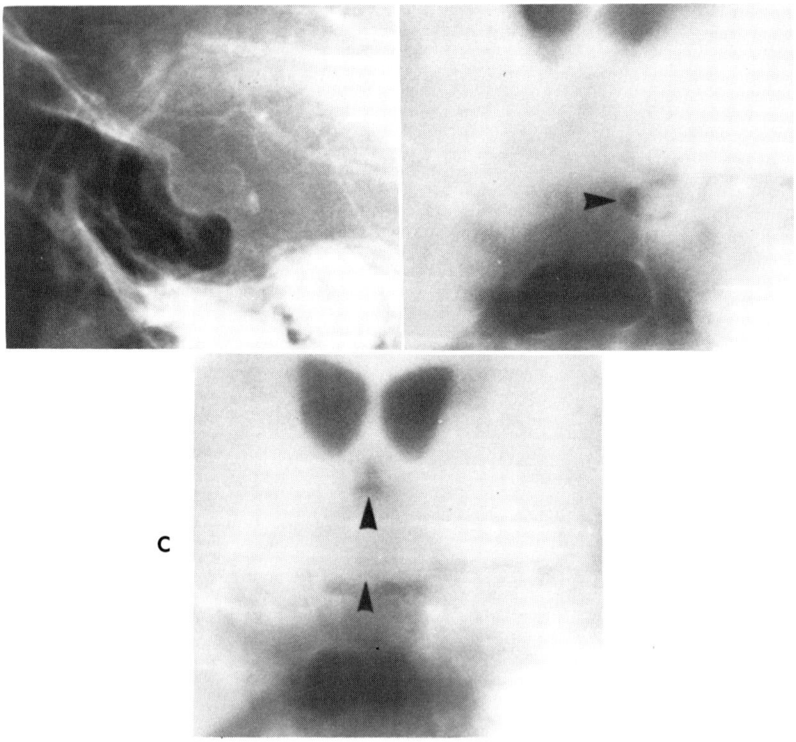

B

C

A, Lateral view of venous phase of arteriogram shows sella of normal size and mineralization. **B,** AP polytomographic cut from pneumoencephalogram through midportion of sella shows complete obliteration of suprasellar and suprachiasmatic cisterns. Arrow points to conjunction between mass and diaphragma sellae. This configuration suggests that metastatic lesion was to pituitary gland with subsequent upward growth in patient with developmentally deficient diaphragma sellae. **C,** Farther posterior, at level of dorsum, AP polytomographic cut at this level shows separation of mass from dorsum (inferior arrow) and marked effacement of anterior recesses of third ventricle (superior arrow).

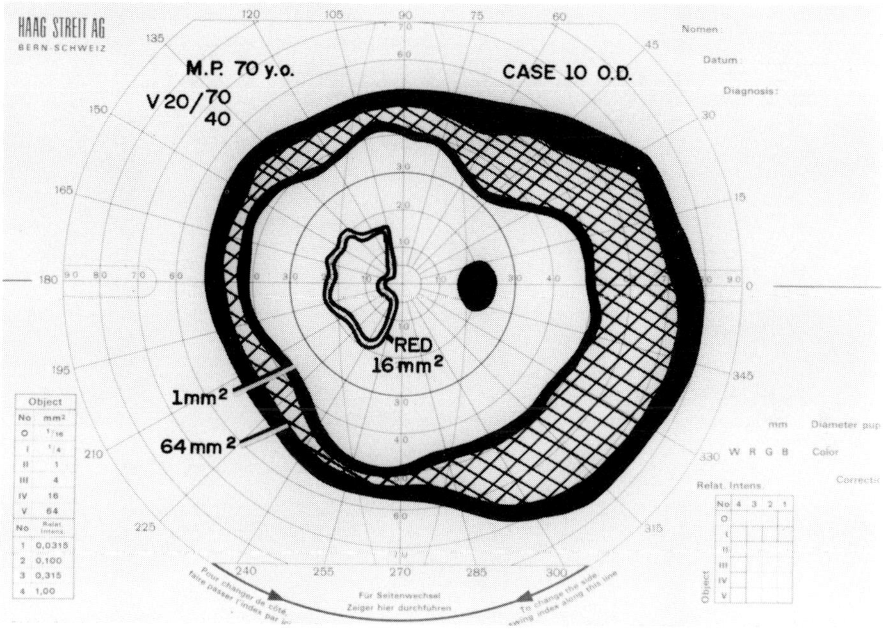
HAAG STREIT AG
BERN-SCHWEIZ
M.P. 70 y.o.
V 20/70 40
CASE 10 O.D.
RED
16 mm²
1mm²
64 mm²

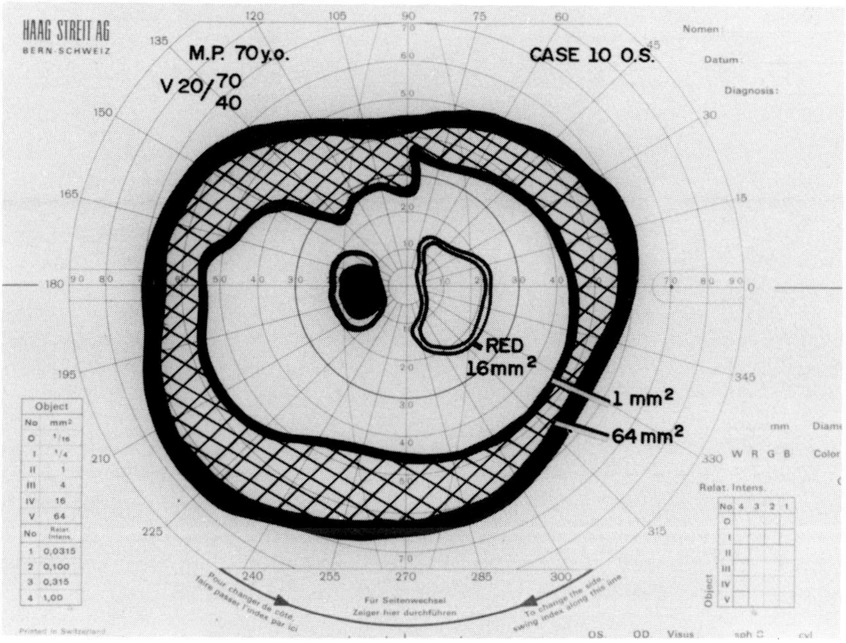
HAAG STREIT AG
BERN-SCHWEIZ
M.P. 70 y.o.
V 20/70 40
CASE 10 O.S.
RED
16mm²
1 mm²
64 mm²

Case 11. J. L., a 47-year-old Negro laundress, was seen in August 1974 complaining of decreased vision OU for two years.

Past history included diabetes (1956), amenorrhea (1962), sarcoidosis (1962), cataract surgery OS (1972), and anemia (1974).

Visual acuity was count fingers OD, hand movements OS. There were nasal remnants to the visual fields OU, suggesting a bitemporal hemianopia. The optic discs showed bilateral optic atrophy. Also noted was orthostatic hypotension.

Plain films, brain scan, and angiogram were normal. The PEG was abnormal, revealing an enlarged chiasm.

Frontal craniotomy demonstrated dense fibrous sheathing of the chiasm. Biopsy of this material revealed optochiasmatic arachnoiditis.

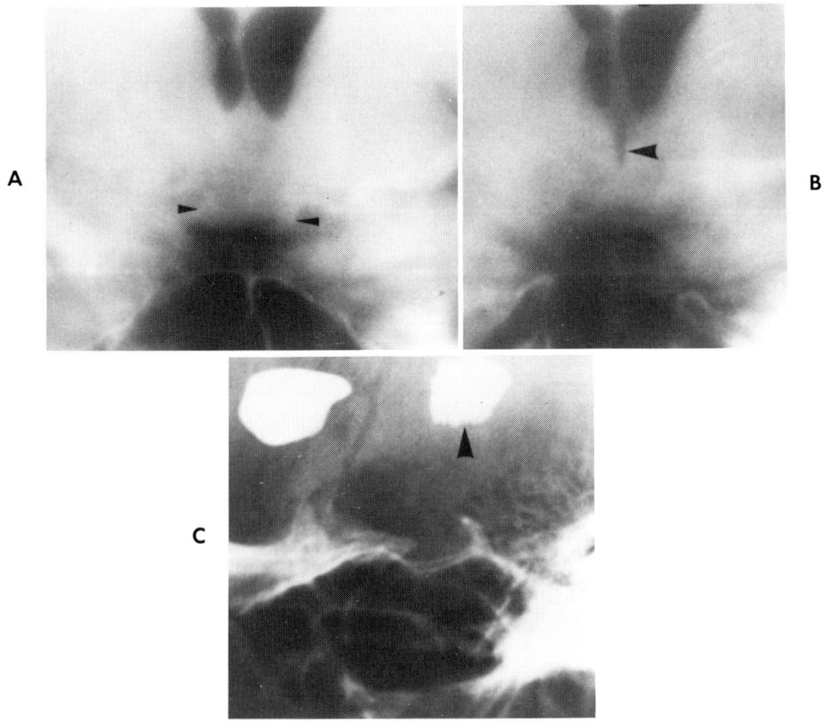

A, Brow-up, AP polytomographic cut from pneumoencephalogram at level of midportion of sella shows shadow of optic chiasm (arrows) to be enlarged. At this level, anterior recesses of third ventricle are not filled at all. **B,** Farther posterior, just behind level of dorsum, minimal filling of third ventricle is seen. **C,** Lateral films from Pantopaque ventriculogram confirms lack of filling of anterior recesses of third ventricle. At surgery, chiasm was found to be encased in fibrous tissue. In addition to arachnoiditis, lack of filling of anterior recesses of third ventricle suggests ventriculitis.

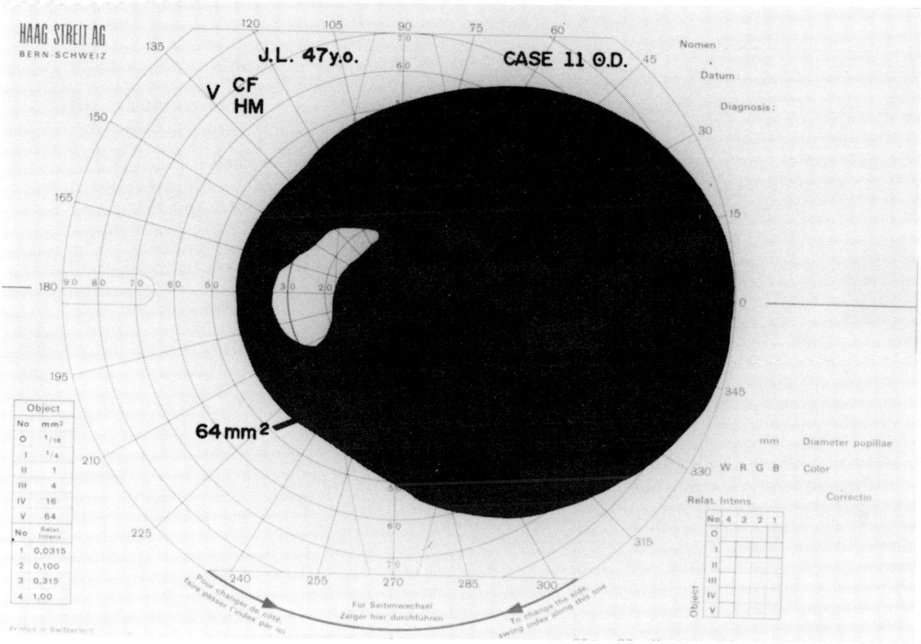
HAAG STREIT AG
BERN SCHWEIZ
J.L. 47y.o.
CASE 11 O.D.
V CF
HM
64 mm²
Nomen
Datum
Diagnosis:
Für Seitenwechsel
Zeiger hier durchführen

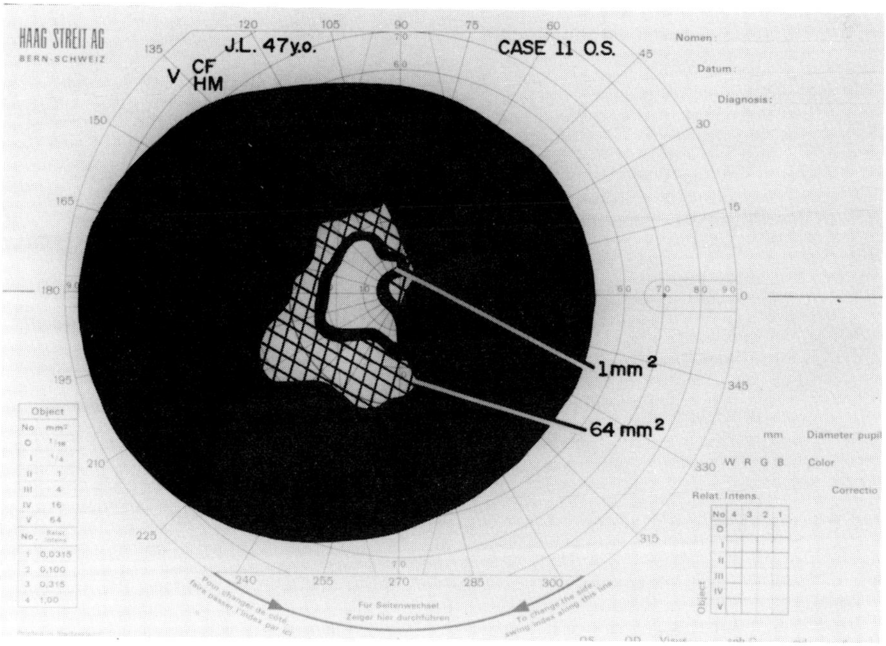
HAAG STREIT AG
BERN SCHWEIZ
J.L. 47y.o.
CASE 11 O.S.
V CF
HM
1 mm²
64 mm²
Nomen
Datum
Diagnosis:
Für Seitenwechsel
Zeiger hier durchführen

ACKNOWLEDGMENT

The technical assistance of Mrs. Shirley Palui and Mrs. Dotty Blackham is gratefully acknowledged.

REFERENCES

1. Vallebona, A.: Una modalita di tecnica per la dissociazione radiografica della ombre applicata allo studio del cranio, Radiol. Med. **17:**1090-1097, 1930.
2. Ziedses des Plantes, B. G.: Examen due troisieme et du quatrieme ventricule au moyen de petites quantites d'air, Acta Radiol. (Stockh.) **34:**399-407, 1950.
3. Schechter, M. M., and De Gutierrez-Mahoney, C. G.: Autotomography showing the normal and abnormal mid-line ventricular structures and basal cisterns, Br. J. Radiol. **35:**438-461, 1962.
4. Bourdon, R.: Cranial tomography in neuroradiology. Tomography of the skull, Acta Radiol. **40:**272-278, 1953.
5. Valentino, V.: Some experiences with tomography in neuroradiology, Acta Radiol. (Stockh.) **45:**101-105, 1956.
6. DiChiro, G.: An atlas of detailed normal pneumoencephalographic anatomy, Springfield, Ill., 1961, Charles C Thomas, Publisher.
7. Amundsen, P.: Gas encephalography with the polytome, Neuroradiology **5:**65-69, 1973.
8. Amundsen, P., Dugstad, P., and Grimsrud, C. K.: Gas encephalography with hypocycloidal tomography: correlation with anatomic cases, Acta Radiol. (Diagn.) (Stockh.) **9** (special issue): 132-134, 1969.
9. Bories, J., Fredy, D., and Rosier, J.: Tomo-encephalography—technique and normal images, Neuroradiology **1:**200-209, 1970.
10. Morris, L., and Wylie, I. G.: Tomography in cerebral pneumoencephalography, Clin. Radiol. **24:**221-230, 1973.
11. Caille, J. M., Piton, J.: La cisterne opto-chiasmatique en tomographie lineaire, Bull. Soc. Ophtalmol. Fr. **70:**1084-1091, 1970.
12. Caille, J. M., Piton, J., Basseau, J. P., et al.: Cisterno tomographie de la region opto-chiasmatique dans l'etude du syndrome chiasmatique, J. Radiol. Electrol. Med. Nucl. **52:**663-668, 1971.
13. Fischgold, H., Bonnemazou, A., Fredy, D., et al.: La cisterne optochiasmatique et son contenu, J. Radiol. Electrol. Med. Nucl. **50:**121-134, 1969.
14. Hanafee, W. N., Lecky, J. W.: Planography during pneumoencephalography, Arch. Ophtalmol. (Paris) **80:**161-165, 1968.
15. Harwood-Nash, D. C.: Optic gliomas and pediatric neuroradiology, Radiol. Clin. North Am. **10:**83-100, 1972.
16. Metzger, J.: Lesigne du chiasma de face en pneumotomographie hypocycloide, Rev. Neurol. (Paris) **117:**666-672, 1967.
17. Metzger, J., Fredy, D., Bonnemazou, A., and Fischgold, H.: La citerne optochiasmatique et son contenu, J. Radiol. Electrol. Med. Nucl. **50:**125-134, 1969.
18. Montaut, J., Picard, L., Raspiller, A., and Remarck, G.: Interet de la tomographie frontale dans le diagnostic du gliome des bandelettes optiques, Rev. Otoneuro-ophtalmol. **40:**31-36, 1971.
19. Johnson, J. C., Lubow, M., and Stears, J.: Polytomoencephalography of the optic chiasm and adjacent structures, Radiology **114:**629-634, 1975.
20. Neelon, F. A., Goree, J. A., and Lebovitz, H. E.: The primary empty sella: clinical and radiographic characteristics and endocrine function, Medicine (Baltimore) **52:**73-92, 1973.
21. Hoyt, W. E.: Correlative functional anatomy of the optic chiasm. In Clinical neurosurgery, Baltimore, 1970, The Williams & Wilkins Company.
22. McLachlan, J. P., Lavender, J. P., and Edwards, C. R. W.: Polytome encephalography in the investigation of pituitary tumors, Clin. Radiol. **22:**361-369, 1971.
23. Wong, I. G., and Lubow, M.: Management of optic glioma of childhood. In Smith, J. L., editor: Neuro-ophthalmology, vol. 6, St. Louis, 1972, The C. V. Mosby Co., pp. 51-59.

Chapter 6

Ischemic chiasmal syndrome

K. Francis Lee
Norman J. Schatz
Peter J. Savino

INTRODUCTION

The majority of lesions that produce chiasmal visual field defects are the result of chiasmal compression by a mass lesion located in the vicinity of the sella turcica. However, an identical clinical picture may likewise be produced by a variety of nontumorous processes involving the chiasm.

Arteriosclerosis is accepted as one such cause.[1] At the sixth annual meeting of the American Society of Neuro-radiology (1968), we reported 12 patients with a chiasmal syndrome related to arteriosclerosis.[2] Since then, we have evaluated 22 patients with chiasmal syndromes attributable to a variety of progressive ischemic processes.

This chapter is intended to define the clinical and neuroradiologic manifestations of the ischemic chiasmal syndrome (ICS) and to point out several pathogenetic factors.

ANATOMIC RELATIONSHIP BETWEEN THE CHIASM, OPTIC NERVE, AND ADJACENT VESSELS

The chiasm lies medial to the internal carotid arteries, with the anterior cerebral arteries passing above the junction of the optic nerves and chiasm. The chiasm itself is in the floor of the third ventricle, forming the optic and infundibular recesses. These structures are easily demonstrated by pneumoencephalography.[3] The position of the chiasm in relation to the tuberculum sellae turcicae and pituitary stalk is variable.[4, 5] Bull[6] studied 117 normal pneumoencephalograms to locate the chiasm, and on the basis of this and other data, Walker[7] calculated the mean length of the intracranial portion of the optic nerve to be 17.1 ± 2.5 mm (10-23 mm), and the height of the chiasmal point (between the optic and infundibular recesses) to be 10.7 ± 2.4 mm (4-17 mm) above the nasotubercular line.[7] With the combined use of pneumoencephalography and polytomographic techniques, a detailed anatomic study of this region is possible radiologically.

NORMAL BLOOD SUPPLY TO THE OPTIC NERVE, CHIASM, AND PITUITARY GLAND

The blood supply of the pituitary gland, optic nerve, and chiasm has been studied by many investigators.[5, 8, 8a, 9] The pituitary gland receives its arterial supply from two groups of vessels, the right and left superior hypophyseal arteries and the right and left inferior hypophyseal arteries.

The superior hypophyseal artery arises from the medial aspect of the internal carotid artery at the level of the origin of the ophthalmic artery. Each superior hypophyseal artery divides into two main branches that pass respectively to the anterior and posterior aspects of the pituitary stalk. The anterior superior hypophyseal artery sends branches to the pituitary gland as well as to the optic nerve, the ventral surface of optic chiasm, and the hypothalamus. The posterior superior hypophyseal artery nourishes the pituitary gland, optic tract, and tuber cinereum.

The anastomotic plexus surrounding the infundibular stalk is supplied by the ipsilateral and contralateral connecting branches of these vessels of the internal carotid arteries and supplies the posterior lobe of the pituitary and adjacent dura. The periinfundibular anastomosis, therefore, has three components: (1) the superior hypophyseal arteries, (2) the infundibular arteries from the posterior communicating arteries, and (3) a prechiasmal anastomosis from the anterior cerebral arteries.

The vascular supply to the intracranial optic nerve is likewise multiple, with the ophthalmic artery supplying its inferomedial aspect and the superior hypophyseal artery its inferior surface. The dorsal portion of the optic nerve and chiasm are nourished by the anterior cerebral artery.

The ophthalmic, anterior cerebral, anterior communicating, internal carotid, superior hypophyseal, middle cerebral, posterior communicating, and anterior choroidal arteries all contribute chiasmal branches. However, the inferior surface of the chiasm is supplied predominantly by the anterior superior hypophyseal arteries, directly or via the periinfundibular plexus, while the superior surface of the anterior chiasmal angle is supplied by branches of the carotid, anterior cerebral, and anterior communicating arteries. The lateral chiasm receives blood supply from the internal carotid via the lateral chiasmal arteries, and the posteroinferior chiasmal angle is mainly supplied by the posterior communicating artery.

The vascular supply of the diaphragma sellae is derived from the inferior hypophyseal arteries, the anterior capsular arteries from the cavernous carotid, and, occasionally, branches of the superior hypophyseal arteries.

MATERIALS AND METHODS

The majority of our patients were referred from Wills Eye Hospital to Thomas Jefferson University Hospital for evaluation of visual symptoms. Extensive neuro-ophthalmologic, neuroradiologic, and endocrinologic (pituitary function) investigations were carried out. Radiologic studies included plain skull films with stereoscopic PA and lateral views, optic canal views, and polytomographic sections of the sella turcica and optic canal in various projections, including a basal view.

Cerebral arteriography using the Seldinger technique was performed, and pertinent films subjected to subtraction study. Magnification angiography (×3.0) was used for detailed analysis of minor blood vessels. Pneumoencephalography, using the Philips polytomographic unit, was carried out with the patient in the brow-up and hanging-head positions. After sufficient air was introduced into the lateral ventricles to attain maximum filling of the rostral portion of the third ventricle, sagittal and coronal sections at 2-mm intervals were obtained. An intraventricular pantopaque study was performed in patients where other studies were equivocal.

Table 4. Ischemic chiasmal syndrome

Group	*Number of cases*	*Age range*	*Pathologic features*	*Visual impairment*	*Number with empty sella*	*Pituitary function*
I	6	60-70	Low-lying ectatic anterior cerebral and carotid	Slowly progressive	5	Low normal
II	4	50-70	Atherosclerotic plaque formation	Gradual, or acute onset	3	Usually low
III	8	20-60	Optochiasmatic arachnoiditis and fibrosis	Gradual, progressive	5	Usually low
IV	2	50-70	Arteritis with stenosis and dilatation of vessels	Acute onset	1	Low
V	2	20-30	Postpartum pituitary necrosis and ischemia	Acute onset, slow recovery	2	Depressed
Total	22				16	

RESULTS

Five etiologic categories were identified on the basis of the findings (Table 4). Over 80% of the patients (18/22) showed a slowly progressive impairment of vision, with only patients in groups IV and V experiencing acute episodes.

Approximately three-quarters (16/22) of the patients demonstrated a concomitant empty sella syndrome. This diagnosis was made when pneumoencephalography demonstrated air below the diaphragma sellae.

Pituitary function was depressed in each group, with patients in group I giving values closer to normal.

GROUP I: MECHANICAL COMPRESSION OF THE OPTIC NERVE AND CHIASM DUE TO REDUNDANT SCLEROTIC ANTERIOR CEREBRAL ARTERIES

Case 1. The patient, a 74-year-old man with known neurofibromatosis, complained of progressive visual loss for approximately three years. Visual acuity was 6/9 in the right eye and 6/18 in the left eye. Visual fields showed bitemporal heminanopia and binasal field constriction (Fig. 6-1, *A*). There was bilateral optic nerve pallor. Multiple neurofibromata covered his entire body.

Skull x-rays revealed an enlarged sella. There was a low-positioned tortuous sclerotic anterior cerebral artery on the right (Fig. 6-1, *B*). Pneumoencephalography demonstrated an empty sella, with intrasellar herniation of the infundibular recess. The chiasmal recess was blunted (Fig. 6-1, *C*).

Because of the clinical picture of chiasmal compression, progressive bitemporal field loss, and enlarged pituitary fossa, a right frontal craniotomy was performed. A huge tortuous anterior cerebral artery was seen to notch the anterior aspect of the chiasm (Fig. 6-1, *D*).

COMMENT. This 74-year-old man with neurofibromatosis presented with progressive visual loss and a bitemporal hemianopia. Evaluation, including exploratory craniotomy, revealed only a tortuous anterior cerebral artery compressing the chiasm, and an empty sella.

Five other cases were considered to belong to this group. Compression of the chiasm produces scotomas that may be central, peripheral, or both. Scotomas extending into the nasal field are due to superimposed optic nerve ischemia. Those in the temporal field respect the vertical median, strongly indicating a chiasmal origin.

Typical vascular chiasmal syndrome may rarely be seen in cases of intracranial aneurysm, although variable visual field loss may develop depending on the site of aneurysmal impingement on the visual apparatus.[10, 11]

In the presence of upward growth of pituitary tumor, the anterior cerebral artery may act as a restrictive cord on the dorsal surface of the prechiasmal optic nerve, with the resultant notching or grooving[12, 13] accounting for chiasmal visual field defects.[4, 14] Infarction of the chiasm may develop as the result of focal ischemia produced by an intrinsic or extrinsic tumor.[15] It is conceivable that a similar but milder compressive effect may be produced temporarily in the absence of tumor by the upward bulging of

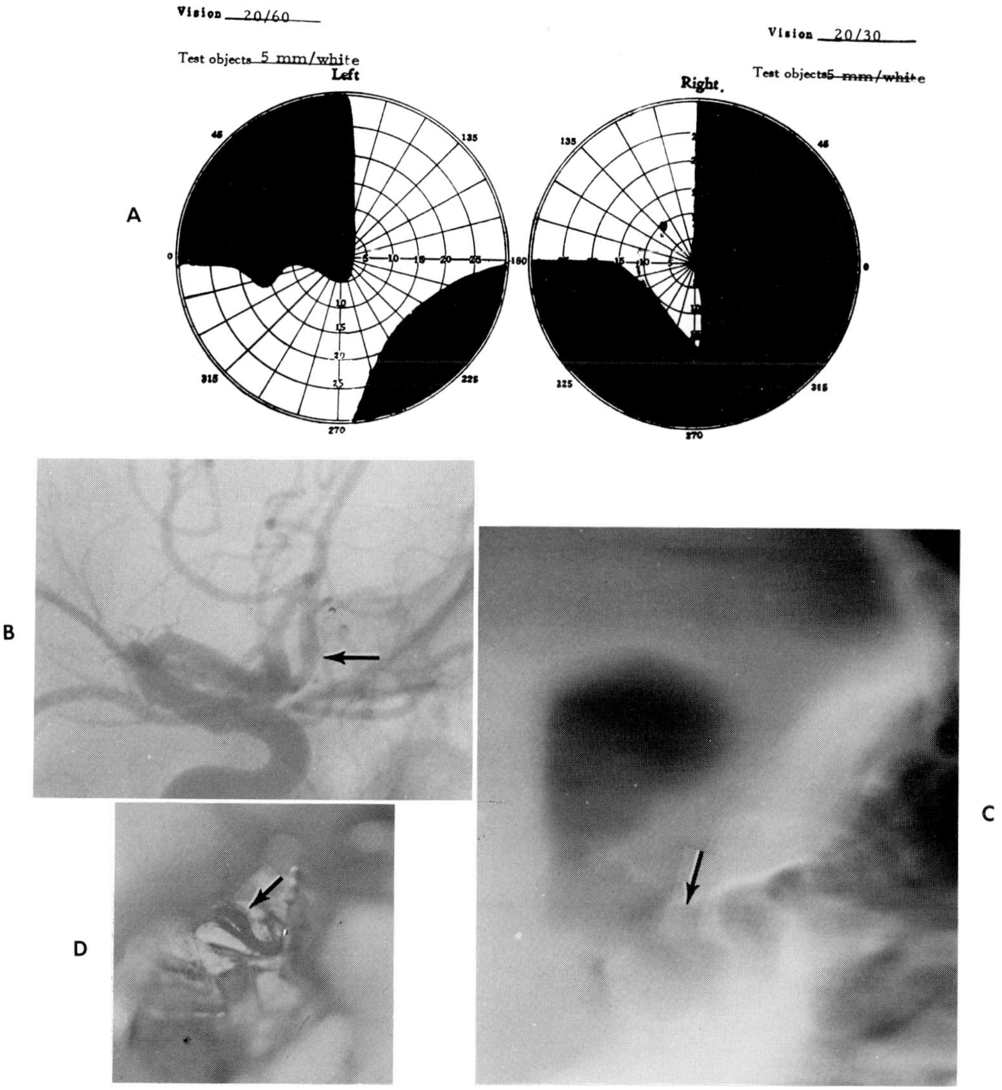

Fig. 6-1. A, Visual field of 74-year-old man with mechanical compression of the optic nerve–chiasmal junction by a redundant right anterior cerebral artery showed a bitemporal hemianopia with binasal field constriction. **B,** Right carotid arteriogram revealed a low-lying tortuous anterior cerebral artery (arrow). **C,** Midsagittal tomogram of pneumoencephalogram revealed enlargement of the pituitary fossa with intrasellar herniation of the rostral end of the third ventricle. The optic recess is blunted with a low-lying chiasm (arrow). **D,** At surgery a dolichoectatic anterior cerebral artery was found to be causing a groove at the optic nerve–chiasmal junction (arrow).

the diaphragma sellae due to enlarged pituitary gland during pregnancy or menstruation.*

Hilton and Hoyt[16] reported a case of progressive chiasmal syndrome in a 68-year-old man who had bitemporal field defects and tortuous dilated anterior cerebral arteries on angiography. The pneumoencephalogram showed no evidence of tumor, and no surgery was performed. The angiographic findings in this patient resembled the necropsy specimen shown by Walsh and Gass,[17] which demonstrated an anterior chiasmal indentation by sclerotic elongated anterior cerebral arteries. Unfortunately, however, no premortem clinical information was available. Similar cases have documented compression and atrophy of the optic nerves or chiasm or both, resulting from abnormal dolichoectatic anterior cerebral or carotid arteries.[1, 18-20]

Hilton and Hoyt[16] expressed the view that the pathologic changes in the anterior cerebral arteries in their patient probably impaired circulation in the prechiasmal arterial anastomotic network; traction, stretching of minor vessels, and obliteration of their ostia in the diseased carotid and anterior cerebral arteries may be the cause of chiasmal ischemia.

Indentation or grooving of the optic nerve by a low-lying anterior cerebral artery does not necessarily cause visual field loss, presumably because an adequate vascular anastomosis is present despite a focal compression.

GROUP II: ISCHEMIC CHIASMAL SYNDROME SECONDARY TO ATHEROSCLEROTIC NARROWING AND OCCLUSION OF VESSELS

Case 2. The patient, a 56-year-old man known to be hypertensive, presented with a three-year history of frontal headaches. Two months before admission, the patient experienced visual difficulty, noting that words would run together. The patient was a heavy drinker, and 24 hours after a binge of drinking he would have convulsions. He was admitted for control of seizures.

Evaluation upon admission revealed 6/6 visual acuity in the left eye. The right eye had been enucleated following a childhood injury. There was a dense temporal hemianopia in the left eye (Fig. 6-2, *A*) and pallor of the left optic nerve head. The neurologic examination was normal. Blood pressure was 170/110, and a grade-2 aortic systolic murmur was heard. The physical examination was unremarkable.

---

*EDITOR'S NOTE. Visual disturbances in the form of field defects during pregnancy require comment. A disorder as common as optic neuritis will eventually occur during pregnancy, but a direct relationship remains tenuous. On the other hand, intracranial tumors (e.g., meningiomas) are known to undergo growth spurts during pregnancy. Distinction must be made between mild temporal field constriction of a functional nature and true temporal hemianopic defects; with the latter, neurodiagnostic studies are indicated. Hypertrophy of the pituitary gland during pregnancy has been suggested as a cause of bitemporal defects, but if one considers the distance between the diaphragma sellae and the chiasm, this mechanism seems most unlikely and has, to my knowledge, never been substantiated. The possibility of *functional* visual loss should be kept in mind. J. S. G.

A

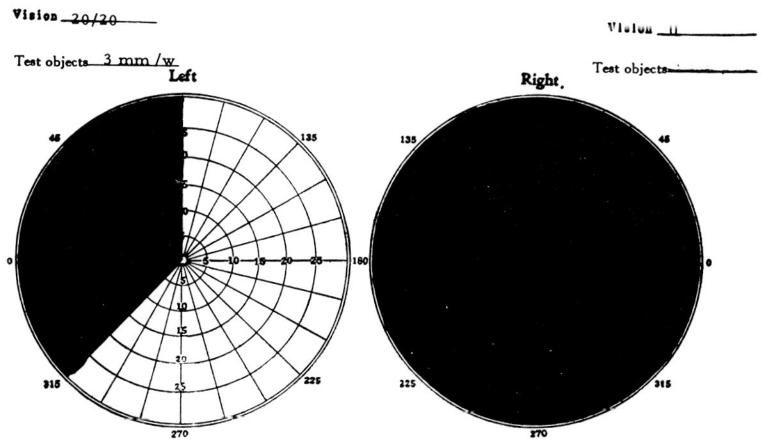

B

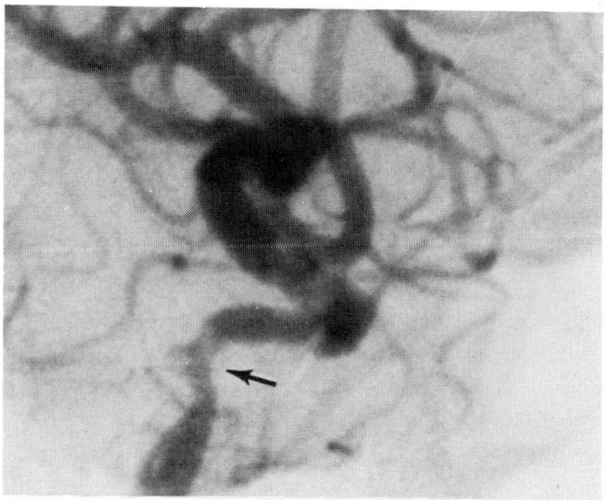

Fig. 6-2. A, Visual field examination of 50-year-old man showed a dense temporal hemianopia in the left eye. The right eye had been enucleated. **B,** Carotid arteriogram showed marginal serrations of the internal carotid artery due to atheromatous plaques (arrow).

Skull x-ray films revealed an enlarged pituitary fossa. Pneumoencephalogram and bilateral carotid arteriogram revealed intrasellar extension of the suprasellar cisterns and low-positioned tortuous anterior cerebral arteries. Magnification arteriogram revealed thin atheromatous plaques in the cavernous and supraclinoid segments of the left internal carotid artery (Fig. 6-2, *B*).

COMMENT. This 56-year-old man was admitted for evaluation of a "rum fit." He was found to have a chiasmal visual field defect with an enlarged and empty sella demonstrated on pneumoencephalogram. Atherosclerotic plaques in the carotid siphon with stenosis or obliteration of the ostia of chiasmal arteries and Dawson's plexus were demonstrated angiographically. This patient represents a combined mechanism of ischemic process with atherosclerotic carotid arteries and dolicoectatic anterior cerebral arteries producing a chiasmal syndrome. In four of our patients the clinical and neuroradiologic findings were similar.

A few instances of pituitary ischemia associated with cerebrovascular disease have been recorded. Hobbs[21] presented a patient with hypopituitarism related to insufficient carotid artery blood supply. The patient, a 43-year-old women, showed evidence of acute pituitary insufficiency. The right carotid artery was totally occluded, and the left carotid artery was almost obliterated at the level of the cavernous sinus. The vascular origin in this case seems quite clear. Gilroy and Meyer[22] described a "new clinical syndrome," pituitary insufficiency with cerebrovascular symptoms. These authors related postural hypotensive episodes manifested by ataxia, vertigo, dimness of vision, and diplopia to hypopituitarism. The symptoms were alleviated by exogenous steroid replacement. Although atherosclerotic changes of severe degree were demonstrated by arteriography, no theory for the origin of hypopituitarism was postulated. An ischemic cause seems likely.

The employment of magnification angiography with subtraction is essential to demonstrate the subtle arteriosclerotic plaque formation in the carotid siphon and its branches that is responsible for this form of ischemic chiasmal syndrome.

GROUP III: VASCULAR ENCASEMENT AND OCCLUSION SECONDARY TO DIFFUSE ARACHNOIDAL ADHESION AND THICKENING

Case 3. The patient was a 31-year-old man who had a history of decreasing vision bilaterally, greater in the right eye for six months.

He was first examined in January 1974, when general neurologic examination was normal. The visual acuity was 6/15 in both eyes. Visual field examination demonstrated central scotomas and bitemporal hemianopic field defects (Fig. 6-3, *A*).

Laboratory studies revealed the following values: hemoglobin 13.4 gm/100 ml; hematocrit reading, 39.9%; and a normal white blood cell count. RPR and FTA were nonreactive.

X-ray films revealed shortening of the dorsum sellae. Cerebral arteriograms were normal except for a segmental narrowing of the supraclinoid portion of the right internal carotid artery (Fig. 6-3, *B*). Pneumoencephalogram revealed obliteration of the optic and infundibular recesses, but no elevation or actual indentation of the rostral end of the third ventricle was present. No air reached the chiasmatic cistern (Fig. 6-3, *C*). Brain scan was normal.

A craniotomy was performed on February 1, 1974. The carotid arteries were normal. Dense adhesions were noted between the frontal lobes. Between the thickened arachnoid and the optic nerves a meshwork of fine vascular adhesions was noted and removed. Pathologic examination revealed nonspecific chronic inflammation. Postoperatively the vision and visual fields were unchanged.

COMMENT. This 31-year-old man had a progressive chiasmal syndrome secondary to basal arachnoiditis of unknown cause. The only positive finding was chronic arachnoiditis.

Optochiasmatic arachnoiditis is considered by some to be a distinct entity, while others view it as a nonspecific sequela of a variety of causes.[20, 23-25] The optic nerves and chiasm may be encased in a mass of dense adhesions of thickened arachnoid following either basal meningitis (bacterial or syphilitic), hemorrhage from a ruptured aneurysm, or trauma. Similar adhesions, however, may be found independent of a preceding causal episode. In these instances, the fibrotic subarachnoid tissue may show no inflammatory component. However, Lindenberg and co-workers[20] state that a similar pathologic picture may be seen following a persistent low-grade inflammatory process, frequently of an unspecific nature, and Walsh and Hoyt[1] consider all such cases as inflammatory in nature.

Visual loss is the primary disturbance associated with this entity, the loss being attributed to interference with the blood supply to the optic nerve and chiasm.[26]

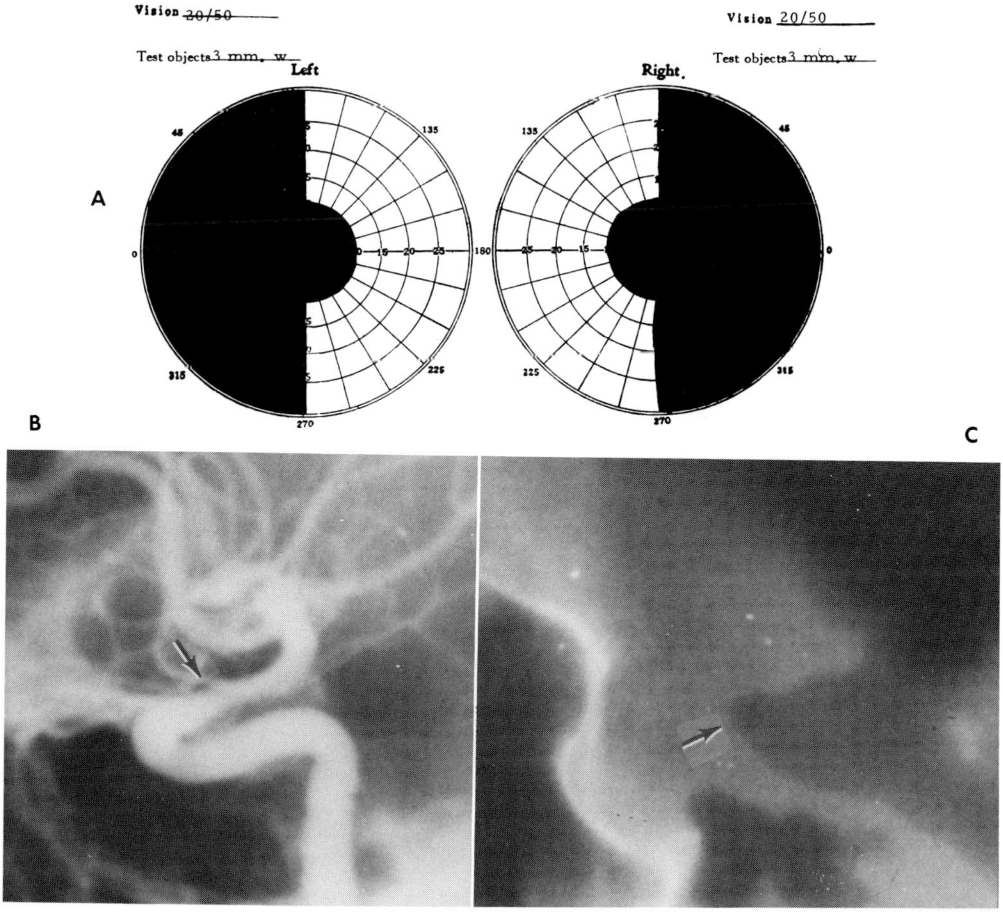

Fig. 6-3. A, Visual field of 31-year-old man with optochiasmatic arachnoiditis revealed central scotomas and bitemporal hemianopic field defects. **B,** Right carotid arteriogram revealed an irregular segmental narrowing of the supraclinoid portion of the internal carotid artery (arrow). **C,** A midsagittal tomogram of pneumoencephalogram in brow-up position revealed blunting of the recesses of the third ventricle (arrow) with encasement of air in the interpeduncular fossa. No air is seen in the chiasmatic cistern or cisterna lamina terminalis. At surgery, dense arachnoidal adhesions and fibrosis were noted involving the chiasm and optic nerves, and anterior cerebral arteries.

GROUP IV: ARTERITIS OF VARIOUS ORIGINS

Case 4. The patient, a 62 year old woman, was first seen in 1968. Two years before she had developed pain over the left eye and blurred vision that progressed to no light perception in several days. Over the next six to eight weeks her vision improved, but she was aware of a "haze" temporally in her left eye.

Examination revealed a visual acuity of count-fingers at 180 cm in the left eye and 6/7.5 in the right eye. Visual field examination revealed a large central scotoma in the left eye and a superior temporal defect in the right eye (Fig. 6-4, *A*). The optic fundi showed pallor of both discs.

On the eighth hospital day she developed severe left orbital pain. Visual acuity decreased to no light perception in the left eye, with development of a complete temporal hemianopia in the right. Ophthalmoscopy revealed congested retinal veins with an area of hemorrhage near the left optic disc. Sedimentation rate was 40 mm/hr. Carotid arteriograms revealed irregular beadings of the ophthalmic and anterior cerebral arteries, compatible with giant cell arteritis (Fig. 6-4, *B*). Prednisone therapy was begun and the

A

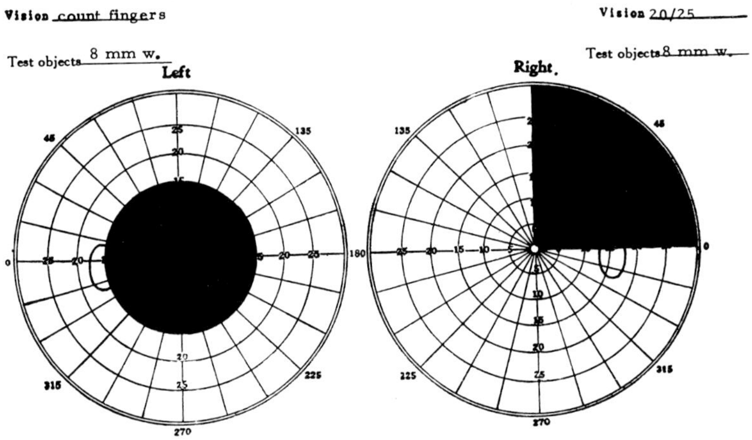

B

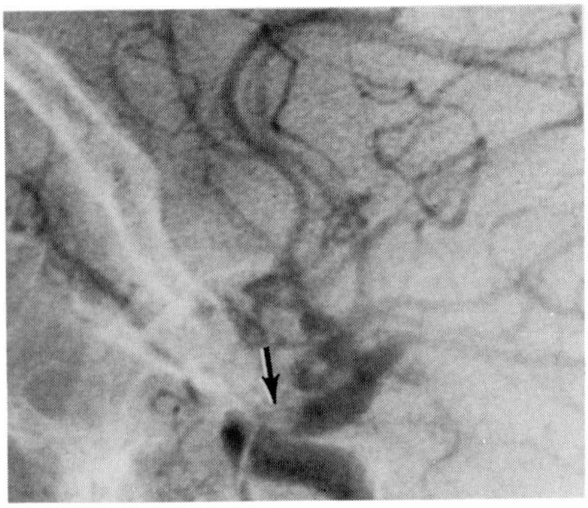

Fig. 6-4. A, Visual field of 62-year-old woman with giant cell arteritis revealed a large central scotoma in the left eye and a superior temporal defect in the right eye. **B,** Carotid arteriogram revealed an irregular narrowing of the supraclinoid segment of the carotid artery (arrow) associated with beading of the ophthalmic artery.

pain subsided. The vision returned to 6/6 in each eye within four days, the only sequela being a temporal hemianopic defect in the left eye.

COMMENT. This woman presented with signs and symptoms of an ischemic process affecting the optic chiasm and optic nerves. She had severe and protracted headaches associated with tenderness in the temporal arteries. Carotid arteriogram showed evidence of arteritis. The sedimentation rate was minimally elevated and her vision returned with steroid treatment. The findings are consistent with the diagnosis of giant cell arteritis with involvement of the optic chiasm.

Walsh and Hoyt[1] described a patient with similar angiographic findings who clinically presented with an increased erythrocyte sedimentation rate, panhypopituitarism, and a bitemporal visual field defect associated with a normal-appearing sella. The endocrinologic disturbance responded promptly to steroid therapy. Hinck and co-workers[27] reported a case of giant cell arteritis with carotid arteriograms that demonstrated scattered focal areas of stenosis of varied degrees intermingled with arterial ectasias, giving the appearance of a somewhat irregular string of beads. Arteritis with intracranial ischemia may develop secondary to collagen diseases (lupus erythematosus, scleroderma, dermatomyositis, rheumatoid arthritis, and so on), necrotizing angiitis (periarteritis nodosa, temporal arteritis, Wegener's granulomatosis), and various infectious diseases.[28] Superficial temporal artery arteriography may be of value in demonstrating vascular irregularity secondary to arteritis,[29] although negative arteriogram or biopsy cannot rule out a giant cell arteritis elsewhere.

GROUP V: POSTPARTUM ISCHEMIC CHIASMAL SYNDROME ASSOCIATED WITH PITUITARY NECROSIS

Case 5. A 27-year-old woman, gravida II para 2, presented in July 1971 with complaints of hazy vision in the right eye for three months. Her first pregnancy was full term, but the infant died because of an omphalocele. Her second pregnancy terminated in a full-term healthy infant. Four months after delivery, she became aware of cloudy vision in her right eye. She described images as being dull and hazy. She had been experiencing headaches over the right eye and postural lightheadedness during this period. Following delivery, her menses became irregular and she had several months of amenorrhea.

General physical examination revealed a thin female. Blood pressure was 95/60, pulse 68, respiration 20. She weighed 80 pounds (36.4 kg). Milk could be expressed easily from her breasts, although she was not nursing.

Neurologic examination was normal except for visual findings. The visual acuity was 6/15 in the right eye and 6/6 in the left eye. Visual fields demonstrated a central scotoma in the right eye and a superior bitemporal field defect (Fig. 6-5, *A*). There was a right afferent pupillary defect and pallor of the right optic nerve head.

Laboratory studies revealed the following values: Hgb, 14.1 gm/100 ml; Hct, 40.6%. Results of urinalysis were normal. Plasma cortisol value at 8 AM was 21.6 μg/100 ml. PBI level was 6.6 μg/100 ml. In a 24-hour urine study 17-OH and 17-ketosteroids were low, but results of repeat study were normal. Metyrapone test showed a fair rise. Spinal fluid examination revealed 9 white cells with normal protein and IgG levels.

Skull x-ray films showed the pituitary fossa to be normal in size but ballooned in configuration. Carotid arteriogram showed a low-lying A-1 segment with no evidence of mass lesion (Fig. 6-5, *C*). Pneumoencephalogram revealed an empty sella with a depressed pituitary gland (Fig. 6-5, *B*).

Vision gradually improved, and visual acuity returned to 6/6 in both eyes. There was a residual paracentral scotoma in the right eye. The patient's menstrual irregularity and galactorrhea disappeared.

COMMENT. This 27-year-old woman noted the onset of visual loss, hypomenorrhea, and galactorrhea in the postpartum period. Endocrine studies showed a mild disturbance of pituitary reserve.

X-ray examination demonstrated low-positioned anterior cerebral arteries and an empty sella. There was gradual improvement in her endocrine status and resolution of her visual symptoms and signs. Vascular disease of the pituitary gland and chiasm could account for her clinical picture.

According to Sheehan,[30] postpartum necrosis of the anterior lobe of the pituitary is not uncommon. A small necrotic lesion is innocuous, but severe hypopituitarism may develop if a patient with a large lesion survives. Shee-

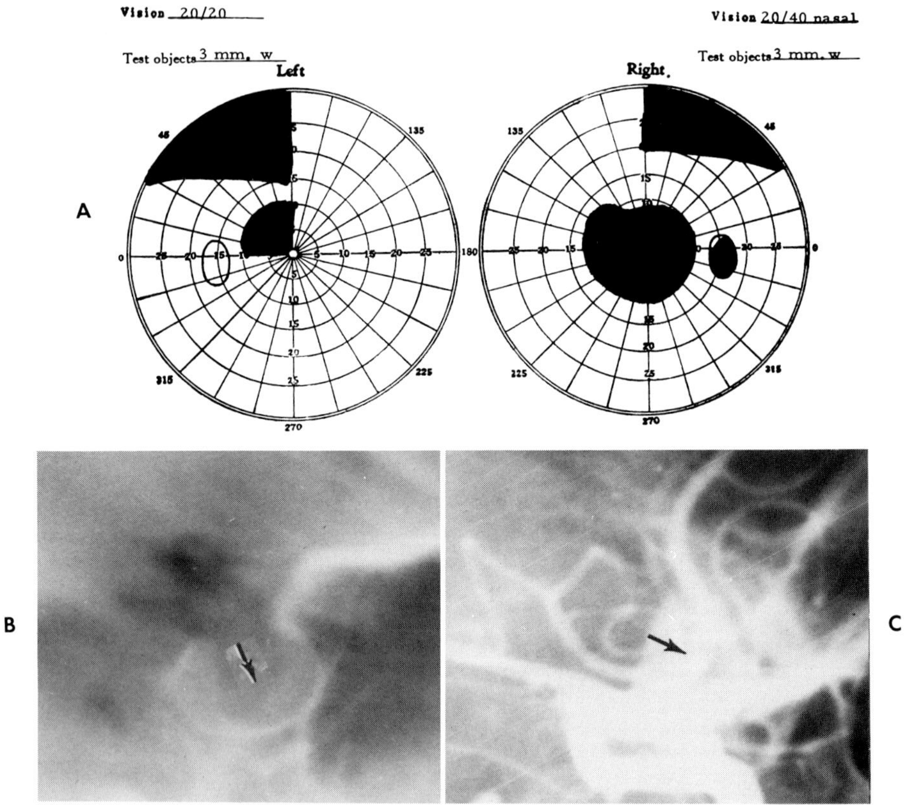

Fig. 6-5. A, Visual field of 27-year-old woman with postpartum pituitary necrosis demonstrated a central scotoma in the right eye and a superior bitemporal field defect. **B,** Pneumoencephalogram revealed an empty sella with a depressed pituitary gland (arrow). **C,** Carotid arteriogram showed a low-lying anterior cerebral artery (arrow) with no evidence of mass lesion.

han and Summers[31] found that the acute necrotic lesions were mostly related to postpartum necrosis, but diabetes, cranial arteritis, and cavernous sinus thrombosis were also etiologic factors; subacute lesions were secondary to tuberculosis, syphilis, and giant cell granuloma, while chronic fibrous lesions were due to either healed postpartum necrosis or scarring of undetermined cause.*

DISCUSSION

The optic chiasm is composed of afferent nerve fibers that transmit visual impulses. Consequently, any disturbance in the integrity of the chiasm results in visual field defects,[32] the most characteristic of which is a bitemporal hemianopia.[33] The chiasmal syndrome is usually produced by compression. A variety of juxtasellar mass lesions, including neoplasms, granulomas, aneurysms, foreign bodies, and hematomas, may be responsible. Nontumorous lesions such as demyelinating disease and trauma are rarer but definite causes.

The ischemic chiasmal syndrome (ICS) is believed to be secondary to various ischemic processes without evidence of mass lesion. Therefore, *a mass lesion should be categorically excluded by neuroradiologic procedures before the diagnosis of ICS is considered.*[34-36]

Ectatic arterial dilation may compress the adjacent structures, producing neurologic symptoms.[37-39] Similarly, ICS may develop secondary to mechanical compression of the optic chiasm or optic nerve junction, or both, by a tortuous ectatic anterior cerebral artery.[14, 16, 18] Consequently, minor twigs supplying the chiasm may be compressed or occluded, or ishemia of the optic nerve and chiasm may be produced by atheromatous plaques in the circle of Willis with partial or complete occlusion of the arterial twigs supplying the optic structures. Other causes of ischemia include diffuse arachnoiditis and dense fibrosis secondary to a granulomatous process or postirradiation change. Arteritis of various origins may also produce ICS.

We have noted a very high association of empty sella syndrome with ICS and particularly with sclerotic tortuous anterior cerebral arteries (group I). An incompetent diaphragma sellae may be purely developmental, as demonstrated on autopsy specimens.[5, 40] It is conceivable, however, that a deficient diaphragma sellae may be caused by ischemic necrosis with resultant intrasellar extension of subarachnoid space, thus producing the empty sella syndrome.

The ischemic chiasmal syndrome may be classified into five pathogenetic groups: (1) mechanical indentations of the chiasm secondary to dilated, sclerotic, and tortuous vessels, (2) vascular occlusion secondary to atherosclerotic plaque formation, (3) arachnoiditis with fibrosis, (4) arteritis, and (5) postpartum necrosis.

---

*EDITOR'S NOTE. See also Chapter 8 regarding spontaneous pituitary necrosis ("apoplexy"). J. S. G.

The chiasmal syndrome is most frequently produced by the compressive effect of a mass lesion. Thorough neuroradiologic investigation will differentiate the ischemic causes from chiasmal compression. The recognition of this clinical and radiologic entity has been stressed.

SUMMARY AND CONCLUSIONS

1. Ischemic chiasmal syndrome (ICS) is manifested by progressive visual field deficit, usually bitemporal hemianopia, thus clinically simulating a juxtasellar mass lesion.

2. The following conditions appear to play important roles in producing this syndrome, although its exact pathogenesis often may be difficult to establish:

a. Mechanical compression of the optic chiasm or optic nerve or both by a dolichoectatic anterior cerebral artery or carotid artery or both, with resultant occlusion of minor arterioles supplying the optic structure.
b. Vascular occlusion secondary to atherosclerotic plaque formation.
c. Diffuse arachnoidal adhesion and thickening with encasement and occlusion of the minor vessels.
d. Arteritis of various origins, especially giant cell arteritis.
e. Postpartum ICS, associated with pituitary necrosis.

Among these, arachnoiditis (c) of various origins was the most common cause of ICS.

3. Sophisticated neuroradiologic procedures including magnification angiography and detailed pneumoencephalography with polytomography are essential in ruling out a mass lesion and correlating the clinical and radiologic findings of this syndrome.

4. A very high incidence of empty sella syndrome with ICS has been demonstrated. Since there is a common blood supply to the pituitary, diaphragma sellae, and optic chiasm, a vascular mechanism of ICS, the empty sella syndrome, and hypopituitarism is strongly suspected.

REFERENCES

1. Walsh, F. B., and Hoyt, W. F.: Clinical neuro-ophthalmology, Baltimore, 1969, The Williams & Wilkins Company, pp. 1778, 2102, 1883.
2. Lee, K. F., Schatz, N. J., and Hodes, P. J.: Arteriosclerotic chiasmal syndrome. Paper presented at the sixth annual meeting of the American Society of Neuroradiology, New Orleans, 1968.
3. DiChiro, G.: An atlas of detailed pneumoencephalographic anatomy, Springfield, Ill., 1961, Charles C Thomas, Publisher, pp. 115, 205, 257, 285.
4. Schaeffer, J. P.: Some points in the regional anatomy of the optic pathways with special reference to tumors of the hypophysis cerebri and resulting ocular changes, Anat. Rec. **28:**243, 1924.
5. Bergland, R. M., Ray, B. S., and Torack, R. M.: Anatomical variations in the pituitary gland and adjacent structures in 225 human autopsy cases, J. Neurosurg. **28:**93, 1968.
6. Bull, J.: The normal variations in the position of the optic recess of the third ventricle, Acta Radiol. **46:**72, 1956.

7. Walker, A. E.: The neurosurgical evaluation of the chiasmal syndromes, Am. J. Ophthalmol. **54**:563, 1962.
8. Dawson, B. H.: The blood vessels of the human optic chiasma and their relation to those of the hypophysis and hypothalmus, Brain **81**:207, 1958.
8a. Foley, J. M., Kinney, T. D., and Alexander, L.: The vascular supply of the hypothalmus in man, J. Neuropath. Exp. Neurol. **1**:265, 1942.
9. Parkinson, D.: Collateral circulation of cavernous carotid artery: anatomy, Canad. J. Surg. **7**:251, 1964.
10. Jefferson, G.: Compression of the optic chiasma, optic nerves and optic tracts by intracranial aneurysms, Brain **60**:444, 1937.
11. Walsh, F. B.: Visual field defects due to aneurysms at the circle of Willis, Arch. Ophthalmol. **71**:15-27, 1964.
12. Fay, T., and Grant, F. C.: Lesions of the optic chiasm and tracts with relation to the adjacent vascular structures, Arch. Neurol. Psychiat. **9**:739, 1923.
13. Rucker, C. W., and Kernohan, J. W.: Notching of the optic chiasm by overlying arteries in pituitary tumors, Arch. Ophthalmol. **51**:161, 1954.
14. de Schweinitz, G. E.: Concerning certain ocular aspects of pituitary body disorders, mainly exclusive of the usual central and peripheral heminanopic field defects, Trans. Ophthalmol. Soc. U. K. **43**:12, 1923.
15. Schneider, R. C., Kriss, F. C., and Falls, H. F.: Prechiasmal infarction associated with intrachiasmal and suprasellar tumors, J. Neurosurg. **2**:197, 1970.
16. Hilton, G. F., and Hoyt, W. F.: An arteriosclerotic chiasmal syndrome; bitemporal hemianopia associated with fusiform dilation of the anterior cerebral arteries, J.A.M.A. **196**:200, 1966.
17. Walsh, F. B., and Gass, J. D.: Concerning the optic chiasm; the de Schweinitz lecture, Am. J. Ophthalmol. **50**:1031, 1960.
18. Sacks, J. G., and Lindenberg, R.: Dolicho-ectatic intracranial arteries, Johns Hopkins Med. J. **125**:95-105, 1969.
19. Lee, K. F., Lin, S. R., and Schatz, N. J.: Neuroradiology of juxtasellar mass lesions, CRC Crit. Rev. Radiol. Sci. **3**: 105, 1972.
20. Lindenberg, R., Walsh, F. B., and Sacks, J. G.: Neuropathology of vision. Philadelphia, 1973, Lea & Febiger, pp. 174-180, 200, 212, 246.
21. Hobbs, K. E. F.: A case of Sheehan's syndrome with almost complete bilateral internal carotid occlusion, Guys Hosp. Rep. **108**:87, 1959.
22. Gilroy, J., and Meyer, J. S.: Pituitary insufficiency with cerebrovascular symptoms. A new clinical syndrome, N. Engl. J. Med. **269**:1115, 1963.
23. Vail, D.: Optochiasmic arachnoiditis, Arch. Ophthalmol. **20**:384, 1938.
24. Hausman, L.: Syphilitic atrophy of the optic nerve and papilledema due to optochiasmal arachnoiditis, Arch. Ophthalmol. **23**:1107, 1940.
25. Bruetsch, W. L.: Surgical treatment of syphilitic primary atrophy of the optic nerves (syphilitic optochiasmatic arachnoiditis), Arch. Ophthalmol. **38**:735, 1947.
26. Oliver, M., Beller, A. J., and Behar, A.: Chiasmal arachnoiditis as a manifestation of generalized arachnoiditis in systemic vascular disease, Br. J. Ophthalmol. **52**:227, 1968.
27. Hinck, V. C., Carter, C. C., and Rippey, J. G.: Giant cell (cranial) arteritis. A case with angiographic abnormalities, Am. J. Roentgen. Radium Ther. Nucl. Med. **92**:769, 1964.
28. Ferris, E. J., and Levine, H. L.: Cerebral arteritis: classification, Radiology **109**: 327, 1973.
29. Gillanders, L. A.: Temporal arteriography, Clin. Radiol. **20**:149, 1969.
30. Sheehan, H. L. Post-partum necrosis of the anterior lobe of the pituitary, Lancet **2**:321, 1940.
31. Sheehan, H. L., and Summers, V. K.: The syndrome of hypopituitarism, Q. J. Med. **18**:319, 1949.
32. Hoyt, W. F., and Luis, O.: The primate chiasm, Arch. Ophthalmol. **70**:69, 1963.
33. Scott, G. I.: Traquair's clinical perimetry, London, 1957, Henry Kimpton Publisher.
34. Chase, N. E., and Taveras, J. M.: Cerebral angiography in the diagnosis of suprasellar tumors, Am. J. Roentgenol. Radium Ther. Nucl. Med. **86**:154, 1961.
35. Udvarhelyi, B., Langfitt, T. W., and Cox, A.: Neuroradiologic diagnostic procedures in suprasellar space-occupying le-

sions with special reference to angiographic measurements, Acta Radiol. (Diagn. (Stockh.) **1**:485, 1963.
36. duBoulay, G., and Trickey, S.: The choice of radiological investigations in the management of tumors around the sella, Clin. Radiol. **18**:349, 1967.
37. Ley, A.: Compression of the optic nerve by a fusiform aneurysm of the carotid artery, J. Neurol. Neurosurg. Psychiatry **13**:75, 1950.
38. Greitz, T., and Lofstedt, S.: The relationship between the third ventricle and the basilar artery, Acta Radiol. (Stockh.) **42**:85, 1954.
39. Mitts, M. G., and McQueen, J. D.: Visual loss associated with fusiform enlargement of the intracranial portion of the internal carotid artery, J. Neurosurg. **23**:33, 1965.
40. Busch, W.: Die Morphologie der Sella turcica und ihre Beziehungen zur Hypophyse, Virchows Arch. **320**:437, 1951.

Chapter 7

Delayed radiation necrosis of the optic nerves and chiasm

Norman J. Schatz
Stephen Lichtenstein
James J. Corbett

Radiation necrosis of the brain following treatment of intracranial and extracranial neoplasms is well recognized,[1-3] though rare. Acute reaction following therapy is seen only after clinically acceptable doses are exceeded.[4] An early "delayed" reaction,[5, 6] also referred to as *transient postradiation effect,*[4] is thought by some to occur a few weeks or months after radiation of the brain or spinal cord, and usually ends in complete recovery.[6, 7] True delayed radiation necrosis represents the most significant complication of brain radiation.[4]

It is the purpose of this chapter to record three patients with delayed radiation brain necrosis. Each patient presented with *visual loss that developed after therapy with currently acceptable radiotherapeutic doses.* The anterior visual system was the only area clinically involved in these patients.

CASE REPORTS

Case 1. A 51-year-old woman presented with carpal tunnel syndrome and acromegaly in 1961. In 1970, following a four-year history of progressively disabling frontal headaches, a skull radiograph revealed an enlarged pituitary fossa. Visual acuity was 20/20 in both eyes, and visual fields were full. In July 1970, 5000 rads of cobalt-60 radiation was delivered to the pituitary fossa in 25 treatments over 34 days. The patient did well until March 1971, when she became aware of a "haze over the right eye." Visual acuity was count-fingers in the right eye. There was an afferent defect of the right pupil on light stimulation and a dense 20° central scotoma (Fig. 7-1). The visual acuity was 20/20 in the left eye with a full field. Pituitary function and neuroradiologic

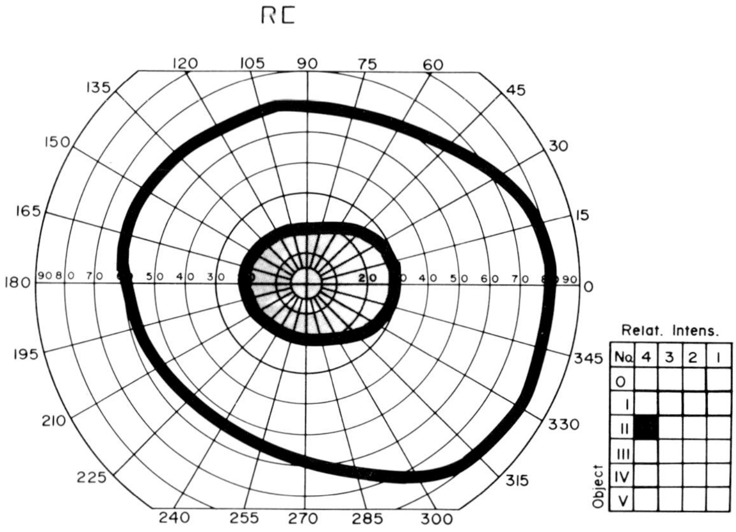

Fig. 7-1. Case 1. March 1971, eight months after radiation therapy. Patient has a dense central scotoma in the right eye. Visual acuity 20/400.

studies were normal. There has been no change in the patient's status to the present time.

Case 2. A 46-year-old man presented with acromegaly in July 1969. Visual acuity was 20/20 in both eyes with full visual fields. Five thousand rads of cobalt-60 radiation was delivered to the pituitary fossa in 25 treatments over 36 days in November 1969. Six months later the patient became aware of sudden loss of vision in the superior field of his right eye. Repeat examination of the right eye revealed a diminished pupillary light response, visual acuity of count-fingers in the inferior visual field, a superior altitudinal field defect with a central scotoma, and a pale optic disc. Visual acuity was 20/20 in the left eye, with a superior temporal field defect to the color red (Fig. 7-2, *A*). Results of carotid arteriography and pneumoencephalography were normal. Despite intensive steroid therapy, vision in the right eye continued to deteriorate. One month later the patient experienced sudden loss of vision superiorly in the left eye. Visual acuity in the left eye was 20/25 with a dense superior temporal quadrantanopia. Vision in the right eye had further deteriorated to count-fingers inferonasally (Fig. 7-2, *B*). At exploratory craniotomy the chiasm was normal and no mass was seen. Vision continued to decrease. At examination in 1974, right eye vision was count-fingers inferonasally only, while the left eye was 20/200 with a dense temporal hemianopia and central scotoma (Fig. 7-2, *C*).

Case 3. A 12-year-old girl presented with multiple right-sided cranial nerve palsies including the oculomotor, trigeminal, facial, auditory, vagus, and spinal accessory nerves. She underwent craniotomy in February 1972, with resection of an angioblastic meningioma of the clivus. Postoperative cobalt-60 radiation of 5400 rads in 27 treatments over 36 days was delivered to the clivus. When reevaluated in May 1973, visual acuity was 20/20 in both eyes with full visual fields. Hearing loss in the right ear secondary to surgery was her only remaining neurologic disorder. In January 1974 the patient noticed decreasing vision in the right eye. Examination of the right eye revealed visual acuity of 20/25, a diminished pupillary light response, and an inferior altitudinal field defect. Visual acuity in the left eye was 20/20 with a full field (Fig.

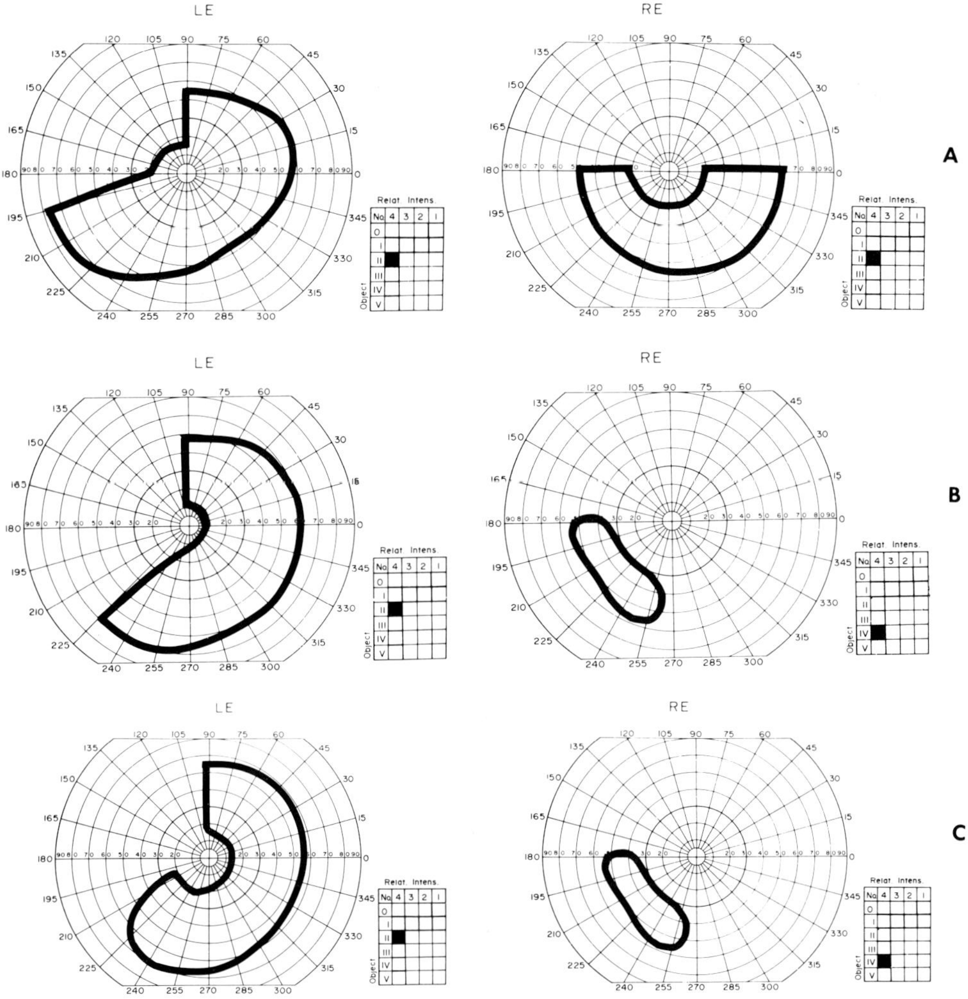

Fig. 7-2. Case 2. **A,** May 1970, six months after radiation therapy. Patient has a central scotoma and superior altitudinal defect in the right eye and a visual acuity of 20/400. A superior temporal defect was seen in the left eye. **B,** June 1970, seven months after radiation therapy. Patient has a striking loss of field with preservation of only finger-counting vision inferonasally in the right eye. A dense superior temporal quadrantanopia is seen in the left eye with a 20/20 visual acuity. **C,** June 1974. Identical visual field in the right eye as in June 1970, with a dense temporal hemianopia, central scotoma, and visual acuity of 20/200 in the left eye.

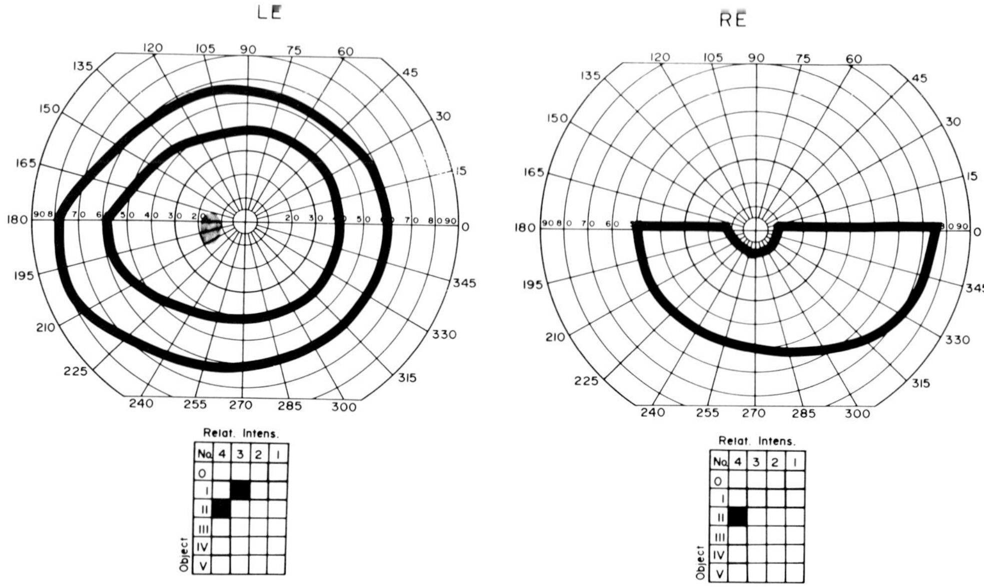

Fig. 7-3. Case 3. Twenty-two months after radiation therapy. Patient has a superior altitudinal field defect and visual acuity of 20/25 on the right, and a full field with 20/20 visual acuity on the left.

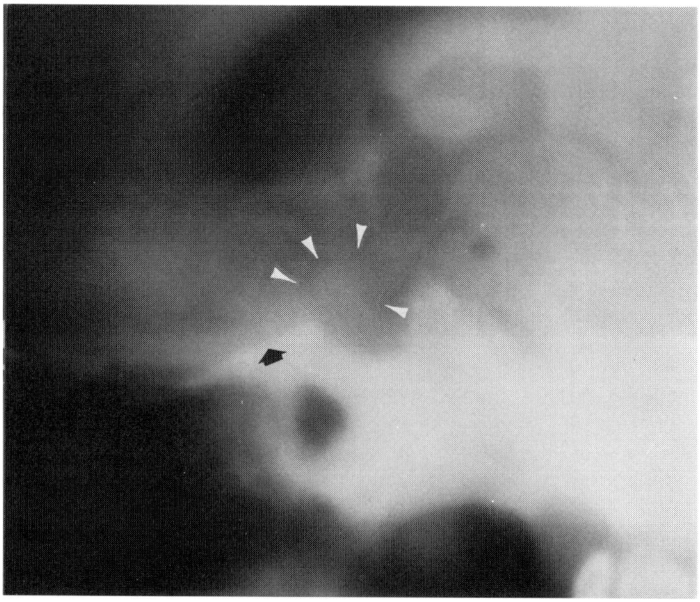

Fig. 7-4. Case 3. Pneumoencephalogram revealing a mass lesion thought to be tumor recurrence (white arrows). The planum sphenoidale is marked with a black arrow.

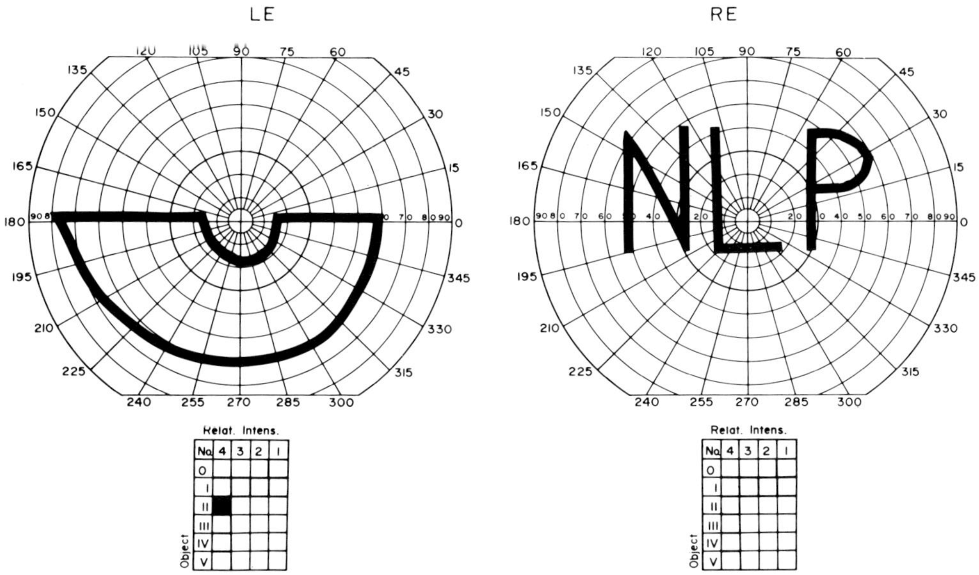

Fig. 7-5. Case 3. Thirty months after radiation therapy. The right eye has no light perception and the left eye has a superior altitudinal defect and central scotoma with visual acuity of 20/400.

7-3). Results of carotid arteriography and pneumoencephalography were interpreted as demonstrating a mass thought to be tumor recurrence (Fig. 7-4). Exploratory craniotomy demonstrated no recurrence, but dense opticochiasmatic adhesions were found. Despite steroid therapy right eye vision progressively deteriorated to hand movements superonasally over a period of four months. As the right eye progressively lost field, the temporal field of the left eye became desaturated to color red. Over the next four months visual acuity deteriorated in the left eye. A superior altitudinal defect appeared abruptly (Fig. 7-5). Despite steroid therapy, the patient continued to lose acuity, and at present has no light perception in the right eye and finger-counting vision inferiorly on the left.

DISCUSSION

Kramer[8] reviewed 85 patients with pituitary adenomas irradiated at Thomas Jefferson University Hospital and found no clinical evidence of delayed radiation necrosis. He concluded that this problem is rare using current radiotherapeutic dose levels given in a single course over an adequate time span. These levels of radiation range between 4500 and 5000 rads in 4½ to 5½ weeks for tumors in the region of the sella turcica.[8] According to Kramer,[8] normal brain can tolerate a tissue dose of 6500 to 7000 rads delivered in 6½ to 8 weeks in five daily fractions per week with an "acceptable" small risk of delayed brain necrosis. Symptoms of delayed necrosis vary depending on the site of the lesion. Radiologic studies are rarely definitive in the differentiation between recurrent tumor, infection, and necrosis.[4, 8]

A review of cases of radiation brain necrosis reported from 1931 to 1967 revealed a total of 57 cases.[8] The majority of these cases received either excessively high doses of radiation with multiple treatment courses or large doses administered over short treatment times. The time interval between treatment and necrosis in these cases peaked between one and three years, with only rare occurrences after seven years. Of seven patients with delayed necrosis following radiotherapy of pituitary tumors, five received excessively high doses delivered over repeated treatment periods. In the two patients not subjected to excessive radiation, delayed necrosis was seen in one patient after a single course of 4500 rads delivered in 28 days for a chromophobe adenoma of the pituitary. The second patient received 6250 rads in 42 days for a probable tumor of the hypophysis. Both patients died following progressive neurologic deterioration. Loss of visual acuity and visual field began 12 to 19 months after irradiation. There was clinical evidence and pathologic documentation of radiation damage to the hypothalamus, optic chiasm, and frontal and temporal lobes.[9] Crompton and Layton[9] noted the difficulty with which tumor recurrence and radiation necrosis were differentiated. They did, however, point out that visual field defects which developed following radiation in their second patient were unlike those expected with recurrence of pituitary adenoma and more suggestive of a vascular cause.[9]

There are a few reports of radiation necrosis involving the visual system following excessive doses of radiation. High total doses delivered in short periods of time or high doses of radiation delivered by radon seeds implanted in the pituitary gland were characteristic of these reports.[10-14] In two reports, two patients received doses that were within acceptable limits but dosage schedules were not included in the clinical information.[15, 16] Our cases are similar to those reported by Crompton and Layton[9] in that radiation damage of visual structures developed in patients subjected to currently acceptable doses of radiation. For the details of these case reports refer to Table 5.

The pathogenesis of delayed radiation necrosis of the brain has not yet been elucidated clearly. The evidence points to a microvascular cause, with a pathologic picture of endothelial proliferation, fibrinoid necrosis and basal lamina thickening.[3, 17] Colby and Kearns[18] suggested that the empty sella is a mechanism for delayed visual loss in patients radiated for neoplasm in the region of the pituitary gland. Visual loss is attributed to dense scar tissue drawing the optic nerves and chiasm into the sella.[18] Subsequent reports have confirmed the association of postradiation empty sella with visual loss.[4, 19]

SUMMARY

Three patients are presented who developed delayed radiation brain necrosis 6, 8, and 11 months following irradiation with currently acceptable radiotherapeutic doses. Throughout their clinical course to the present time

Table 5. Details of case reports of radiation necrosis involving visual system following excessive doses of radiation

Author	*Reason for treatment*	*Radiation dose*	*Location of damage and visual defect*	*Interval of necrosis*	*Result*
Crompton and Layton[9]	Chromophobe adenoma	4500 rads/28 days	Necrosis of hypothalamus, uncus, optic chiasm. J-16 acuity OU and bilateral inferior altitudinal defects	12 months	Death
Crompton and Layton[9]	Probable tumor of hypophysis (unverified)	6250 rads/42 days	Necrosis of hypothalamus, optic tract, and temporal lobes. 6/18 OD and 6/60 OS with bitemporal inferior quadrantic defects	19 months	Death
Buys and Kearns[10]	Advanced malignancy	7000 rads/14 days; repeated one year later	Necrosis of temporal lobe, hypothalamus, optic nerves, tract, and chiasm. Blindness OU	1 month after second course of radiation	Death
Buys and Kearns[10]	Advanced malignancy	12,500 rads/ 12 days	No autopsy. Superior arcuate field defect and temporal hemianopia progressing to blindness	14 months	Death
Forrest[11] (4 cases; no details of individual cases)	Advanced malignancy	10,000-15,000 rads/28 days	Optic nerve and chiasm clinically affected	1-4 months	Not reported
Ghatak and White[12]	Craniopharyngioma	7995 rads to pituitary, 28 treatments over 70 days	Hypothalamus and optic tract. Right inferior incongruous hemianopia	4 months	Death
Peck and McGovern[13]	Acromegaly	10,126 rads to pituitary in four courses over 3½ years	Temporal lobe necrosis. Optic nerve normal. Arachnoid around chiasm thickened	8 months	Surgical cure

Continued.

Table 5. Details of case reports of radiation necrosis involving visual system following excessive doses of radiation—cont'd

Author	*Reason for treatment*	*Radiation dose*	*Location of damage and visual defect*	*Interval to necrosis*	*Result*
Shukovsky and Fletcher[14] (3 cases)	Ethmoid sinus and nasal cavity neoplasm	6900-7500 rads over 6 weeks	No autopsy. Optic disc pallor on examination	4-5 years	Radiotherapeutic cure
Rosengren[15]	Thyroid exophthalmos	900 rads to hypophysis; 3250 rads to hypophysis 2½ years later	Craniotomy: left optic nerve thin and atrophic, right optic nerve gray and edematous	8 months after second course of radiation	Blindness OU
Rosengren[15]	Tuberculosis	5000 rads to chiasm; 6000 rads to optic nerves over 117 days	Left optic nerve. Optic atrophy and "loss of vision"	5 years	Amaurosis OS
Ross, Rosenberg, and Friedman[16]	Epidermoid carcinoma of maxillary antrum	6000 rads	Anterior segment changes and necrosis of intraorbital optic nerve	2½ years	Not reported
Schatz Lichtenstein Corbett					
Case 1	Acromegaly	5000 rads in 25 treatments over 34 days	See Fig. 7-1	8 months	Optic atrophy OD
Case 2	Acromegaly	5000 rads in 25 treatments over 36 days	See Fig. 7-2	6 months OD 7 months OS	Chiasmal syndrome
Case 3	Angioblastic meningioma of clivus	5400 rads in 27 treatments in 36 days	See Figs. 7-3 to 7-5	21 months OD 25 months OS	Bilateral optic nerve and chiasm syndrome

only the visual system has been involved. Contrast studies were negative in the two cases of acromegaly and were misleading in the patient with angioblastic meningioma of the clivus. The visual field defects in two of these patients were identical to the so-called vascular patterns of ischemic optic nerve and chiasmal disease. Visual loss as a delayed manifestation of radiation to the brain is rarely associated with any radiotherapeutic technique. At currently employed doses it is particularly uncommon. This complication must be considered along with recurrence of intracranial tumor and infection in the differential diagnosis of visual loss following radiation therapy.

ACKNOWLEDGMENT

Grateful acknowledgment to Peter Savino, M.D., and Goeffrey R. Barger, M.D., for editorial assistance.

REFERENCES

1. Bouchard, J.: Radiation therapy of tumors and diseases of the nervous system, Philadelphia, 1966, Lea & Febiger, pp. 29-55.
2. Minckler, J.: Pathology of the nervous system, vol. 1, New York, 1968, McGraw-Hill Book Company, pp. 910-912.
3. Pennybacker, J., and Russell, D. S.: Necrosis of the brain due to radiation therapy. Clinical and pathological observations, J. Neurol. Neurosurg. Psychiatry **11:**183-198, 1948.
4. Kramer, S., and Lee, K. F.: Complications of radiation therapy: the central nervous system, Semin. Roentgenol. **9:** 75-83, 1974.
5. Lampert, P. W., and Davis, R. L.: Delayed effects of radiation on the human central nervous system: "early" and "late" delayed reactions, Neurology (Minneap.) **14:**912-917, 1964.
6. Rider, W. D.: Radiation damage to the brain—a new syndrome, J. Can. Assoc. Radiol. **14:**67-69, 1963.
7. Lampert, P. W., Tom, M. I., and Rider, W. D.: Disseminated demyelination of the brain following Co^{60} (gamma) radiation, Arch. Pathol. **68:**322-330, 1959.
8. Kramer, S.: The hazards of therapeutic irradiation of the central nervous system, Clin. Neurosurg. **15:**301-318, 1968.
9. Crompton, M. R., and Layton, D. D.: Delayed radionecrosis of the brain following therapeutic X-radiation of the pituitary, Brain **84:**84-101, 1961.
10. Buys, N. S., and Kearns, T. C.: Irradiation damage to the chiasm, Am. J. Ophthalmol. **44:**483-486, 1957.
11. Forrest, A. P. M.: Pituitary radon implant for advanced cancer, Lancet **1:** 399-401, 1956.
12. Ghatak, N. R., and White, B. E.: Delayed radiation necrosis of the hypothalamus, Arch. Neurol. **21:**425-430, 1969.
13. Peck, F. C., Jr., and McGovern, E. R.: Radiation necrosis of the brain in acromegaly, J. Neurosurg. **15:**536-542, 1966.
14. Shukovsky, L. J., and Fletcher, G. H.: Retinal and optic nerve complications in a high dose irradiation technique of ethmoid sinus and nasal cavity, Radiology **104:**629-634, 1972.
15. Rosengren, B.: Two cases of atrophy of the optic nerve after previous roentgen treatment of the chiasmal region and optic nerves, Acta Ophthalmol. (Kbh.) **36:**874-877, 1958.
16. Ross, H., Rosenberg, S., and Friedman, A.: Delayed radiation necrosis of the optic nerve, Am. J. Ophthalmol. **76:**683-686, 1973.
17. McDonald, L. W., and Hayes, T. L.: The role of capillaries in the pathogenesis of delayed radionecrosis of brain, Am. J. Pathol. **50:**745-758, 1967.
18. Colby, M. Y., Jr., and Kearns, T. P.: Radiation therapy of pituitary adenomas with associated visual impairment, Mayo Clin. Proc. **37:**15-24, 1962.
19. Lee, W. M., and Adams, J. E.: The empty sella syndrome, J. Neurosurg. **28:** 351-356, 1968.
20. Almquist, S., Dahlgren, S., Notter, G., and Sundbom, L.: Brain necrosis after irradiation of the hypophysis in Cushing's disease, Acta Radiol. (Stockh.) **2:** 179-188, 1964.

Chapter 8

Pituitary apoplexy in clinical perspective

Noble J. David
Fredie P. Gargano
Joel S. Glaser

INTRODUCTION

Pituitary apoplexy is generally regarded as a rare clinical event, judging by the small series sporadically reported by individual neurosurgeons, ophthalmologists, and pathologists. The student of this disorder may find it difficult to extract consistent principles for recognition and management from the limited clinical descriptions available. Reports derived from necropsy experience[1] understandably stress the more serious consequences, including hyperpyrexia, coma, and death. Recorded cases from ophthalmologic clinics[2, 3] emphasize involvement of the anterior visual pathways and ophthalmoplegia. Although surgical intervention is strongly urged by some clinicians who stress the high incidence of blindness and death resulting from neglect of this situation,[4-6] a substantial fraction of patients with pituitary apoplexy have had a benign course after irradiation therapy or supportive treatment alone. Spontaneous arrest and regression of both tumor growth and hormone secretion following this syndrome has been well documented.[7-9]

Unfortunately, because of the intriguing variations in its clinical course, pituitary apoplexy is still commonly misdiagnosed. During the past eight years we have had the opportunity to study 13 patients who fulfill our diagnostic criteria for pituitary apoplexy. This chapter includes brief descriptions of nine patients. Particular regard is paid to ocular motor and radiographic features that have not been adequately stressed previously. All patients had sufficient clinical evidence to indicate a preexisting expanding intrasellar tumor, and each had a clinical course indicative of sudden enlargement of the pituitary mass lesion. Especially noteworthy in this series is the high incidence of postadrenalectomy pituitary apoplexy, as reviewed by Rovit and Duane,[10] and the high rate of profound ophthalmoplegia without significant impairment in visual function. The existing literature is somewhat misleading regarding disordered motility in pituitary apoplexy, and the need for surgical intervention to relieve these manifestations is in our view much less imperative.

The patients described herein were examined by one or more of us. They were added to this series from a consecutive experience wtih 123 hypophyseal adenomas, indicating an incidence of approximately 10%, roughly similar to that quoted in previous reports. Patient material was not obtained retrospectively from review of charts by diagnosis or manifestations. Although nonoperative management occasionally precluded histologic confirmation of the diagnosis, the chance of error seems small considering the reliability of the clinical criteria to be discussed later.

CASE REPORTS

Case 1. A 54-year-old laborer was admitted to the VA Hospital, Miami, Florida, complaining of blindness in his right eye, and right ptosis. Two days before admission he had noted "splitting headaches" beginning in the right side of his face and neck and becoming frontoparietal. The following night he noted drooping of the right eyelid and rapidly decreasing visual acuity in the right eye. On examination the patient displayed a total right ophthalmoplegia (third, fourth, and sixth cranial nerves), the eye was fixed downward and out, and the pupil was dilated and fixed to light. A bitemporal field defect was demonstrated to confrontation finger-counting. Over the next four days he developed a total third nerve palsy on the left with preservation of abduction and trochlear function. At this time his visual acuity had diminished to finger-counting at 4 feet in both eyes, with dense bitemporal field loss. Lumbar puncture revealed an opening pressure of 240 mm H_2O and yielded xanthochromic and acellular fluid, with a protein concentration of 112 mg/100 ml. Plain skull roentgenograms were not taken. The patient was thought to have suffered subarachnoid hemorrhage due to ruptured berry aneurysm. Bilateral carotid arteriograms revealed lateral displacement and uncoiling of both carotid siphons, embracing a mass in an enlarged and eroded sella turcica. There was no tenting of the proximal segments of the anterior cerebral arteries to suggest prominent anterior suprasellar extension. On the fifth hospital day the patient underwent a right frontotemporal craniotomy. The optic chiasm was compressed from beneath by a large necrotic chromophobe adenoma arising out of the sella turcica. The optic chiasm was thoroughly decompressed. Postoperatively the patient received 4500 rads to the area of the tumor. His field defects persisted in the immediate postoperative period, with the appearance of papilledema, but eight days after the operation the ptosis and ocular movements began to improve. Before discharge he had fully recovered from his ocular motor paralyses. One year later his vision was 20/20 in both eyes and his visual fields were full.

COMMENT. This highly characteristic example of pituitary apoplexy displays its cardinal features: (1) onset of the classic triad of headaches, ophthalmoplegia, and evidence of subarachnoid hemorrhage, the patient commonly admitted to the ward with a misdiagnosis of ruptured aneurysm; (2) correct diagnosis indicated by roentgenographic evidence of an enlarged sella and supported by appropriate visual field defects, hypopituitarism, or some odd constellation of ocular motor impairment. There is little question that emergency craniotomy is justified to decompress the optic chiasm when vision is obviously failing. As we shall see, the indications for so formidable an enterprise are not always so clear, as the next case demonstrates. The patient had unquestionable pituitary apoplexy but showed little or no involvement of the visual system.

Case 2. A 37-year-old white accountant was admitted to the hospital complaining of headaches and rhinorrhea for 1½ days. Frontal pain had been sudden in onset, severe, constant, and unrelieved by patent analgesics. The discharge of clear, colorless fluid from the right nostril accompanied the onset of headache. Within hours this discharge became progressively more bloody. Twelve hours before admission the patient noted double vision and could not "focus his eyes." There was no history of fever, chills, or infection.

Eight years previously the patient consulted a physician for obesity and diminished libido and was found to be hypothyroid, for which he was given 1 grain of desiccated thyroid daily.

Physical examination revealed a slightly obese man complaining of severe headache. There was complete ptosis on the left and near-total ptosis on the right. Bilateral third nerve palsies were observed, complete on the left but incomplete on the right, with partial preservation of adduction and elevation. The pupils were fixed to light. Convergence could not be tested. The fourth and sixth nerves were intact as were corneal and facial sensation. Visual fields were full to confrontation and on tangent screen with a 5-mm white projection light; visual acuity was 20/20 bilaterally. No optic atrophy was detected. The right nostril was caked with clotted blood that pulsated with each cardiac systole. There was blood in the posterior oropharynx. The neck was supple, the thyroid small. The testes were atrophic. The remainder of the neurologic examination was within normal limits. Roentgenograms of the skull revealed a ballooned sella turcica with obliteration of the sphenoid sinus by the inferior convexity

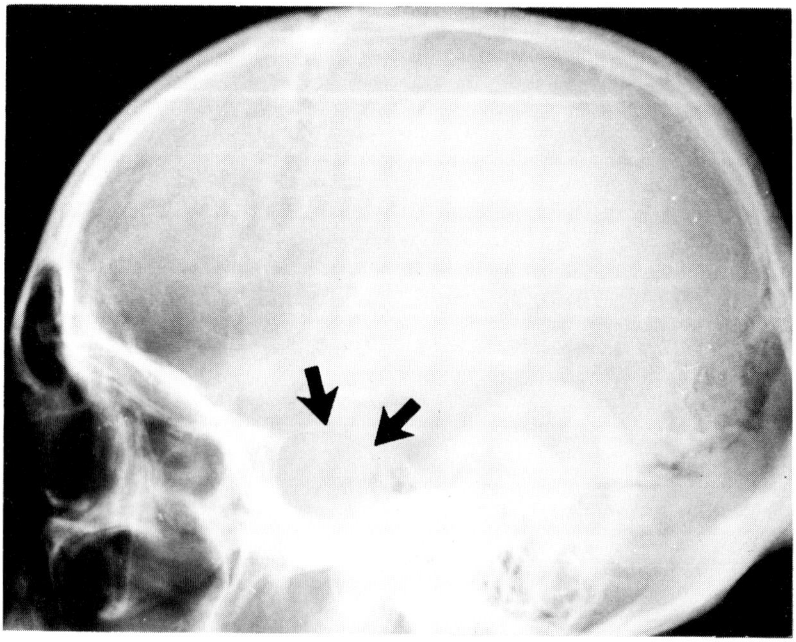

Fig. 8-1. Patient 2. Lateral skull film shows ballooning of the sella turcica. There is undercutting of both anterior clinoids. The dorsum is thinned and posteriorly displaced. Calcification of the diaphragma sellae extends from the dorsum to the anterior clinoids (arrows). Marked infrasellar extension is noted. A definite nasopharyngeal mass is not identified.

of the tumor. Laminograms revealed two defects in cortical bone of the sphenoid sinus that allowed communication to the nasopharynx. Calcification of the diaphragma sellae delineated the convex dome of the tumor (Fig. 8-1). Carotid arteriograms revealed uncoiling and anterolateral displacement of the carotid siphons but no evidence of suprasellar extension in the first segments of the anterior cerebral arteries. Results of urinalysis, serum electrolyte study, and hemogram were all within normal limits. Lumbar puncture revealed an opening pressure of 350 mm H_2O and yielded clear but slightly xanthochromic, acellular cerebrospinal fluid, with a protein concentration of 196 mg/100 ml. Although the patient changed little in the next eight days, his physicians feared recurrence of the apoplectic episode. The patient underwent right frontal craniotomy, which revealed a large dark bleb of tumor between the right internal carotid artery and the cavernous sinus. Necrotic and bloody tissue removed from the tumor within the sella turcica was identified microscopically as chromophobe adenoma. Subsequent treatment included irradiation to the tumor and replacement of steroid, thyroid, and androgenic hormones. At no time did any visual impairment except for diplopia manifest itself. One year later misdirection of the right third nerve was apparent. Visual acuity was 20/20 with full fields.

COMMENT. This patient is unique in our experience, and no counterpart can be found in the literature. His tumor had usurped the sphenoid sinus and allowed the escape of cerebrospinal fluid and blood at the time of apoplexy through a defect into the nasopharynx. The lateral skull x-ray films (Fig. 8-1) show a convex rim of calcified tumor at the level of the diaphragma sellae and indicate that this upward thrust had not yet compromised the optic chiasm. It is amusing in retrospect to recall the consternation of physicians attempting to explain how a bleeding intracranial aneurysm could have produced bilateral mixed ocular motor palsies. That pituitary apoplexy often masquerades as ruptured aneurysm still is not widely appreciated, nor is it recognized that it can easily be confused with other causes of acute sensorial deterioration, particularly meningitis. The following patient, previously reported by Jacobi and coworkers,[9] illustrates beautifully this aspect of the disorder.

Case 3. A 26-year-old white man entered the hospital complaining of severe headaches with nausea and vomiting of two days' duration. He described progressive enlargement of the hands and thickening of the facial features over a period of five to eight years. His shoe size had increased from 10B at the time of discharge from the armed forces eight years before to 12EEE at the time of admission. Easy fatigability, clumsiness, decrease in visual acuity, increasing oiliness of the skin, and intermittent paresthesias of the fourth and fifth fingers were noted during the year preceding admission. The patient had also experienced constipation, intermittent depression, and decreased sexual interest, but had attributed these symptoms to the use of narcotics.

Physical examination on admission showed a mildly febrile young man, alert and oriented but in obvious discomfort from severe headache. Coarse facial features and large broad hands and feet were noted. Visual field examination to confrontation showed bitemporal superior quadrantic defects. The optic discs were normal. The remainder of the examination was unrevealing.

Laboratory studies on admission disclosed the following values: hematocrit reading, 53%; hemoglobin, 18.4 gm/100 ml; white blood cell count, 5400/cu mm, with normal differential; serum sodium, 142 mEq/liter; serum potassium 4.5 mEq/liter; serum carbon dioxide, 28 mEq/liter; serum chlorides, 95 mEq/liter; BUN, 18 mg/100 ml; serum calcium, 10.3 mg/100 ml; serum phosphorus, 6.4 mg/100 ml; serum alkaline phosphatase, 30 (normal 4 to 17) King-Armstrong units/100 ml; SGOT, 110 (normal <40) units, SGPT, 200 (normal <35) units; total bilirubin, 3.4 mg/100 ml; prothrombin time, 53% of normal. Skull roentgenograms showed a markedly enlarged and balloon-shaped sella turcica, extensive pneumatization of the paranasal sinuses, and prominence of the mandible. The heel pads were 24 mm thick. A lumbar puncture shortly after admission yielded clear, colorless fluid. Laboratory studies showed the following values: opening pressure, 140 mm H_2O; mononuclear cells, 2/cu mm; red blood cells, 1/cu mm; protein, 45 mg/100 ml; glucose 63 mg/100 ml;

VDRL, nonreactive; culture, negative. Twenty-four hours after admission the patient suddenly became obtunded, and his temperature increased to 103°. His neck was stiff; bilateral Babinski signs were present. Repeat lumbar puncture revealed cloudy fluid and the following laboratory values: pressure, 260 mm H_2O; white blood cells, 270/cu mm; red blood cells, 135/cu mm; protein, 129 mg/100 ml; glucose, 42 mg/100 ml; Gram stain, negative; culture, negative. Blood and urine cultures were also negative. A diagnosis of bacterial meningitis was considered, and parenterally administered chloramphenicol (Chloromycetin) and erythromycin therapy was begun. During the next 24 hours, the patient's level of consciousness decreased, his temperature rose to 105°, and his pulse rate was 144, his blood pressure, 110/70. The following laboratory values were found: BUN, 46 mg/100 ml; serum sodium, 130 mEq/liter; serum potassium 4.9 mEq/liter; serum carbon dioxide 16 mEq/liter; serum chlorides, 87 mEq/liter. Pituitary apoplexy with secondary adrenal insufficiency was suspected and treatment with corticosteroids administered parenterally in large doses was begun. The patient's clinical status improved dramatically, and 36 hours later he was alert oriented, ambulatory, and had normal vital signs.

Intermittently severe headache gradually abated and the cerebrospinal fluid showed progressive decrease in protein and clearing of pleocytosis. Visual fields two weeks after the acute episode failed to demonstrate any defects. A pneumoencephalogram showed a normal anterior third ventricle with no evidence of a suprasellar mass.

Three weeks after the acute episode, insulin-glucose tolerance test produced hypoglycemia and did not cause any elevation of basal growth hormone level (less than 1 ng/100 ml). Over the next two years there was a decrease in the size of the patient's hands and feet and in the coarseness of his facial features. He resumed full activity. Laboratory studies showed persistent subnormal basal growth hormone levels and no detectable urinary gonadotropin excretion.

COMMENT. A "meningitic" picture in pituitary apoplexy has been well described[11-13] but is still not generally appreciated. Although acromegaly and enlargement of the sella turcica were recognized in this man, his abrupt febrile episode was first taken for narcotic withdrawal and thereafter for meningeal suppuration. Prompt treatment with steroid hormones probably saved his life. The similarities of his acute illness to addisonian crisis coupled with his known pituitary disease led to the correct diagnosis. Craniotomy was deferred day by day because of his dramatic improvement on steroid therapy and the absence of impressive visual involvement.

Absence of elevated growth hormone levels in the postoperative studies documents this patient's automatic acromegalic cure following apoplexy in the tumor and adds him to a sizeable list of similar descriptions.[9, 14] The next patient was not so fortunate.

Case 4. Three weeks before admittance a 36-year-old white man had noticed the sudden onset of a central scotoma in his left eye, which resolved completely in a day or so. A headache developed on the day before admittance and gradually became more severe. Six years before he had been diagnosed as having acromegaly. Symptoms referable to this disease probably began at age 23 years, at which time he weighed 132 pounds, and wore size 8 shoes. By the age of 30 years his weight had increased to 232 pounds and his shoes were size 12. He was not treated.

Examination revealed a large man with massive hands and feet and facies typical of acromegaly. He was alert, oriented, and cooperative but complained of a severe, ill-defined headache. Vision was recorded as 20/40 in both eyes, but formal field studies were not done nor was any confrontation testing of his fields recorded. Roentgenograms of the skull showed an irregular expansion of the sella turcica and erosion of the clinoid processes anteriorly and posteriorly. The frontal sinuses were enlarged.

After three days of worsening headache in the hospital, the patient developed fever, dimness of vision, and photophobia. His headache then improved. Visual acuity was again 20/40 OU, but a relative bitemporal field defect to finger confrontation was present. He had severe paresis of the right sixth nerve and a mild right third nerve paresis, chiefly adductive insufficiency. Later that afternoon the bitemporal hemianopia was absolute, as was the right third nerve palsy with complete right ptosis and a dilated fixed pupil. Intravenously administered hydrocortisone therapy was begun. The next day his fever rose abruptly to 107° and he developed nuchal rigidity and hot dry skin. He died of cardiac arrest during induction of anesthesia for an emergency transfrontal craniotomy. Autopsy revealed a spherical extension, 2.5 cm in diameter, of an intrasellar tumor rising above the diaphragma sellae and invaginating the hypothalamus and mamillary bodies (Fig. 8-2). Histologically, hemorrhagic necrosis was found in a chromophobe adenoma provoking an intense inflammatory response, chiefly of polymorphonuclear cells, in the perivascular spaces of the hypothalamus and in the basal meninges.

COMMENT. Evidence of progressive involvement of the visual system or of the hypothalamus demands emergency transfrontal craniotomy and decompression. This patient would probably have been saved by earlier surgical attack.

Another peculiar endocrinopathy was well represented in our series. Three of our patients had earlier undergone bilateral subtotal adrenalectomy for classic Cushing's syndrome. They all had lateral skull roentgenograms taken at the time of adrenalectomy that were found to be normal. All developed subsequent expansion of the sella turcica by a pituitary adenoma and eventually suffered pituitary apoplexy. The following description is classical.

Case 5. A 34-year-old white married man had developed signs and symptoms of Cushing's disease 2½ years before admittance and had been treated successfully with bilateral subtotal adrenalectomy followed by maintenance cortisone. At the time of adrenal surgery the sella turcica was normal (Fig. 8-3, *A*). Subsequently the patient was followed uneventfully for 13 months, at which time he noted that his skin was becoming diffusely hyperpigmented. Repeat skull roentgenograms (Fig. 8-3, *B* and *C*) revealed that he had developed deepening and enlargement of the sella turcica typical of an intrasellar neoplasm. He was not treated but remained well until six days before admittance, when he developed sudden, severe, left-sided headache and lateral diplopia. He was admitted to another hospital, where his cerebrospinal fluid was found to be completely within normal limits. Two days later repeat lumbar puncture revealed turbid xanthochromic fluid under increased pressure. There were 35 white blood cells, 33 of which were polymorphonuclear, and 600 red blood cells per cubic millimeter. The protein concentration was 160 mg/100 ml. Routine laboratory data were otherwise normal. The patient was transferred to Jackson Memorial Hospital for irradiation therapy of a pituitary tumor. On admission he was an alert, deeply pigmented man in mild distress from headache. His scars, particularly in the abdomen and neck, showed increased pigmentation. The right pupil was larger than the left but both reacted to light. The left eye turned inward due to a total left abducens palsy. Visual fields by confrontation showed an irregular bitemporal field defect that did not affect central acuity. Corneal reflexes were normal, as was facial sensation. Bilateral carotid arteriograms revealed uncoiling and lateral displacement of both carotid siphons without evidence of suprasellar extension. The patient underwent a course of radiation (5400 rads) to the pituitary. His headache remained severe, and after the third day of treatment he was shown by tangent screen examination to have more obvious irregular bitemporal field defects without impairment of central visual acuity. Thereafter the fields improved and his headache subsided. His fields were normal 15 days after admission and within the next three months his abducens palsy had resolved. Skin pigmentation has gradually lightened. He now works regularly as a clerk, is free of headache, and has normal visual and ocular motor function. Nine years after the event there are no symptoms of relapse of any endocrine disorder. The sella turcica has recalcified (Fig. 8-3, *D*).

COMMENT. This young man's course is in all respects similar to the syndrome first clearly described by Nelson,[15] the development of a chromophobe adenoma after subtotal adrenalectomy for Cushing's syndrome. Indeed, the histologic diagnosis in Nelson's case was established in the course of emergency craniotomy for pituitary apoplexy that occurred during irradiation of the tumor. Our patient's hyperpigmentation, which accompanied the rapid sellar enlargement, is apparently related to hypersecretion of either corticotropin or melanocyte-stimulating hormone from the pituitary adenoma. In spite of

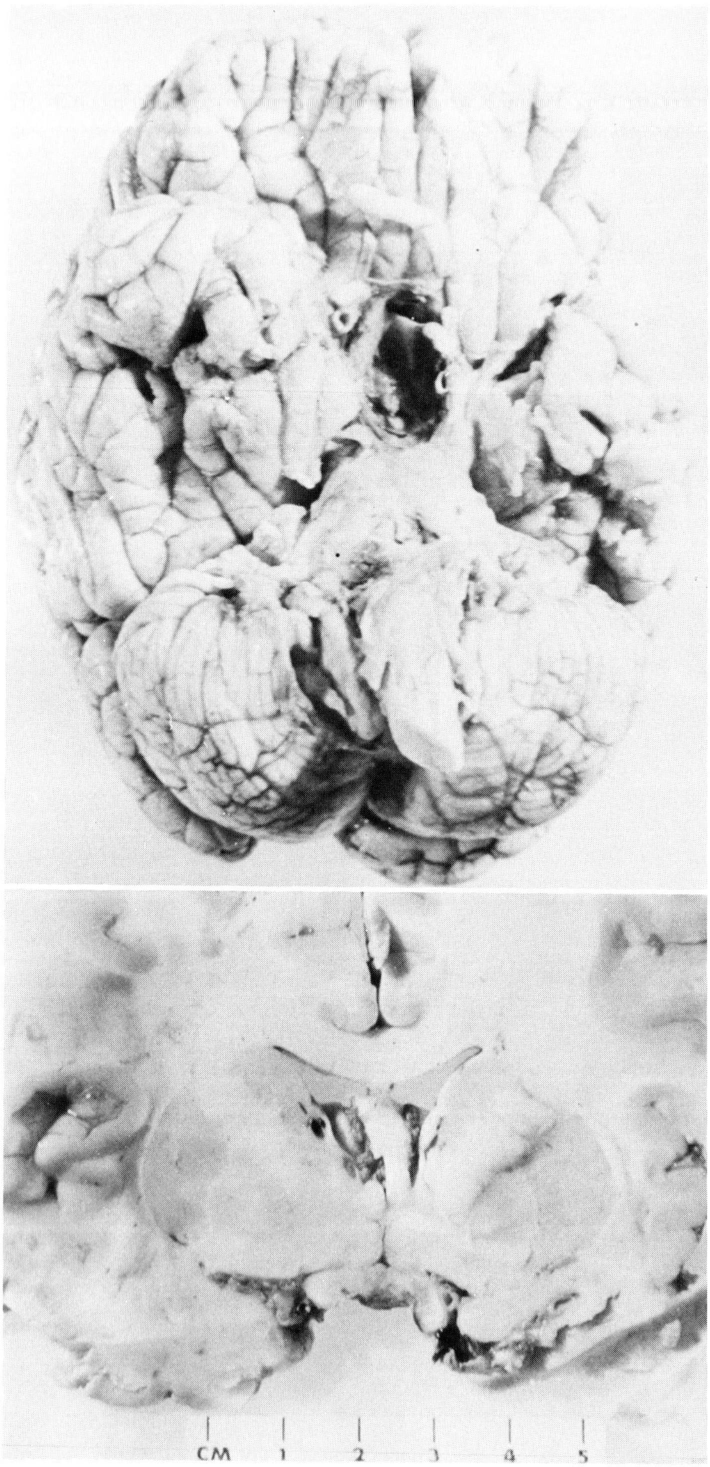

Fig. 8-2. Patient 4. Inferior surface of the brain at autopsy reveals excavation of the hypothalamus and midbrain caused by upward thrust of the swollen pituitary tumor. Cerebral vessels show marked inflammatory response. Optic chiasm and pituitary tissue have been removed.

A C

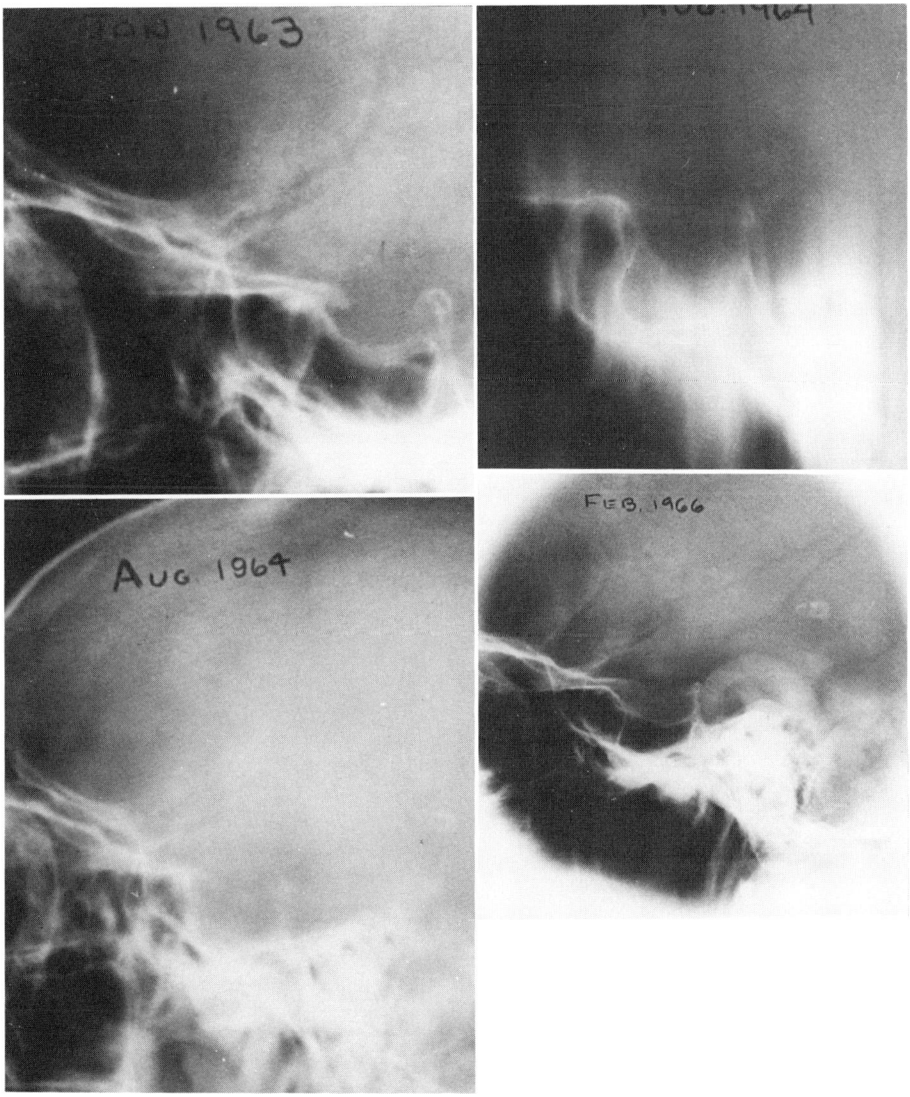

B D

Fig. 8-3. Patient 5. **A,** Lateral skull film. The size of the sella turcica is normal. The anterior and posterior clinoids are normal. The sellar floor is demineralized with suggestive early bulging into the sphenoid sinus. **B,** Lateral skull film. There is now gross distortion of the normal sellar contours. There is anterior extension indicated by clinoid erosion and soft tissue density below level of tuberculum sellae. The dorsum is erected. The floor of the sella is eroded. **C,** Midline laminographic section shows marked infrasellar extension. **D,** Lateral skull film. The sella turcica has returned to its normal appearance.

clear evidence of a pituitary hemorrhage this patient never had visual complaints or more than a mild bitemporal hemianopia, in contrast to the total sixth nerve palsy. Treatment by irradiation alone not only spared the patient a craniotomy but was followed by prolonged remission, a result that must be kept in mind when surgery is urged in this situation.

Case 6. A 67-year-old white man of Cuban birth entered the hospital complaining of headache. The history was obtained from his daughter, who stated that the patient had been well until four days before, when he had awaked with a headache followed that day by anorexia and vomiting. The next day he had still complained of severe, unremitting occipital headache and had had intractable vomiting; the following day he had taken no food, complained of increased headache, and developed a fever. At that time he had not been able to walk without assistance, and the daughter had noticed that his left eye "turned in and became red." Later in the day he had become unresponsive to verbal communication and had behaved in a confused and agitated manner. Three years previously mild diabetes mellitus had been diagnosed and treated with diet.

Physical examination revealed an agitated, confused, and stuporous elderly man. Pulse rate was 120, blood pressure 80/60, and temperature 101°. His general appearance, genitalia, and deep tendon reflexes did not suggest endocrinopathy. He was hypotensive, but serum electrolyte levels did not reflect any evidence of addisonian crisis. The optic discs were pink and showed no evidence of atrophy. When first seen he had a left sixth nerve paralysis with injection of the left conjunctiva. Both pupils measured 3 mm and reacted to light. The remainder of the extraocular apparatus was normal, but within several hours he developed a profound *right* sixth nerve paralysis. Immediately thereafter he began to develop bilateral ptosis. Lateral skull roentgenograms revealed an enlarged sella (Fig. 8-4, *A*). He was treated intravenously with a combination of insulin, dexamethasone, fluids, electrolytes, and pressor amines. His urinary output became adequate once his dehydration was corrected. Laboratory studies disclosed the following values: hemoglobin 18.0 gm/100 ml; hematocrit reading 53%; WBC, 10,000/cu mm, with 85% segs, 3% stabs, and 12% lymphocytes; blood gases (CO_2 and O_2) within normal limits; SMA-12 results all normal; serum sodium, 132 mEq/liter; serum potassium, 3.6 mEq/liter; serum chlorides, 92 mEq/liter; serum carbon dioxide, 20 mEq/liter; serum total protein, 6.5 gm/100 ml; remainder normal except for blood glucose 470 mg/100 ml; BUN, 30 mg/100 ml; RAI uptake, 33%; cerebrospinal fluid —pressure not recorded; colorless and clear; 4 WBC, 2 polys, 2 monos, 27 RBC; protein, 51 mg/100 ml; VDRL, non-reactive; India ink, negative. Pneumoencephalogram was normal (Fig. 8-4, *B*). Carotid arteriography revealed that both carotid siphons were displaced forward and laterally, uncoiled by the bulging tumor (Fig. 8-4, *C*).

The patient was treated with radiation therapy, begun ten days after admittance. He improved and became asymptomatic except for the abducens palsies, which cleared slowly. When he could be tested, the visual acuity and fields were normal and remained so.

COMMENT. This patient was initially regarded as a problem in differential diagnosis of disturbed sensorium in an elderly man. Torula meningitis was highly suspect when fever, signs of increased intracranial pressure (bilateral sixth nerve palsies), and pleocytosis were found. The enigma unraveled after lateral skull roentgenograms were examined. Once the diagnosis was established and his condition was improving, the patient as well as his doctors became reluctant to proceed with craniotomy. Although in this case it was a felicitous decision, we wish to stress that this management is justified only if visual acuity is normal and the sensorium clear.

Case 7. A 36-year-old woman was admitted to the hospital for the second time for regulation of complex medical problems. Fourteen years earlier she had been discovered to have juvenile diabetes mellitus and was treated with insulin. Twelve years before this admission she had been noted to have hypertension, "buffalo hump" obesity, purple striae, and hirsutism characteristic of Cushing's syndrome. The sella turcica had not been enlarged. Signs and symptoms of her Cushing's disease had remitted after bilateral subtotal adrenalectomy. Subsequently she had noted impressive darkening of the pigment of her body, particularly dense in the nipples and scars. Seven

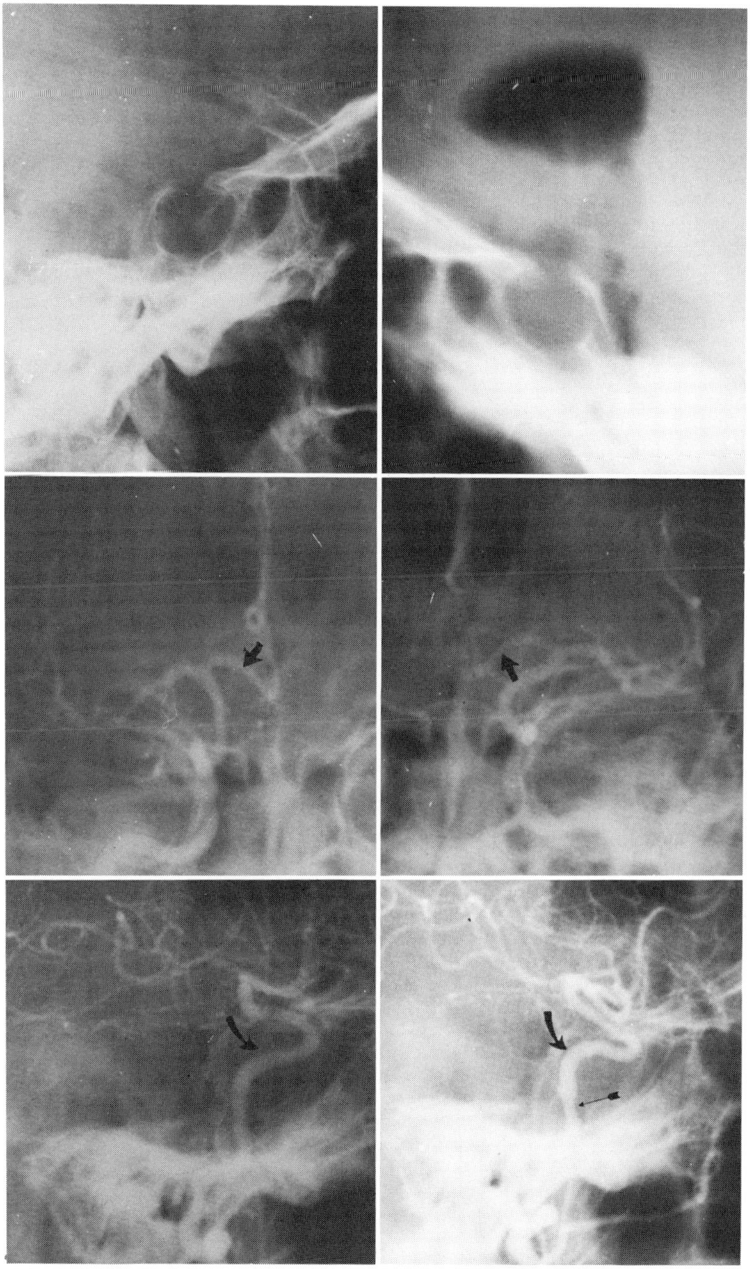

A B C_1 C_2 C_3 C_4

Fig. 8-4. Patient 6. **A,** Lateral skull film. The sella is enlarged. There is undercutting of the anterior clinoids. The midportion of the sella floor is eroded. **B,** Lateral brow-up pneumoencephalogram. The optic and infundibular recesses are normal. The chiasmatic cistern is normal. There is no evidence of suprasellar extension. The demineralization of the sella floor is well demonstrated. **C,** Anteroposterior and lateral views of right and left carotid arteriograms. There is bilateral displacement of the intracavernous portions of the internal carotid on the AP views ($\mathbf{C}_1$ and $\mathbf{C}_2$). The supraclinoid vessels (arrows) are normal. On the lateral view the right carotid siphon ($\mathbf{C}_3$) is open (arrow). On the left side ($\mathbf{C}_4$) there appears to be encasement of the internal carotid in the precavernous (small arrow) and intracavernous (large arrow) portions.

years before admission, skull roentgenograms had revealed an asymptomatic enlargement of the sella turcica. She had received 4000 rads of therapeutic radiation without subsequent change. Four years later there had been no change in the size of the sella, but her pigmentation had greatly increased.

Physical examination revealed a hypertensive, anxious, deeply pigmented woman with a hirsute chin and sparse scalp hair. Vision and extraocular movements were normal. Studies of her adrenal, diabetic, and hypertensive states were begun. Fortuitously, on the eleventh hospital day she suddenly complained of a sensation of swelling in her right forehead and blurring of vision. She had ptosis of the right eye with a total ophthalmoplegia, including the right third, fourth, and sixth nerves, and an unreactive pupil. The corneal reflex on the right was diminished, as was the perception of light touch over the forehead on that side. There were no abnormalities of ocular motility on the left, but obvious superior bitemporal field defects were detected with a projection light on a 1-meter screen. Visual acuity was 20/20 bilaterally. Bilateral carotid arteriograms and a pneumoencephalogram delineated lateral expansion of the tumor with uncoiling and lateral displacement of the carotid siphons and protrusion of a nubbin of tumor into the interpeduncular space (Fig. 8-5). There was no roentgenographic evidence of suprasellar expansion. She was observed for two days, after which a right frontotemporal craniotomy was performed with decompression of the optic chiasm and partial removal of a hemorrhagic pituitary tumor that displaced the chiasm superiorly and thinned the right optic nerve.

Although the immediate postoperative course was stormy and convalescence slow, her eventual course was salutary. Regression of the pigmentation ensued and her normal skin tone returned. She felt well and her diabetes was easily controlled thereafter. Replacement medications were continued as before without incident. The ophthalmoplegia cleared, as did the right trigeminal sensory defect. The visual field defects also remitted. All this occurred within six months. She was followed for seven years and remained asymptomatic with respect to her pituitary tumor.

COMMENT. This is another example of complex endocrinopathy culminating in "Nelson's syndrome," that is, growth of a corticotropin-producing pituitary adenoma

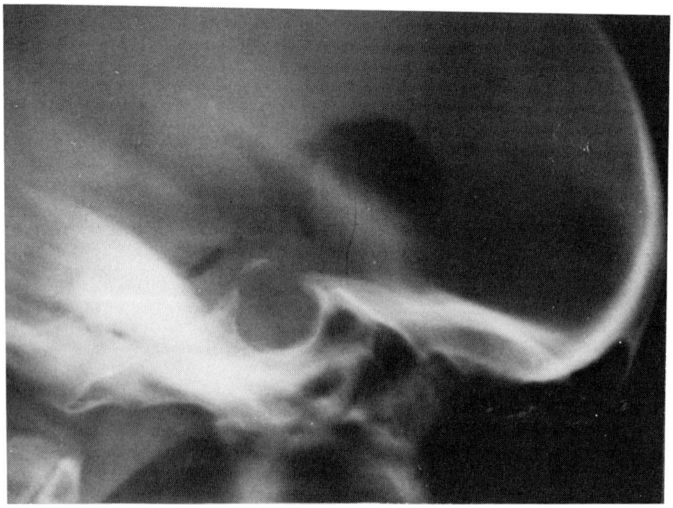

Fig. 8-5. Patient 7. Lateral brow-up pneumoencephalogram autotomogram. The sella turcica is enlarged. There is a defect in the dorsum. The optic recess is normal. The infundibular recess is blunted. There is extension of tumor into the prepontine space with posterior displacement of the prepontine cistern. Subtemporal extension was demonstrated by elevation of the right temporal horn and right basal vein of Rosenthal.

after bilateral adrenalectomy. This is one of two patients in this series who showed mild but definite involvement of the fifth cranial nerve.

Case 8. A 48-year-old white woman was admitted to the hospital for progressive acute visual loss in the right eye. She dated the onset of symptoms of acromegaly to the delivery of her third and last child 17 years before, when lassitude, fatigability, and "arthritis" of the hands and feet had made it impossible for her to care for the infant. The patient had then noted increasing shoe size and acral overgrowth of the fingers, but her endocrinopathy had first been recognized only eight years later when skull roentgenograms had revealed an enlarged sella turcica. Symptoms and signs of acromegaly had persisted in spite of a course of cobalt irradiation four years, and proton beam (Bragg peak) irradiation seven years prior to admission to the hospital. Signs and symptoms of acromegaly had persisted after treatment and growth hormone levels had remained high. One year prior to admission she had developed persistent aching pain in the left ophthalmic division of the trigeminal nerve with mild diminution of the corneal reflex on that side. This had been relieved slightly by diphenylhydantoin therapy. Six days prior to admission she had awaked with blurred vision in the right eye and had thought she had "gotten makeup in it." Four days later she was examined and found to have a right superior temporal field defect and visual acuity of 20/50 in that eye (Fig. 8-6). She was scheduled for admittance for study several days later, but the next day noted further worsening of the vision in her right eye associated with photophobia and the sensation of aching fullness of the right eye. She was admitted directly to the hospital with a diagnosis of "pituitary apoplexy."

Examination revealed a small, spare, hirsute woman with obvious coarse physiognomy and spadelike hands of acromegaly. Blood pressure was 110/70. Vision in the right eye had fallen to 20/80 with persistence of the temporal field defect. A slight abduction paresis of the right eye was present. The remainder of the examination was unremarkable. Skull films revealed enlargement of the sella turcica and thinning of the dorsum and posterior clinoids, which were elevated. The diploë were enlarged, and the paranasal sinuses huge.

She was treated with large doses of hydrocortisone administered parenterally and dexamethasone administered orally. Two days after the patient was admitted, cerebral angiography revealed "tenting" of the right anterior cerebral artery interpreted as upward displacement by a suprasellar mass. On the fourth hospital day a *left* superior temporal depression to small targets was heralded as the appearance of a junctional scotoma. On the fifth hospital day right subfrontal craniotomy was performed; 5 cc of bloody, turbid fluid was aspirated through the dome of a pituitary adenoma extending upward, stretching the right optic nerve and anterior chiasm over its dome. The visual pathways were decompressed and removal of tumor carried into the sella turcica, all visible remnants being removed. The patient's postoperative course was gratifying, with

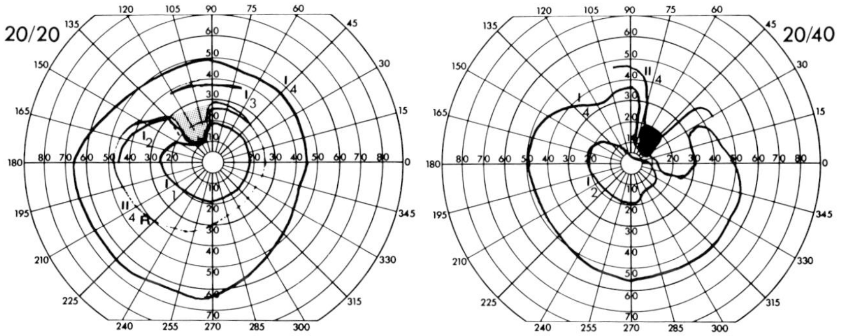

Fig. 8-6. Patient 8. Visual fields two days prior to admission demonstrated defect in right eye only. Subtle defect in left temporal field evolved over four days.

relief of both the chronic left headaches and the acute right retroorbital pain. Right eye vision rapidly recovered although some temporal field defect remained. The patient also believed that her acromegalic features had regressed somewhat.

Case 9. A 64-year-old woman, previously in excellent health, awoke with an extremely severe headache accompanied by nausea and vomiting but no visual disturbance. Later that day she was told that her situation was due to a "sinus condition" and was treated with pain medication and antibiotics. The patient continued to suffer from severe head pain and became dehydrated, for which she was admitted to the hospital. On the way to the hospital she noted bilateral "blurred vision" that rapidly worsened over 24 hours. The patient recalled that "as my vision got worse, the head pain got better." A diagnosis of bilateral optic neuritis was made, prednisone therapy, 90 mg daily was begun. There apparently was some improvement in vision. Nine days later vision was recorded at 5/200 in the right eye and 20/20 in the left. Ocular motility was normal but visual field examination revealed bilateral temporal field loss as well as central depression on the right. Plain skull films showed no abnormality, but carotid angiography and pneumoencephalography revealed a suprasellar mass lesion with elevation and blunting of the anteroinferior portion of the third ventricle. Brain scan was normal. At craniotomy a large sellar mass was found, displacing the right optic nerve laterally and anteriorly. This was confirmed histologically as a chromophobe adenoma, with evidence of previous hemorrhage, and radiation therapy (4400 rads) was accomplished following decompression of the chiasm and incomplete resection of the tumor. Although the temporal defect of the left field improved, the right field defect and acuity were unchanged after five years.

COMMENT. This patient presented with severe head pain followed by rapid loss of vision. The bitemporal pattern of the field loss was initially overlooked and a diagnosis of optic neuritis was made. This diagnostic error was also made in a recently published case,[16] wherein bilateral diminished vision returned to normal during one month of systemic steroid therapy; after a 14-month interval, bitemporal field defects led to the discovery of a large suprasellar cystic adenoma. Fortunately, in the present case, large doses of corticosteroids were prescribed, albeit for the wrong reasons. Rapid bilateral visual loss with severe head pain is not likely to be caused by optic neuritis. The pattern of the visual field defect is, as always, critical, and a parachiasmal mass lesion should have been suspected. Plain skull films at both the initial and referral hospitals were considered normal.

DISCUSSION

Although Bliebtreu[17] is credited with the initial description of intra-adenomatous bleeding in a young acromegalic patient, the term *pituitary apoplexy* was formally introduced by Brougham and co-workers[1] in a clinicopathologic review of five fatal cases. The use of this term presents no problems with reference to the syndrome attendant to sudden upward irruption of a pituitary mass into the optic chiasm and hypothalamus, causing blindness, hyperpyrexia, tachypnea, shock, coma, and death. But, reflecting on our own experience and the literature on the subject, we find many cases in which a variety of clinical manifestations provide excellent evidence for sudden expansion of a pituitary tumor. Until recently,[4, 11] most of these clinical variants have not been called pituitary apoplexy, probably for the following reasons: (1) lack of proof of intrapituitary bleeding, (2) mildness or absence of visual or sensorial symptoms, and (3) tendency for spontaneous recovery or regression of the tumor mass.

Neither clinical nor anatomic evidence of hemorrhage within the neoplasm is essential to the diagnosis. Spinal fluid examination, when performed, has often shown an inflammatory response or none at all. Nor has hemorrhagic change invariably been found at surgical exploration or autopsy examination, bland infarction with necrosis or simply edema of the adenomatous tissue being common findings. Such was the case in one of five patients in Brougham's classic description.

Occasional sparing of the optic chiasm and hypothalamus in pituitary apoplexy is easily explained by the proclivity of this tumor to extend in other directions in the course of its gradual enlargement: laterally into the cavernous sinuses, inferiorly into the sphenoid sinus, or posteriorly into the prepontine cistern. If upward tumor growth were limited by a tough diaphragma sellae with small aperture,[18] we would not be surprised to observe damage to other parasellar structures as a cause for the presenting syndrome of apoplexy.

That postapoplectic cure occurs with regression of visual loss, ocular motor palsies, and tumor hypersecretion is clear from numerous reports.[7, 9, 19] One begins to believe that pituitary apoplexy in itself is excellent treatment for the tumor were it not so hazardous to the sight and life of the patient. Most hypophysologists believe that the yellow or chocolate fluid filled "cysts" found routinely at operation or autopsy in pituitary adenomas are remnants of earlier focal tumor necrosis. Their presence suggests that patients, if questioned assiduously, might describe abrupt changes in symptoms correlating with the occurrence of "miniapoplectic" episodes.

For these reasons, we have cause to regard pituitary apoplexy as *a syndrome produced by any sudden enlargement of a preexisting pituitary adenoma.* This broad definition follows the justifiable trend in this decade to rely more and more on careful clinical interpretation rather than to base diagnosis on demonstration of pathologic anatomy.

Vision

Abrupt deterioration of vision is regarded as a hallmark of pituitary apoplexy. However, 5 of the 13 patients in our series with pituitary apoplexy had no visual involvement whatsoever in spite of excellent evidence for sudden enlargement of the tumor. Although such patients warrant the diagnosis of pituitary apoplexy, there seems little reason to counsel immediate craniotomy, especially if the clinical course stabilizes before any significant chiasmal compression can be detected. In one of these patients (case 2, Fig. 8-1), the upper border of the tumor could be seen as a gentle calcified upward convexity of the stretched diaphragma sellae, a conclusion that was confirmed at craniotomy. A thick, competent sellar diaphragm with a small aperture for the pituitary stalk would be expected to protect the optic chiasm and to predispose to expansion of an enlarging pituitary mass into the cavernous and sphenoid sinuses.

One further point deserves mention. When chiasmal compression from suprasellar growth of the tumor occurs gradually, visual function may be relatively well preserved in spite of gross chiasmal distortion and thinning of the optic nerves. Conversely, blindness or severe visual deficit may occur in pituitary apoplexy with but meager radiographic evidence of upward tumor extension. The chiasm will not tolerate sudden elevation and compression. In the latter circumstance, the optic chiasm must be decompressed immediately by surgical intervention if vision is to be restored.

Headache

Headache, usually severe and abrupt in onset, was present in all 13 patients with pituitary apoplexy in our series. The pain was most often described as frontotemporal or retroorbital sensation of fullness and pressure accompanying deep intractable aching. Six of the thirteen patients had clearly lateralized headaches, a symptom that showed excellent correlation with lateralization of visual and, particularly, ocular motor deficit. The character of the unilateral headache and its association with extraocular motor palsies strongly suggests that upper trigeminal involvement in the cavernous sinus may be its mechanism, although only one patient (case 7) ever demonstrated diminution of corneal reflex and cutaneous sensibility in the ophthalmic trigeminal distribution. Patient 4, who had been acromegalic for 17 years, was free of headache for four days after the abrupt onset of monocular visual diminution. A second bout of further visual deterioration brought with it severe retroorbital aching and photophobia on the affected side. This saltatory progression of symptoms and signs in pituitary apoplexy is common and probably reflects sudden expansion of the tumor from infarction or bleeding. The clinician should keep in mind that the march of events in pituitary "apoplexy" may take place over a period of hours or days and not in one sudden complete stroke as this term suggests.

Disorders of ocular motility

The cavernous sinuses form the lateral borders of the sella turcica and are compromised by any lateral growth of a pituitary adenoma. In spite of their traverse through this sinus, the third, fourth, and sixth cranial nerves rarely suffer detectable damage from an insidiously enlarging intrasellar tumor. Among the 123 consecutive cases of pituitary neoplasms we have studied, there was only one patient whose cranial nerves were damaged, a man with a huge adenoma causing bilateral abducens palsies (report in preparation). Jefferson[20] first pointed out that extensive gradual encroachment upon the ocular motor nerves caused little dysfunction, where rapid compression of these nerves in pituitary apoplexy is responsible for the profound ophthalmoplegia, often bilateral and occasionally total,[2, 25] cited in every published report of the syndrome.

Foix[21] is generally regarded as the first author to describe ocular motor paralysis in pituitary adenoma. His patient suffered abrupt onset of third, fourth, and sixth cranial nerve palsies with headache and normal visual acuity and fields, thoroughly fulfilling the clinical criteria for the syndrome of pituitary apoplexy without visual involvement. The splendid article by Weinberger and co-workers[22] on the cavernous sinus syndrome in pituitary adenomas emphasized what they regarded as a neglected but important clinical event. Their group I is a collection of six patients, all of whom obviously suffered pituitary apoplexy, although this term was not used, a conclusion made possible by their thorough clinical descriptions and surgical reports. They pointed out that sixth nerve palsy in this disorder results from direct pressure on the nerve in the cavernous sinus and is not a nonspecific reflection of intracranial hypertension. They quoted Schaeffer's[23] observation that marked anatomic variations in substance and size of the aperture of the diaphragma sellae undoubtedly influenced the growth pattern of pituitary adenomas, as mentioned above. If the pituitary tumor is removed or regresses, either through operation, irradiation, or postapoplectic necrosis, the ocular motor functions return rapidly. In our series, only patient 2 retained a severe right third nerve paralysis followed by symptoms of misdirected regeneration. We believe that this nerve was damaged at the operation, since the palsy was incomplete and resolving prior to his surgery.

Endocrinopathy

The 13 patients in our series presented primarily with signs and symptoms referable to encroachment of the tumor upon parasellar structures. Two patients (cases 3 and 6) acutely developed some features of addisonian crisis, with hypotension, azotemia, and obtundity; they responded dramatically to steroid therapy. Syndromes of acute hypopituitarism may not be well represented by reason of selection of these patients from neurologic and ophthalmologic clinics. One patient (case 2) was hypothyroid eight years before his apoplectic episode. Six other patients with nonsecreting pituitary adenomas showed no impressive clinical or chemical evidence of hypophyseal insufficiency.

In contrast to the hypersecretory adenomas discussed below, none of the seven patients with nonsecreting adenomas was known to have a pituitary adenoma prior to the apoplectic episode. Nonetheless, patients harboring these "silent" tumors often appear to have pasty skin and a slightly eunuchoid habitus but reveal no frank aberration in quantitative chemical tests that might corroborate the clinical impression of endocrinopathy.[19] Such patients often feel better on replacement hormones but do not demonstrate frank deficiencies that are common after pituitary apoplexy, irradiation therapy, or surgical removal of the tumor.

Three of the 13 patients with pituitary apoplexy had acromegaly. The literature suggests that pituitary apoplexy is good therapy for this disorder. Regression of acromegalic soft tissue changes is recorded,[14] as well as dramatic decreases in levels of plasma growth hormone. Young and associates[24] have made the interesting observation that histologic examination and bioassay of adenomas associated with acromegaly indicate that classic eosinophilic granulation and high content of growth hormone are characteristic of the small tumors found in elderly acromegalic males who suffer no symptoms of local encroachment and who die of other causes. In patients with expanding tumors who are operated upon for relief of chiasmal compression, the biopsy specimen yields atypical adenomas, often indistinguishable from the small cell chromophobe tumors and containing much smaller amounts of growth hormone per unit of tumor weight. In 1960 Nelson and co-workers[15] published their findings in a patient who developed signs and symptoms of a pituitary tumor two years after bilateral subtotal adrenalectomy for Cushing's syndrome. Before this surgery the sella turcica had been normal in size. Amelioration of the patient's hyperadrenalism was followed by deepening pigmentation of skin, amenorrhea, headache, and the gradual emergence of visual field defects. The sella turcica was enlarged, and bioassay revealed markedly elevated levels of plasma corticotropic hormone, an uncommon finding in Cushing's syndrome prior to adrenalectomy. During roentgen therapy "sudden hemorrhage into the tumor led to urgent operative intervention." Removal of the bloody, tense, necrotic tumor mass restored the patient's vision and led to regression of skin pigmentation and a decrease in plasma corticotropin levels. The biopsy specimen was interpreted as chromophobe (not basophilic) adenoma. Nelson and associates estimated that some 10% of adrenalectomized patients would eventually develop a pituitary mass.

Among the 13 patients in our series, there were three with histories remarkably similar to that described above. Although the outcome in all three was favorable, only one required surgery. One patient carried a normal pregnancy to term after the apoplectic episode.

In this peculiar endocrinopathy, rate of growth of the tumor can be estimated, since lateral skull films are routinely obtained in the course of investigation for Cushing's syndrome. Our impression is that pituitary tumors enlarge rapidly in this situation, an attribute that Jefferson[20] considered the strongest single factor predisposing to pituitary apoplexy.

Cerebrospinal fluid

Cerebrospinal fluid obtained at lumbar puncture in patients suffering pituitary apoplexy is usually abnormal and will generally fall into one of three categories:

1. Xanthochromic, with red blood cells, high protein content, and elevated opening pressure.

2. Pleocytic, variable as to intensity and composition, usually with increased protein content and high opening pressure.

3. Normal, or nearly normal, fluid as to color, clarity, cellular composition, and opening pressure.

1. Hemorrhagic fluid. Pituitary apoplexy is one of the causes of subarachnoid bleeding. Cerebral aneurysm is the commonest misdiagnosis and is more readily advanced if ophthalmoplegia is present. Bloody contamination of the cerebrospinal fluid is encountered in patients who show little or no evidence of suprasellar extension of the tumor (cases 2 and 3). Thus, bloody fluid does necessarily bespeak an ominous prognosis.

2. Meningitic fluid. Although pituitary adenomas have harbored fatal abscess and have been associated with fulminant purulent meningitis,[26] the pleocytosis of pituitary apoplexy is almost always sterile. Documentation of a meningitic clinical picture can be found in the reports of Rushworth,[11] Argires and Nelson,[13] and Jacobi and co-workers.[9] They described the mistaken initial clinical impression of meningeal infection, a natural diagnostic pitfall in patients with this type of cellular response. The pleocytosis is presumably provoked by the spillage into the meninges of necrotic tumor debris from an infarcted adenoma. Both the bloody and inflammatory abnormalities of cerebrospinal fluid tend to resolve quickly as the patient recovers from the apoplectic episode.

3. Normal fluid. Patients with pituitary apoplexy who have normal, or nearly normal, cerebrospinal fluid are definitely a minority. Even when fluid appears to be clear and not under increased pressure, mild elevation of the protein content and the finding of 10 to 50 white blood cells per cubic millimeter are common. Completely normal spinal fluid was found initially in two of our 13 patients (cases 3 and 5); repeat examination a day or two later revealed evidence of bleeding or pleocytosis in the cerebrospinal fluid.

Radiology

Roentgenographic abnormalities encountered in patients with pituitary apoplexy are the same as those of chronic intrasellar growth and extrasellar extension of hypophyseal adenomas. Conceivably, recent preapoplectic contrast studies might be available for comparison with the postictal roentgenograms, and this comparison might reveal sudden enlargement of the tumor. We have not had such an opportunity.

Skull roentgenography. The sella turcica was abnormal in the lateral skull roentgenograms in all but one of the 13 patients in our series. Although dyspituitarism associated with hypophyseal adenomas is often seen without sellar enlargement, extrasellar expansion rarely occurs without causing characteristic bony changes. The sella enlarges as the size of the tumor increase, and may deepen uniformly or develop a double floor due to asymmetric enlargement. This may be discernible in the anteroposterior as well as the lateral films. With moderate enlargement the sellar cortex may be preserved, but with further ventral growth the tumor enters the sphenoid sinus and thence the nasopharynx, causing rhinorrhea. The tumor may grow anteriorly and destroy the tuberculum sellae and chiasmatic sulcus; undercutting of the anterior clinoids, erosion of the optic strut, and enlargement of the superior orbital fissures may occur. Posterior extension may cause erosion of the dorsum sellae, permitting tumor to present in the prepontine space. Lateral extension of the tumor cannot be determined on plain film study. Chromophobe adenomas may reach enormous size, destroying the floor of the middle fossa. Usually, however, the dorsum is preserved and is displaced posteriorly in an erect position. Laminography may be necessary to fully evaluate the sellar contours and consistently reveals greater change than do plain films.

Calcification in chromophobe adenomas is rare, occurring in about 3% of the cases. It is usually finely granular in appearance. Occasionally the diaphragm of the sella is calcified, delineating the superior extent of the tumor. This calcification is linear or arcuate at the upper pole of the adenoma.

Cerebral angiography. Cerebral angiography is often performed in patients with pituitary apoplexy in an effort to find a source of intracranial bleeding. Intrasellar adenomas will show no vessel displacement but may show a vascular stain. If there is lateral extension, the posterior portion of the intracavernous internal carotid will be displaced laterally. The vascular displacement accompanying suprasellar extension depends on the size and direction of growth of the tumor. For convenience we will divide the changes in the carotid system into anteroposterior and lateral view abnormalities.

Anteroposterior view

1. Elevation and upward displacement of the anterior cerebral artery.
2. Elevation of the internal carotid bifurcation.
3. Lateral displacement of the supraclinoid portion of the internal carotid.
4. Lateral displacement of the anterior choroidal and posterior communicating arteries.
5. Elevation and lateral displacement of the basal vein of Rosenthal.
6. Lateral displacement of the thalamostriate vein.

Lateral view

1. Opening of the carotid siphon.
2. Upward displacement of the cavernous internal carotid artery.
3. Elevation of the internal carotid bifurcation.
4. Elevation and stretching of the cisternal portion of the anterior choroidal artery.
5. Elevation of the basal vein of Rosenthal.
6. Elevation of the internal cerebral vein.
7. Changes in the thalamostriate and ependymal veins with hydrocephalus.
8. Pathologic stain. Powell and co-workers[26] have demonstrated that the majority of the chromophobe adenomas will stain. The blood supply is from the intracavernous internal carotid, the supraclinoid carotid, and the posterior communicating arteries.

Posterior fossa angiography rarely shows changes except posterior displacement of the basilar artery in prepontine extensions. Also, the perforating thalamogeniculate arteries may be displaced posteriorly.

Cavernous sinus venography should help to delineate the extent and contour of lateral tumor expansion. We have not yet employed this technique.

Pneumoencephalography. With a purely intrasellar lesion the air study will show no abnormality. If there is upward bulging of the diaphragm, there may be upward displacement of the chiasmatic cistern and slight upward lifting of the optic and infundibular recesses.

With a suprasellar extension the pneumoencephalographic appearance will depend on the size and direction of growth of the tumor. Infrasellar extension will not be disclosed by the air study. It is essential to study the optic and infundibular recesses in the hanging head position with air only in the ventricular system to appreciate small suprasellar extension. Lateral midline tomography may be necessary for full evaluation. The usual pneumoencephalographic findings range from blunting or obliteration of the recesses, to complete replacement of the third ventricle. Superior lateral extension may be determined by indentation of the floors of the lateral ventricles. Occasionally, the foramina of Monro may be blocked, necessitating ventriculography. The third ventricle may be displaced laterally by the tumor. Rarely, the aqueduct of Sylvius may be blocked. Subtemporal extension is indicated by elevation of the temporal horns.

Once the ventricular system is evaluated, the air is introduced into the subarachnoid cisterns. Since the tumor is extraaxial, the margins of the mass will be delineated by the subarachnoid air. The posterior and lateral borders of the mass are usually well demarcated by the subarachnoid air. Less commonly, the anterior and superior margins are capped with air. Prepontine air will define extension posteriorly underneath the brain stem.

Treatment

Most reports in the literature have emphasized the need for emergency craniotomy in pituitary apoplexy to preserve vision and life. Surgical intervention is certainly indicated if the tumor has expanded upward into the optic chiasm or hypothalamus or both, in which situation blindness and hyperpyrexic coma may swiftly supervene. Zervas and Mendelson[27] have questioned the need for transfrontal craniotomy in a report of three patients whose intrapituitary hematomas were treated by transsphenoidal needle aspiration. Stressing the minimum of surgical trauma inflicted by this technique, they indicate, as have others,[28] that the transsphenoidal approach is their choice in the mangement of this complication, even when suprasellar extension and involvement of vision are pronounced. In fairness it must be stated that most neurosurgeons still prefer to visualize the optic chiasm and basal structures of the brain through the subfrontal approach in this as in most other suprasellar neoplasms. Future experience will no doubt assist us in sorting out the proper indications for each technique. It seems clear that steroid and fluid therapy combined with conventional therapeutic radiation are sufficient to control patients whose tumors expand laterally and inferiorly,[19] at least until follow-up examination indicates clear need for more aggressive treatment.

Table 6. Thirteen cases of pituitary apoplexy

	Age	*Sex*	*Clinical presentation*	*Visual acuity/ fields*	*Ocular motility*	*Endocrine status*	*Cerebrospinal fluid*
1.	54	M	Splitting headache, R face, neck, 2 days; progressive R ptosis, R visual loss	Finger count OU; bitemporal hemianopia	R III, IV, VI, L III	Normal	OP 240; xanthochromic; no cells; prot. 112
2.	37	M	Sudden severe frontal headache, diplopia, bloody rhinorrhea	Normal	R III, L III	Hypothyroid 8 yrs; on thyroid	OP 350; xanthochromic; no cells; prot. 196
3.	26	M	Severe frontal headache, nausea, vomiting, fever, stiff neck	Normal acuity; bitemporal superior hemianopia	Normal	Acromegaly 8 yrs; untreated	First tap: OP 140; clear; prot. 45; second tap: OP 260; 270 WBC; prot. 129; sterile
4.	36	M	Severe frontal headache, transient L scotoma, then hyperthermia	20/40 OU; then progressive bitemporal hemianopia	Normal, then R VI, partial III	Acromegaly 6(13) yrs; untreated	Not examined
5.	34	M	Severe L headache, diplopia, hyperpigmentation	Normal acuity; slight bitemporal field depression	L VI	Cushing's syndrome 3 yrs; bilateral adrenalectomy; then Nelson's syndrome	First tap normal; second tap: increased pressure; xanthochromic; turbid; 33 polys; 600 RBC; prot. 160
6.	67	M	4 days headache, anorexia, vomiting; then confused, agitated, L eye turned in; fever, BP 80/60	Normal (bedside)	L VI, then R VI, bilateral ptosis	Diabetes mellitus 3 yrs; normal electrolytes	OP?; colorless; 4 WBC; 27 RBC; prot. 51
7.	36	F	R headache, blurred vision; then R III, IV, VI	Normal acuity; subtle bitemporal defects	R III, IV, VI, R V	Juvenile diabetes 14 yrs; Cushing's syndrome 12 yrs; bilateral adrenalectomy; then Nelson's syndrome	Not examined

X-ray findings	*Initial diagnosis*	*Treatment*	*Result*	*Tissue diagnosis*
Ballooned sella; laterally displaced, uncoiled carotid siphons	Subarachnoid hemorrhage; "aneurysm"	Transfrontal craniotomy, decompression of large necrotic adenoma; 4500 rads postop	Full EOM; normal vision	Necrotic chromophobe adenoma
Ballooned sella; calcified diaphragma; laterally displaced, uncoiled carotid siphons	Subarachnoid hemorrhage	Transfrontal craniotomy, radiation postop	R III, misdirection; diabetes mellitus; working	Hemorrhagic necrosis of chromophobe adenoma
Ballooned sella; enlarged sinuses; normal pneumoencephalogram	Bacterial meningitis	Corticosteroids, fluids	Dramatic clinical response to steroid therapy	Not available
Enlarged eroded sella	Acromegaly; evolving pituitary apoplexy	Attempted craniotomy	Death	Hemorrhagic necrosis of chromophobe adenoma; compression of hypothalamus
Enlarged sella; laterally displaced, uncoiled carotid siphons	Subarachnoid hemorrhage	5400 rads	Resolution; vision, L VI; depigmentation	Not available
Enlarged sella; laterally and forwardly displaced, uncoiled carotid siphons; normal pneumoencephalogram	Fungal meningitis	Steriod and fluid replacement; radiotherapy	Excellent, without detectable residues	Not available
Enlarged sella; laterally displaced, uncoiled carotid siphons; small tumor in interpeduncular space on pneumoencephalography	Pituitary apoplexy	Transfrontal craniotomy, decompression of chiasm; (irradiated 7 yrs previously)	Excellent; depigmentation	Necrotic chromophobe adenoma

Continued.

Table 6. Thirteen cases of pituitary apoplexy—cont'd

	Age	*Sex*	*Clinical presentation*	*Visual acuity/ fields*	*Ocular motility*	*Endocrine status*	*Cerebrospinal fluid*
8.	48	F	Rapid R visual loss, R facial pain	R 20/50; R temporal defect, then bitemporal defects	Normal, then R VI	Acromegaly 15 yrs	Not examined
9.	64	F	Severe frontal headaches, then bilateral visual loss with nausea, vomiting	R 5/200, L 20/20; dense bitemporal defects	Normal	Normal	Not examined
10.	35	F	Progressive severe R headache, 1 day	Acuity not tested, full fields on confrontation	R III, partial	Nelson's syndrome 3 yrs; increasing pigmentation	OP 200; colorless; clear; prot. 48
11.	31	F	L frontal headache, diplopia L gaze	Normal	L VI	Normal	OP?, clear, no cells; prot. 19
12.	49	M	Severe headache for 2 wks Dec. 1973; now acromegaly, panhypopituitarism, distal myopathy, "blurred vision"	Normal acuity; minimal relative bitemporal field defects	Normal	Acromegaly; low GH, normal T_3-T_4	Not examined
13.	37	F	1 day history severe headache, nausea, vomiting, lethargy, diplopia	R 20/20, L 20/25; complete bitemporal defects	R, VI, L III, IV, V, R V—1, 2, 3	Amenorrhea 3 yrs	Not examined

X-ray	*Initial diagnosis*	*Treatment*	*Result*	*Tissue diagnosis*
Enlarged sella; elevation R anterior cerebral artery	Pituitary apoplexy	Corticosteroids; frontal craniotomy with evacuation of pituitary with hematoma	Regression of field defects	Hemorrhagic chromophobe adenoma
Normal sella; suprasellar mass on angiography pneumoencephalography	"Sinusitis," then optic neuritis	Corticosteroids; frontal craniotomy with chiasmal decompression, incomplete tumor resection	Residual R visual deficit; otherwise well	Hemorrhagic chromophobe adenoma
Enlarged sella	Psychiatric admission for "toxic delirium"	Irradiation	Transient diabetes insipidus; normal delivery 2 yrs later; recurrent apoplexy 4 yrs later (sudden headache, R VI); remains well	Not available
Ballooned sella; large suprasellar mass on pneumoencephalography	Unexplained VI palsy	Irradiation	Resolution of headaches, L VI	Not available
Enlarged sella, double floor; lateral displacement R cavernous carotid; slight posterior and L parasellar extension on pneumoencephalography	Acromegaly	Cytomel, cortisone, Delatestryl; 5000 rads	Marked clinical improvement	Not available
Enlarged, destroyed sella; laterally displaced, uncoiled carotid siphons	Subarachnoid hemorrhage	Corticosteroids, then frontal craniotomy	Mild bitemporal defects; depth perception problem	Hemorrhagic necrosis of pituitary

REFERENCES

1. Brougham, M., Heusner, A. P., Adams, R. D.: Acute degenerative changes in adenomas of the pituitary body with special reference to pituitary apoplexy, J. Neurosurg. **7**:421-439, 1950.
2. Walsh, F. B.: Bilateral total ophthalmoplegia with adenoma of the pituitary gland, Arch. Ophthalmol. **42**:646-654, 1949.
3. Chamlin, M., Davidoff, L. M., and Feiring, E. H.: Ophthalmologic changes produced by pituitary tumor, Am. J. Ophthalmol. **40**:353-368, 1955.
4. Rovit, R., and Fein, J. M.: Pituitary apoplexy: a review and reappraisal, J. Neurosurg. **37**:280-288, 1972.
5. Uihlein, A., Balfour, W. M., and Donovan, P. F.: Acute hemorrhage into pituitary adenomas, J. Neurosurg. **14**:140-151, 1957.
6. Montgomery, D. A. D., Welbourn, R. B., and McCaughey, W. T. E.: Pituitary tumors manifested after adrenalectomy for Cushing's syndrome, Lancet **2**:708-710, 1959.
7. Wright, R. L., Ojemann, R. G., and Drew, J. H.: Hemorrhage into pituitary adenomata; report of two cases with spontaneous recovery, Arch. Neurol. **12**:326-333, 1965.
8. Krueger, E. G., Unger, S. M., and Roswit, B.: Hemorrhage into pituitary adenoma with spontaneous recovery and reossification of the sella turcica, Neurology (Minneap.) **10**:691-696, 1960.
9. Jacobi, J. D., Fishman, L. M., and Daroff, R. B.: Pituitary apoplexy in acromegaly followed by partial pituitary insufficiency, Arch. Intern. Med. **134**:559-561, 1974.
10. Rovit, R. L., and Duane, T. D.: Cushing's syndrome and pituitary tumors. Pathophysiology and ocular manifestations of ACTH-secreting pituitary adenomas, Am. J. Med. **46**:416-427, 1969.
11. Rushworth, R. G.: Pituitary apoplexy, Med. J. Aust. **1**:251-254, 1971.
12. Jefferson, M., and Rosenthal, F. D.: Spontaneous necrosis in pituitary tumours (pituitary apoplexy), Lancet **1**:342, 1959.
13. Argires, J. P., and Nelson, J.: Pituitary apoplexy: review of the literature and two case reports, South. Med. J. **59**:785-789, 1966.
14. Taylor, A. L., Finster, J. L., Raskin, P. H., Field, J. B., and Mintz, D. H.: Pituitary apoplexy in acromegaly, J. Clin. Endocrinol. Metab. **28**:1784-1792, 1968.
15. Nelson, D. H., Meakin, J. W., and Thorn, G. W.: ACTH-producing pituitary tumors following adrenalectomy for Cushing's syndrome, Ann. Intern. Med. **52**:560-569, 1960.
16. Senelick, R. C., and Van Dyk, H. J.: Chromophobe adenoma masquerading as corticosteroid-responsive optic neuritis, Am. J. Ophthalmol. **78**:485-488, 1974.
17. Bleibtreu, L.: Ein Fall von Akromegalia (Zerstörung der Hypophysis durch Blutung), Munch. Med. Wochenschr. **52**:2079-2080, 1905.
18. Bergland, R. M., Ray, B. S., and Torack, R. M.: Anatomical variations in the pituitary gland and adjacent structures in 225 human autopsy cases, J. Neurosurg. **28**:93-99, 1968.
19. Meadows, S. P.: Unusual clinical features and modes of presentation in pituitary adenomas, including pituitary apoplexy. In Smith, J. L., editor: Neuro-ophthalmology, vol. 4, St. Louis, 1968, The C. V. Mosby Co., pp. 184-189.
20. Jefferson, G.: Extrasellar extensions of pituitary adenomas. President's address. Section of neurology, Proc. R. Soc. Med. **33**:433-458, 1940.
21. Foix, C.: Syndrome de paroi externe des sinus caverneux (ophthalmoplègie unilaterale a marche rapidement progressive algie du territoire de l'ophtalmique). Amélioration considérable par le traitement radiothérapique, Rev. Neurol. (Paris) **38**:827, 1922.
22. Weinberger, L. M., Adler, F. H., and Grant, F. C.: Primary pituitary adenoma and the syndrome of the cavernous sinus; a clinical and anatomic study, Arch. of Ophthalmol. **24**:1197-1235, 1940.
23. Schaeffer, J. P.: Some points in the regional anatomy of the optic pathways with especial reference to tumors of the hypophysis cerebri and resulting ocular changes, Anat. Rec. **28**:243, 1924.
24. Young, D. G., Bahn, R. C., and Randall, R. V.: Pituitary tumors associated with acromegaly, J. Clin. Endocrinol. Metab. **25**: 24, 1965.
25. Symonds, C.: Ocular palsy as the pre-

senting symptom of pituitary adenoma, Johns Hopkins Med. J. **111:**72-81, 1962.

26. Powell, D. F., Baker, H. L., Jr., and Laws, E. R., Jr.: The primary angiographic findings in pituitary adenomas, Radiology **110:**589-595, 1974.
27. Zervas, N. T., and Mendelson, G.: Treatment of acute haemorrhage of pituitary tumours, Lancet **1:**604-605, 1975.
28. Berti, G., Heisey, W. G., and Dohn, D. F.: Pituitary apoplexy treated with stereotactic transsphenoidal aspiration, Cleve. Clin. Q. **41:**163-175, 1974.

Chapter 9

Meningiomas primary within the orbit and optic canal

Frank B. Walsh

This chapter relates principally to seven cases of meningioma, primary in the orbit of children and juveniles. As an addendum some experiences of other observers with such cases are cited. Also, brief mention is made of meningiomas primary in the orbit of adults. What the paper contains reflects collaboration with Dr. Richard Lindenberg to whom I am grateful for several figures and advice. My experience with meningiomas in the young age group indicates particular features that merit attention. Presently, the chance of preserving useful vision in the eye on the side of the lesion cannot be considered as good.

ANATOMY

An understanding of the symptomatology associated with meningiomas must be based on knowledge of the relevant anatomy and histology.

The term *meningioma* implies that such tumors have originated from meninges that surround the brain and extend to invest the optic nerve in the optic canal and orbit. Here we are considering in particular the behavior of meningiomas that have originated in the orbit and optic canal, and it is

Read in part as the second John McLean Memorial Lecture at The New York Academy of Medicine, Section on Ophthalmology, November 24, 1969. From the Wilmer Ophthalmological Institute of The Johns Hopkins University and Hospital. Supported in part by the Filbert Foundation Laboratories and United States Public Health Service Grant 5 RO1 EY00215-10 through the National Institutes of Health.

EDITOR'S NOTE. This paper was originally published in *Neuro-ophthalmology,* vol. 5, Hallandale, Fla., 1969, Huffman Publishing Co., and as such is no longer available.

significant that the arrangement of the optic nerve sheaths at these sites is different from that within the cranium.

The dura within the cranium consists of two layers of fibrous connective tissue that is rather tough and firm. The outer layer functions as periosteum of the calvarium; it exists and functions similarly within the orbit and optic canal. In the cranium and optic canal the inner layer of dura is firmly attached to the outer layer, but within the orbit it is separated from it and forms the dural sleeve surrounding the optic nerve.

The arachnoid sheath is of great importance in regard to meningiomas. It is a membrane that surrounds the surface of the brain without deeply entering the sulci. It continues forward along the optic nerve, terminating at the sclera. Although thin, it has two layers. The outer layer of the arachnoid consists of cells that resemble epithelium; the cells have characteristic dark-staining nuclei. The inner layer consists of stratified fibrous tissue. The arachnoid is separated from the dura by a natural space, the subdural space, and this space is seen within the cranium and around the optic nerve (Fig. 9-1). Within the skull the arachnoid is fastened to the dura and bone only in the areas adjacent to the dural sinuses, where there are tissue thickenings of the arachnoid that are called villi, or pacchionian granulations. Within the cranium many meningiomas originate in these areas; less often they develop directly over a hemisphere.

The arachnoid forms the outer wall of the subarachnoid space. This space contains the cerebrospinal fluid, blood vessels, and a network of trabeculae or subarachnoid tissue that at the surface of the brain connects with the thin pia mater. The subarachnoid trabeculae consist of a core of fibrous tissue surrounded by a single layer of mesothelial cells. When the

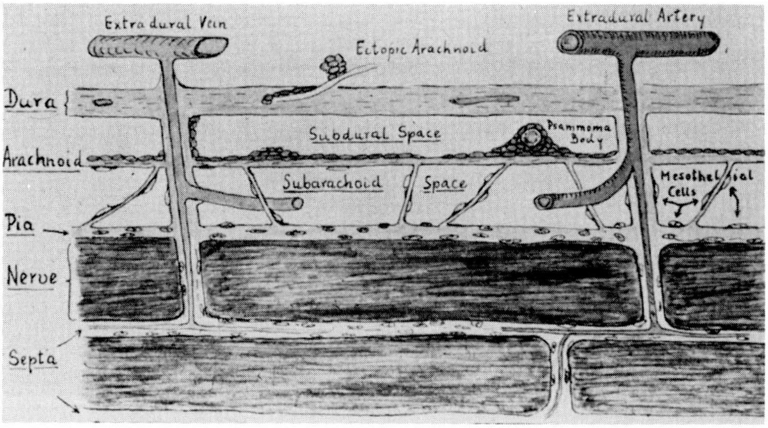

Fig. 9-1. Meninges and blood supply of orbital optic nerve. (Courtesy Dr. Richard Lindenberg.)

mesothelial cells have participated in the development of meningioma, the tumor may become angioblastic or lipoblastic. These mesothelial cells also may give origin to sarcomas of the leptomeninges or to reticuloendothelial tumors.

The histology of meningiomas varies from case to case. If epithelial-like cells predominate (they normally are seen in the outer layer), the tumor may be described as cellular. Densely packed small cells grow in strands that often form whorls. If in addition to whorled strands, psammoma bodies, thought to represent degeneration of the whorled cells, are present, the tumor certainly is a meningioma. In some instances the psammoma bodies become calcified. When cellular elements of the inner layer of the arachnoid are present, as is often the case, the meningioma is of "mixed" type or is a fibromatous meningioma.

Within the cranium, arteries cross the subdural space only where they enter the cranial cavity; these arteries under normal circumstances are the carotid and vertebral arteries. Veins leave the subarachnoid space only near the venous sinuses; they are known as bridging veins before they enter their respective sinuses. Thus, when an autopsy is performed and the dura is incised distant from the dural sinuses, it can be turned over without difficulty, exposing the arachnoid over large areas of the brain. This is significant when considerations are directed to the dura that surrounds the optic nerves.

Now we are in a position to contrast the situation that exists within the orbit and optic canal with that which exists intracranially. The arteries and veins to and from the optic nerves are located extradurally except in the area of the optic canal, where the ophthalmic artery is situated within the subarachnoid space (Fig. 9-1). Within the canal, arterial branches reach the optic nerve. Within the orbit, the ophthalmic artery, which has become extradural, receives collateral supply. The branches of the ophthalmic artery that reach the optic nerve stem must pass through the dura, the arachnoid, and the subarachnoid space. The largest single branch of the ophthalmic artery, the central retinal artery, undoubtedly supplies blood to the optic nerve as well as the retina, but its significance in regard to optic nerve supply is not precisely known. Hayreh's work[1-3] should be consulted. The situation is the same with veins. Also, it should be noted that vessels that enter or leave the orbital optic nerve are accompanied by connective tissue strands that are derived from the dura, pass through the subdural space, the arachnoid, and the subarachnoid space, and form the septa of the optic nerve. Such trabeculae within the orbit are not observed about the intracranial optic nerve or chiasm or in any other part of the brain. It becomes apparent that *an incision through the dural covering of the optic nerve must interfere with the blood supply of the nerve.* Mechanically speaking, the arrangement of trabeculae within the orbit accounts for the meninges and orbital nerve forming a unit that cannot be disrupted without serious consequence to optic nerve functioning.

It has been made clear that meningiomas develop from arachnoid tissue and that the histologic appearance of the tumor varies because it is likely to contain cells that have originated in the external and internal layers of the arachnoid. Either type of cells may predominate. For the purpose of histologic diagnosis, the presence of cells derived from the outer layer of the arachnoid is significant. It relates to early clinicians using the term *dural endothelioma.*

Why meningiomas develop remains unknown. Trauma has been indicted as initiating their development,[4] and pregnancy is known to activate meningiomas. I have observed in a pregnant woman a field defect that was known to have developed during an earlier pregnancy and to have disappeared. With a subsequent pregnancy the field defect reappeared and persisted until an intracranial meningioma was removed. Although we are not considering here meningiomas that may properly be considered as malignant on the basis of distant metastases, it is of interest that the histologic appearance of the meningioma that is primary does not foretell the possibility of its metastasizing. Fortunately such meningiomas are rare.

HISTOLOGY

In many instances meningiomas are recognized without difficulty. In the majority of cases there are epitheliumlike cells in strands and often in

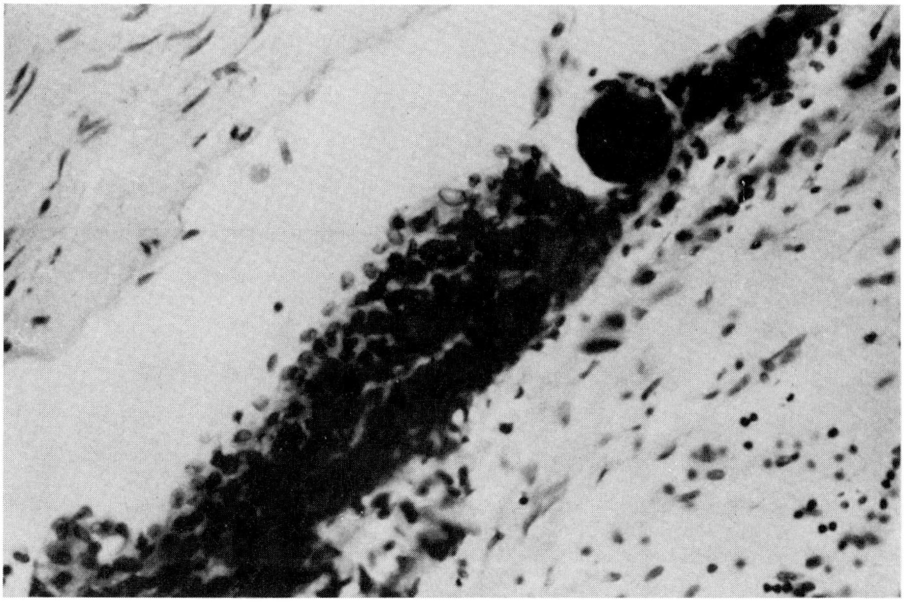

Fig. 9-2. Thickening of arachnoid with psammoma body. Patient was 87-year-old man. Death was due to bronchopneumonia and arteriosclerotic heart disease. There was no history or evidence of ocular involvement.

whorls; when psammona bodies are present with these features the diagnosis is reasonably certain. However, there may be fibrous tissue cells interspersed, as well as varying degrees of vascularity, as may be observed in angioblastic meningiomas. The degree of vascularity may be variable. Russell and Rubinstein[5] have stated that there seems to be no reason to consider meningeal "hemangiopericytoma" as an entity distinct from meningioma and that "capillary hemangioblastoma" cannot be considered as dissimilar to what characterizes angioblastic meningiomas. As already remarked, sarcomas and reticuloendothelial sarcomas may originate from mesothelial cells found about the arachnoid trabeculae. Thus the final diagnosis of meningioma in some instances provides for differences of opinion.

It would seem reasonable that Figs. 9-2 and 9-3 represent only arachnoidal proliferation and not meningioma. In Fig. 9-4, *A* and *B,* there is insufficient evidence to suggest meningioma, but in Fig. 9-4, *C,* taken farther forward from the optic canal region, one can be reasonably certain that the tumor is a meningioma. Fig. 9-5 shows arachnoid tissue that is ectopic within the dura. Such ectopia is important in regard to surgical therapy. Fig. 9-8 holds particular interest. In Fig. 9-8, *A* and *B,* the disc swelling resulting from infiltration of astrocytomas is shown. In Fig. 9-8, *C* and *D,*

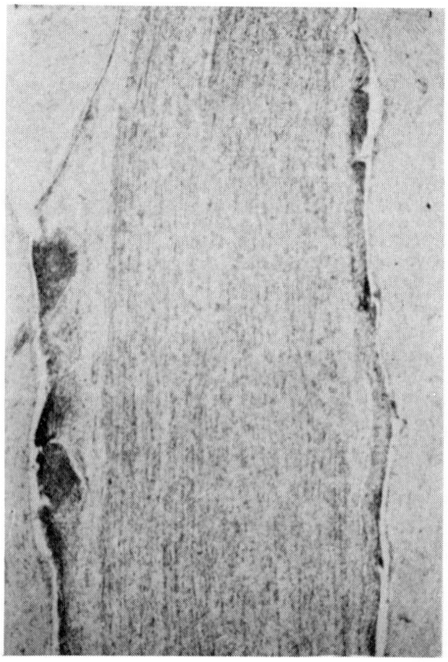

Fig. 9-3. Patient died from rupture of aneurysm that had pressed upon optic nerve. Again there is proliferation of arachnoid, which suggests seeding via optic canal, but arachnoidal alteration is benign. Optic atrophy was not present in other optic nerve.

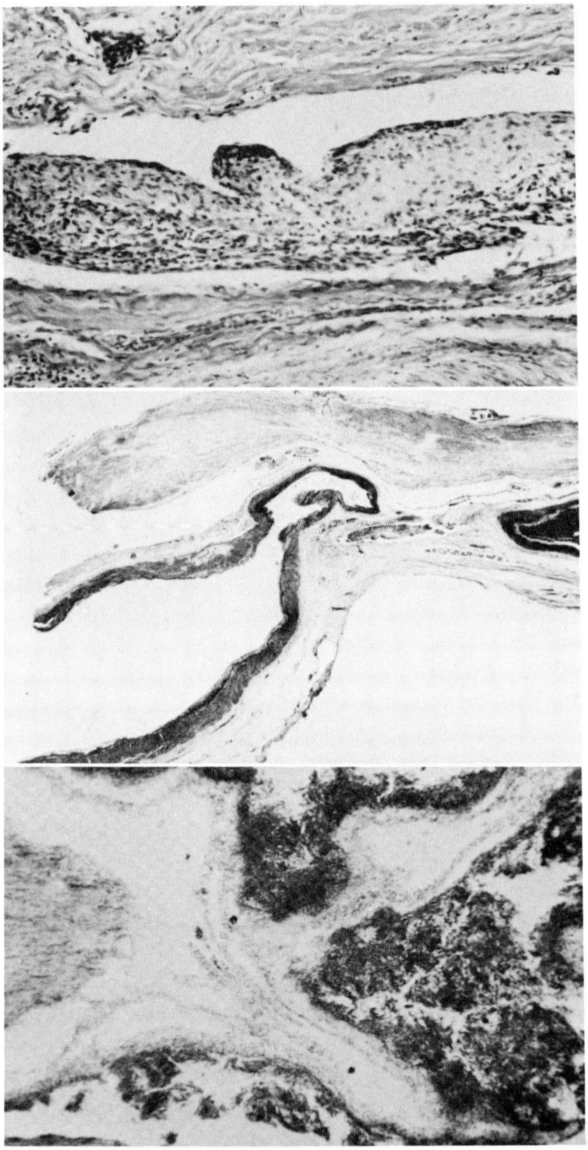

Fig. 9-4. Patient, a 59-year-old man, was known to have been blind in left eye for years. He was struck by an automobile that approached from his left side. Craniocerebral injuries accounted for death. **A,** What appears to be a benign arachnoid villus. **B,** To left is seen carotid artery with commencement of ophthalmic artery, which is again seen on right. A villus is seen above commencement of ophthalmic artery. **C,** Section made more anteriorly. In this case, a diagnosis of meningioma seems to be reasonable.

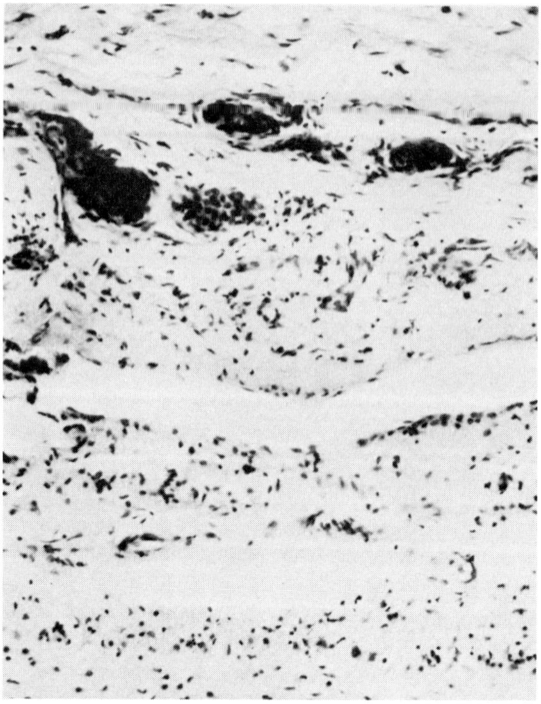

Fig. 9-5. Patient, a 25-year-old Negro female, had never been examined by a physician as far as could be determined. She was dead on arrival at Provident Hospital. Colloid cyst obstructed foramina of Monro, and lateral ventricles were symmetrically dilated. Optic nerves were normal. There was ectopic arachnoid within dura, as shown.

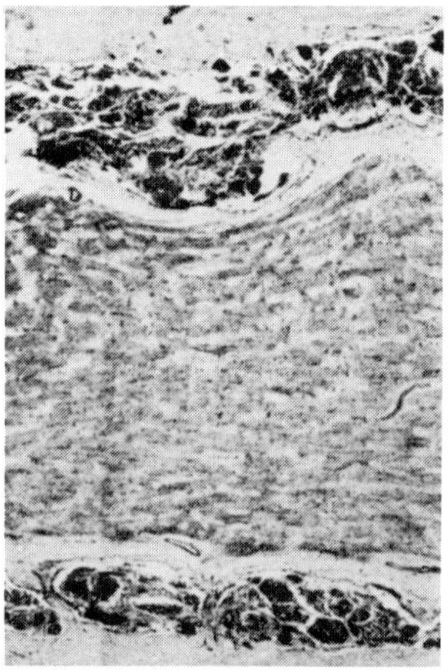

Fig. 9-6. A 55-year-old white woman died from Doriden poisoning. She was essentially blind in both eyes. There was pronounced bilateral optic atrophy. She had refused admission to hospital. At autopsy it was found that meningioma in anterior angle of chiasm had destroyed both optic nerves. Extension of tumor via optic canal is shown. There was atrophy of optic tracts.

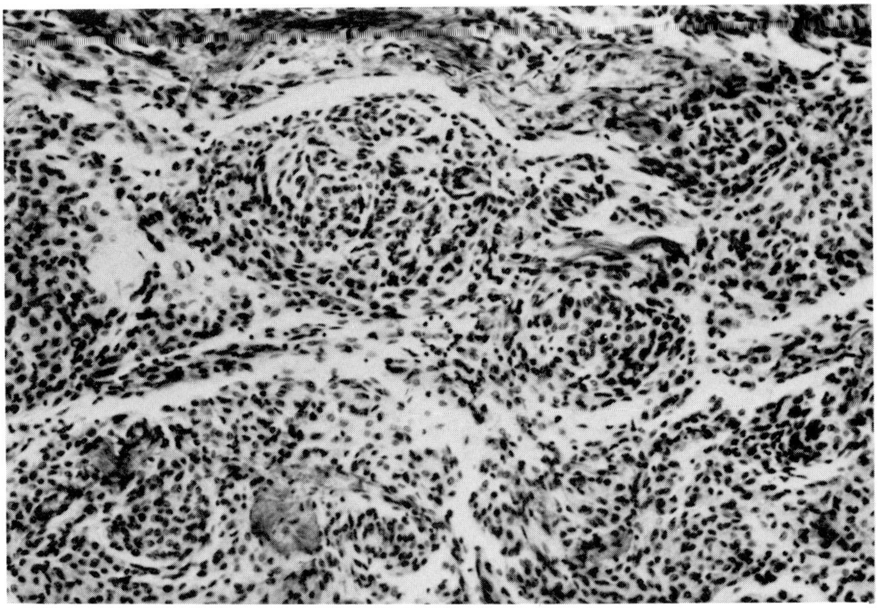

Fig. 9-7. Patient, a 57-year-old white woman, died as result of barbiturate poisoning. Autopsy revealed meningioma over ventral portion of left optic nerve and anterior chiasm. Meningioma shown is classical type without psammoma bodies.

nests of cells that suggest meningioma are found, and such cells are observed on arachnoid villi.

OCCURRENCE

According to Reese,[6] 17% of all tumors of the central nervous system are meningiomas; in a series of 230 consecutive cases of expanding lesions of the orbit with unilateral exophthalmos, in 5% meningioma was responsible. Accepting the 17% occurrence as reasonable, meningiomas, which frequently are characterized by features that interest ophthalmologists, occur more frequently than pituitary adenomas; Russell and Rubinstein[5] remarked that the frequency of such adenomas has in several series varied from 6% to 17.8% of tumors involving the nervous system.

A majority of meningiomas are found in middle-aged adults. They also occur in children and juveniles and in some instances are congenital.[7] They are considered rare in the young age group. From the experience of several observers, including my own, it would be more correct to say that in this last-named group they are relatively infrequent. Within this group a majority are primary within the orbit. Considering all orbital meningiomas, it seems probable a majority have originated within the cranium and have extended to involve the orbit.

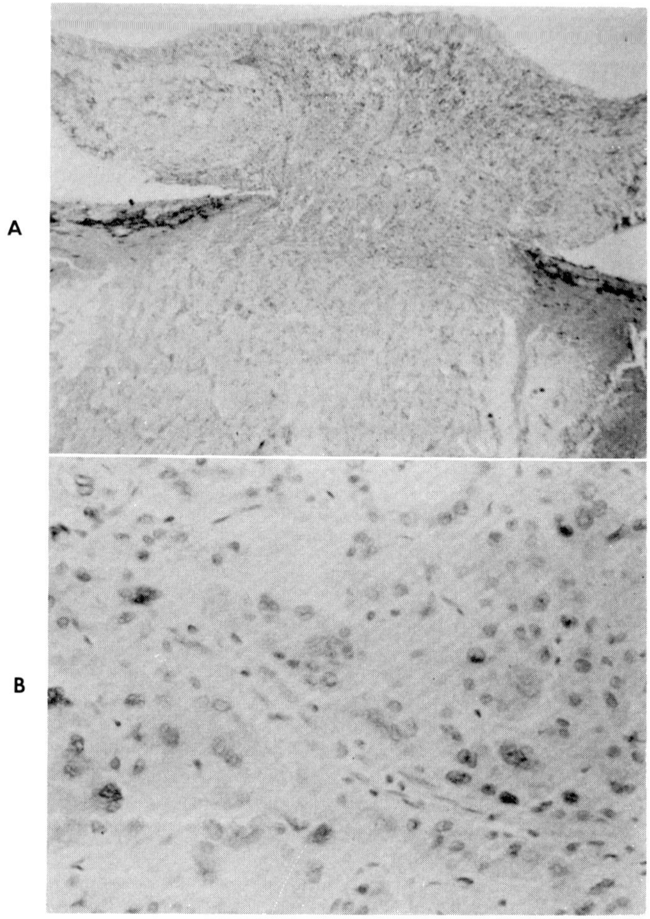

Fig. 9-8. Gliomatous involvement of optic discs. **A,** Appearance of optic discs. **B,** Tumor is astrocytoma. **C,** Nests of cells within dura. **D,** Nests of cells within dura, as in **C,** and also arachnoid villus. In my opinion the optic nerve glioma is associated with what well may be ectopic meningioma formation. (Courtesy Dr. Frank Winters.)

Females are affected more often than males. Ingalls[8] listed ten cases of orbital tumor; nine patients were female and one was male. In the seven cases in children and juveniles described below, six patients were female.

Meningiomas may be associated with other tumors that affect the central nervous system. Neurofibromatosis is sometimes associated. In 1956 I estimated that 15% of primary optic nerve and chiasm tumors (gliomas) were related to neurofibromatosis. Meningioma has been associated with pituitary tumor, glioma of the optic nerve and chiasm, glioblastoma multiforme, and aneurysm.

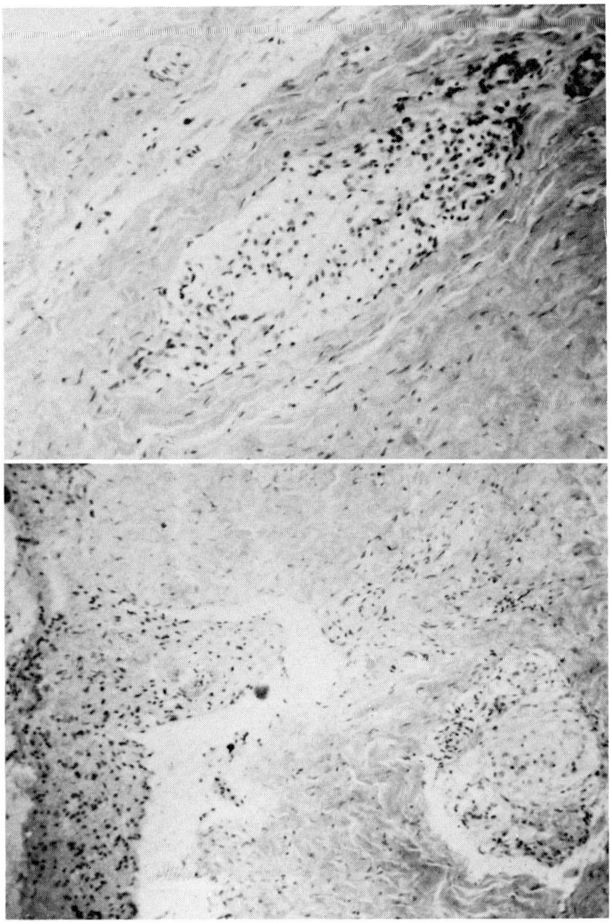

C

D

Fig. 9-8, cont'd. For legend see opposite page.

CLINICAL-PATHOLOGIC STUDIES

The following discussion details my experience with cases of meningioma primary in the orbit. The first section discusses primary orbital meningiomas in children and juveniles. In the second section primary meningiomas involving the optic canal region are briefly described. Ordinarily these would have been included in the discussion of orbital tumors, but I have chosen to discuss them separately because I have not had experience with them in the young age group. In the third section selected cases of primary meningioma in the orbit of adults that seemed particularly instructive are described. The first section, concerned with primary meningiomas of the orbit in the young-age group, is by far the most important part of this contribution.

Primary orbital meningiomas in children and juveniles

Case 1. An 11-year-old white boy was blind in the right eye. The optic disc was pale and swollen. Glioma of the optic nerve was suspected. There was no ophthalmoplegia or proptosis. Enucleation was advised and rejected. Visual acuity in the left eye 17 years later was 20/100. The temporal field was lost. The right eye was enucleated. Meningioma was found (Fig. 9-9); there was infiltration of nerve and choroid. A transcranial operation revealed extension of tumor to the chiasmal region. It was partially removed. The patient was blind in one year.

A

B

C

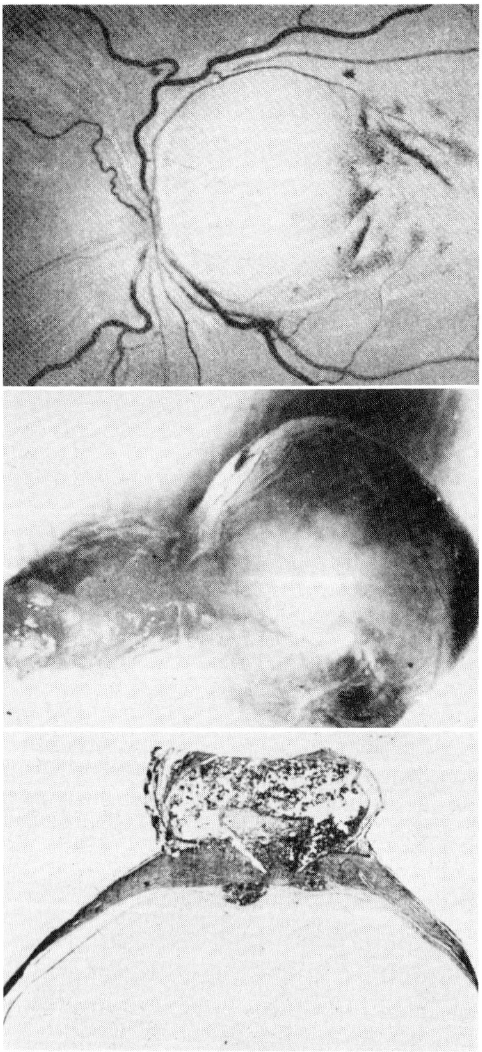

Fig. 9-9. Patient 1. **A,** Appearance of optic nerve head was essentially unchanged after 17 years. I have not observed pigmentation at outer edge of swollen disc extending temporally when glioma has involved optic disc. I do not think this observation is significant, but it is of interest. **B,** Enucleation. Grossly, tumor is within dura. **C,** Invasion of choroid by meningioma.

COMMENT. Slow growth is frequently a feature of meningioma. In this boy it took 17 years for the chiasm to be affected. It is impossible to know whether enucleation and resection of nerve and tumor would have been sufficient treatment. It seems to me that this boy was left completely unprotected and that, in retrospect, even radical surgery such as early exenteration of the orbit was justifiable. In older persons with meningiomas involving the orbit by extension there are sometimes substantial reasons for avoiding almost any type of surgery, as I have learned from sad experience. In some such individuals removal of tumor plus decompression of the orbit is the best that can be done. In the young age group, relying on slow growth does not seem justifiable.

Case 2. E. S., a white girl, developed swelling of the right lower eyelid and complained of slight blurring of that eye. Within weeks proptosis developed. The optic disc was severely swollen, 5 to 6 diopters. There was no ophthalmoplegia. Vision was normal, and the field was normal except for an enlarged blind spot. There were retinal folds between the disc and macula. The suggested diagnosis was glioma of the optic nerve. Through an orbital approach a meningioma was found to surround the nerve immediately posterior to the eyeball. At transcranial operation the tumor was "peeled" off the nerve. The eye was blind when the patient awakened from the anesthesia.

COMMENT. The relatively short history contrasts with that in case 1. The suggestion of glioma was based on the presence of a café au lait spot. That neurofibromatosis is frequently associated with glioma is generally well known. In this patient the normality of the visual acuity suggested to me that an intraneural tumor was an unlikely possibility. I continue to think the point was well taken, although I have been informed by Dr. Robert Penner that normal vision does not always rule out glioma of the optic nerve.

At the Saturday morning clinic the problem concerned treatment. I suggested that the tumor and optic nerve be excised because, grossly, tumor had not passed through the dura. Two neurosurgeons suggested that the tumor could be peeled off the optic nerve. I questioned whether this could be done but was found to be in error, for it was accomplished without difficulty. As might have been anticipated, the eye was blinded by the procedure. Two ophthalmologists who had extensive experience with orbital tumors suggested that the orbit be exenterated.

This patient is being followed by Drs. Melvin Alper and David Berler, who kindly asked me to see her. I agree with them that it is presently impossible to determine whether the operative therapy was adequate or inadequate. The experience with the patients presented in cases 3 and 4 makes us apprehensive about the future of this patient. Our apprehensions do not relate only to possible progressive posterior extension or local recurrence. The possible later development of central neurofibromatosis is a threat whether or not there is any evidence of neurofibromatosis when the meningioma is discovered.

The patient changed her residence, and four years after the operation she was seen by Dr. Joseph A. C. Wadsworth. The tumor had recurred. There was proptosis with limitation of movement of the eye and severe loss of vision. Exenteration of the orbit was performed with transplant of temporal muscles to the orbit. The lids were left intact. Shortly thereafter through a transcranial approach the meningioma was removed from the anterior third of the optic canal. Dr. Wadsworth has seen the patient recently and all appears well.

Case 3. K. J., an 11-year-old white girl, developed loss of vision of the left eye at the age of 11 years. The eye was proptosed 3.5 mm. Retropulsion provided resistance. Visual acuity was 20/20 OD, 12/200 OS. The optic disc was pale temporally. The field contained a central scotoma. X-ray films and arteriographic studies gave normal findings. Orbital exploration failed to show tumor. After several months the proptosis increased and an orbital procedure was repeated. The optic nerve was resected, and meningioma was proven to involve the optic nerve sheaths. Transcranial exploration failed to show intracranial extension. Approximately three years later the patient was operated on elsewhere for suspected dislocated lumbar disc; a plexiform neuroma involving the sacral plexus was partially removed. Thereafter, the patient lost control of the bladder permanently. In another two years she developed deafness of the right ear, ataxia, and falling to the right. There was severe papilledema in the right eye. A right-sided cerebellopontine angle neurinoma was removed at operation. The patient died. At autopsy a second neurinoma was found in the left cerebellopontine angle. Many small meningiomas were attached to the intracranial dura.

COMMENT. An orbital exploration for tumor may be unrewarding even when performed by a skilled operator. The patient never had café au lait spots, nor were there other findings that might have suggested neurofibromatosis.

I wish to emphasize the fact that the first sign of trouble in this patient was the development of an orbital meningioma. The evidence for neurofibromatosis developed subsequently.

It would be impossible to provide two case histories more similar than this one and case 4.

Case 4. B. B., a white girl, had a 5-mm proptosis of the right eye at the age of 4 years. Visual acuity was 20/200 OD. When she was 10 years old the eye was further proptosed, her vision was further reduced, the field contained a central scotoma, and the optic disc had a temporal pallor. The child's mother and a maternal aunt had café au lait spots but the child did not. A transcranial operation revealed a meningioma within the orbit (Figs. 9-10, *A*, and 9-11). The removal was thought to be complete. Following the procedure the eye was blind. Relatively soon afterward, the proptosis, which had lessened, again increased. An orbital operation revealed that the menigioma had recurred within the orbit and had extensively involved the orbital tissues, including the muscles.

Because of the extensive infiltration, Dr. Robert Schimek advised orbital exenteration and forwarded slides to our laboratory. We agreed that orbital exenteration was advisable because of the infiltrative features and suggested that a mesh or plate first be inserted over the operative defect in the orbital roof.

The patient was transferred to Dr. Edgar Housepian, who first removed the recurrence at the apex of the orbit and performed a moderate dural resection. Later, tantalum mesh was inserted over the defect in the orbital roof. Then the orbit was exenterated. Subsequently it became obvious that the right temporalis muscle was infiltrated, and this occasioned several operative procedures. During the same year the patient developed a small lesion on her lip. It was removed and found to be a neurofibroma. Soon thereafter palpable nodules developed on her trunk and scalp. Then, months later, she developed headache, tinnitus, and hearing loss. Technical examinations showed evidence of tumor formation in both cerebellopontine angles. A schwannoma was removed from each angle in successive operations (Fig. 9-10, *B*).

A communication from Dr. Housepian follows: "It is of interest that in my small experience, two of four patients with primary intraorbital meningiomas were children and both of them manifested neurofibromatosis in their period of observation. Further questioning revealed a history of multiple skin lesions in a maternal aunt in Barbara's case. Needless to say, I am concerned about the development of associated tumors of the central nervous system in the future."

COMMENT. Here again is a sequence of delay in diagnosis and of primary orbital meningioma followed by central neurofibromatosis in which identical cerebellopontine-angle tumors developed. In this case as in case 3 there was absence of early evidence of neurofibromatosis.

Case 5. D. R., a 7-year-old white girl, was found to have normal visual acuity OD and 1/200 OS. There was a history of extremely defective vision in the left eye in a paternal uncle and great uncle. The left optic disc was pale temporally. When the patient was 10 years old there appeared to be fibrous tissue protruding from the physiologic cup and an inferior retinal vein was dilated. It was suggested that an angioma might be involving the nervehead. X-ray films were read as normal. In a further 3 years the eye was blind and there was 2 mm of proptosis and slight ophthalmoplegia. X-ray films then showed an increased density of bone in the region of the optic canal. A transcranial operation revealed meningioma in the orbit. The tumor recurred. In subsequent extensive operative procedures the orbit was exenterated and bones of the orbit and left sphenoid ridge were resected (Fig. 9-12).

COMMENT. It is obvious in retrospect that treatment was unduly delayed. I regret having been party to the delay. Would this child have escaped severe extension of the tumor if an orbital exenteration had been undertaken early?

It seems established that in this case invasion of bone became a feature. Nontumorous hyperostosis may develop, notably in the skull, when there is an underlying meningioma. In other instances there may be erosion of bone as a result of pressure. Also, meningiomas may develop within bone, as in this case. How frequently this occurs I do not know.

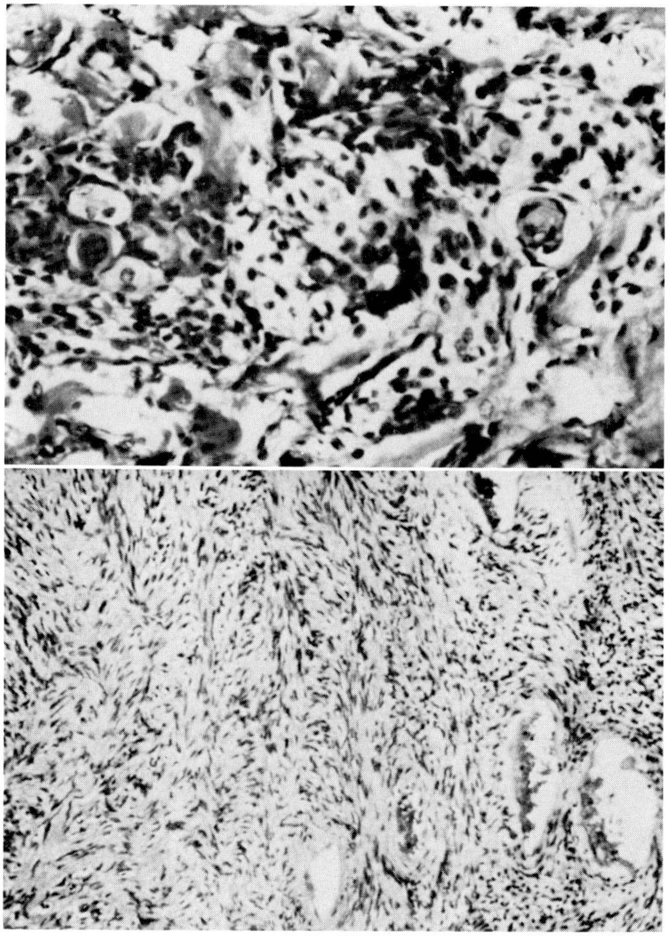

A

B

Fig. 9-10. Patient 4. **A,** Meningioma taken from the orbit. **B,** Schwannoma taken from cerebellopontine angle.

A

B

C

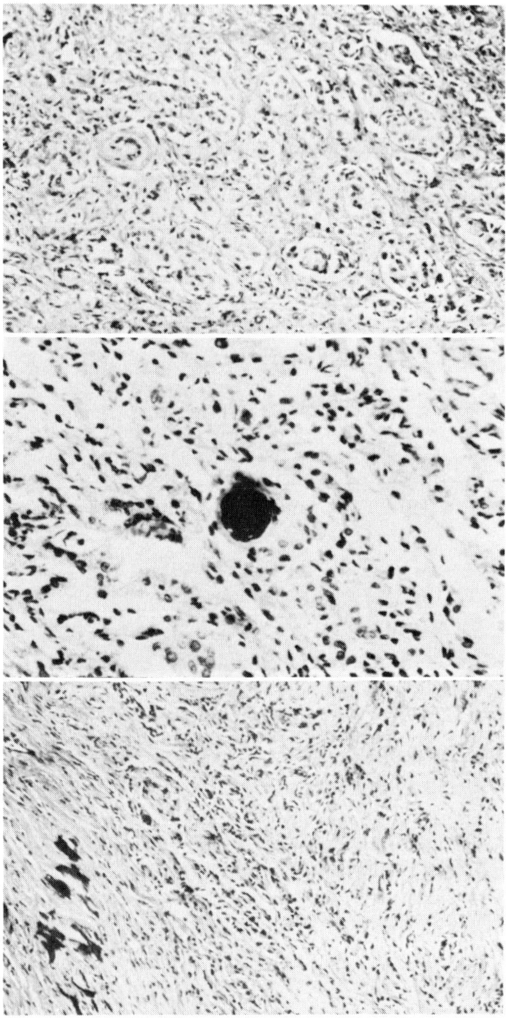

Fig. 9-11. Patient 4. **A,** Moderate magnification of tumor within orbit. Cells are arranged in small and larger groups permeating interstitial tissues of orbit. **B,** Psammoma body believed to result from degeneration of cell nests as seen in **A.** In some areas that appear to be artifacts, red blood cells could be identified, so that these are new formed sinusoid vessels similar to veins but without elastic or muscle tissue. Such an angioma is angioblastic. **C,** Diffuse growth of tumor cells along preformed structures. In lower left corner muscles can be seen to be involved.

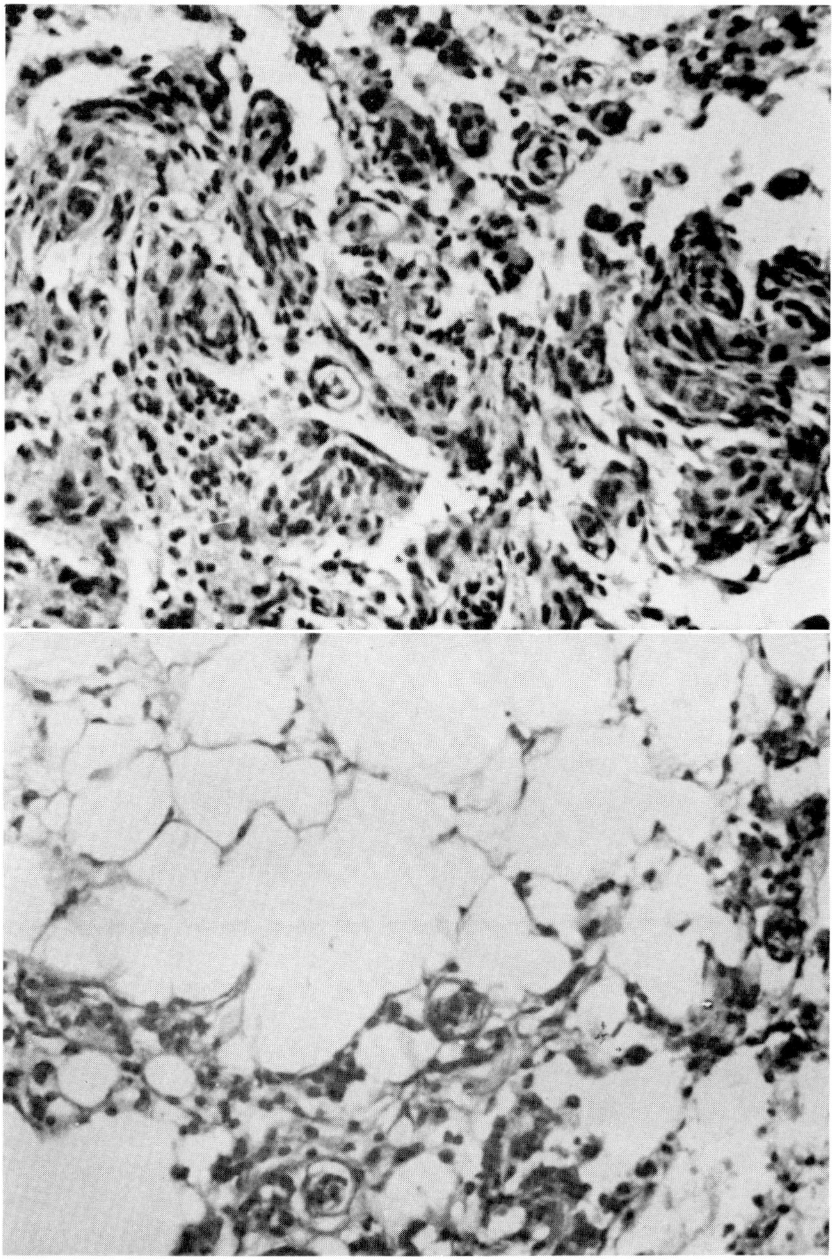

A

B

Fig. 9-12. Patient 5. **A,** Quite cellular tumor showing elongated and circular nuclei. Clefts are artificial and not due to formation of blood vessels. **B,** Tumor infiltrated fat tissue within orbit.

Case 6. B. C., a 6½-year-old white girl, had an intermittent inturning of the left eye following a bout of flu. Two years later she complained of defective vision in the right eye. Visual acuity was 20/200 OD. Ophthalmoscopic examination revealed that the right optic nerve was atrophic. Technical procedures gave normal findings. When the patient was seen at the Johns Hopkins Hospital, the right eye was blind. Transcranial exploratory operation was advised. Several months later this was undertaken

A

B

C

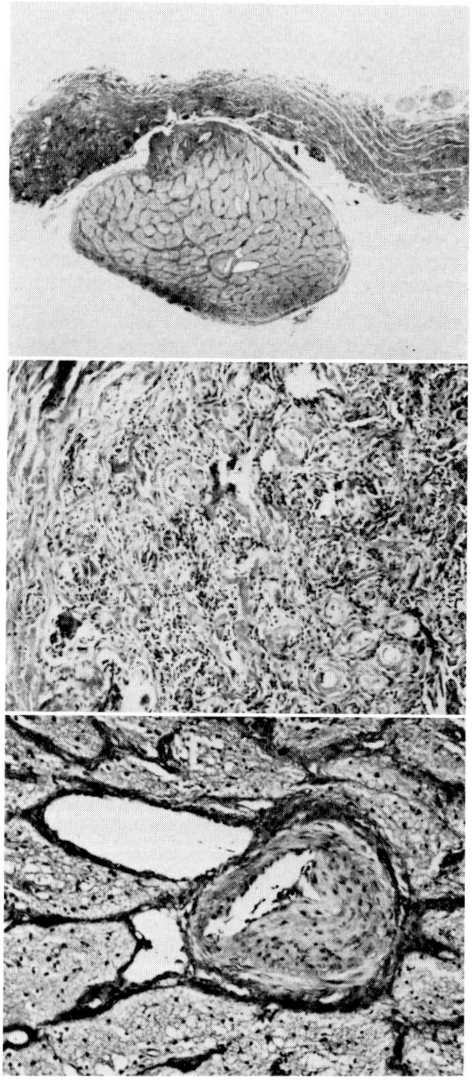

Fig. 9-13. Patient 6. **A,** Optic nerve in cross section. Tumor is in upper left area. Dura is infiltrated. Entire nerve from within orbit and much of it within cranium was serially sectioned and there was no other evidence of tumor. **B,** Tumor at greater magnification. **C,** Presence of central retinal artery indicates that tumor was situated not far posterior to eyeball. What has accounted for the endothelial proliferation within the artery in a child is difficult to explain. Would interference with the blood-carrying capacity of the artery explain the endothelial proliferation?

elsewhere. The operating neurosurgeon was unable to confirm the presence of a tumor but resected the optic nerve from the posterior aspect of the eyeball to a safe distance from the chiasm. At the Armed Forces Institute of Pathology a small meningiothelial tumor was found. The tumor was situated near the eye, because the central retinal artery was included in the slide showing the tumor. In other areas serial sections failed to show tumor (Fig. 9-13).

COMMENT. This case is truly unusual. Two features are decidedly remarkable. The tumor is so small that it is difficult to equate its size with total blindness of the affected eye. The other unusual feature is the appearance of the central retinal artery considering the age of the patient. Probably the endothelial proliferation was dependent upon reduced blood flow over a considerable period of time. Possibly the tumor, although small, in some way strangulated the central retinal artery outside the nerve.

The case that follows cannot be considered closed because it was recorded immediately after having observed Dr. Charles Iliff do an exenteration of the orbit. Retrospective comment stated bluntly may have some merit.

Case 7. A white girl, age 9 years, complained of slight blurring of vision in the right eye, although visual acuity was recorded as normal at that time. Within two years the eye was blind except for perception of light. I do not know the amount of proptosis or other features present at that time. X-ray films and a right carotid arteriogram were taken and according to report were unrevealing. A right frontal craniotomy was performed and a biopsy was taken from a tumor mass at the posterior aspect of the orbit; it was thought the tumor had originated at the anterior opening of the optic canal. It was said that the defect in the orbital roof was covered with a piece of bone. No effort was made to remove all the tumor. Subsequently the eye was enucleated and the tumor was said to have been removed piecemeal; it was thought that the tumor had been completely removed. An artificial eye was inserted. Subsequently it protruded forward. Technical studies were repeated and again were unrevealing.

The patient was then seen by Dr. Iliff, who found a palpable mass within the outer orbit. X-ray films showed what was evaluated as bony thickening. A biopsy seemed in order. Through unavoidable circumstances it was performed elsewhere, and the report was "no tumor."

After the greater part of a year had passed it became obvious that there was a mass that was growing in size, and the patient returned. A biopsy made through the lower eyelid confirmed the recurrence of meningioma. X-ray films including tomograms, failed to show disruption of the orbital roof or implant of bone. The orbit was exenterated without undue difficulty. A defect in the orbital roof was observed; the defect was small, not more than 0.5 cm in breadth and 1 cm in length. Two specimens of bone were removed for study. The area of the bony defect was cauterized.

Pathologic studies showed the meningioma to be extensive. It extended to the apex of the orbit and in places infiltrated the periosteum. There was evidence of cauterization having been performed over the area of the orbital roof defect and at the apex of the orbit.

After the exenteration had been done it was explained to the child's parents that it was impossible to state that there would not be a recurrence. Only passage of time will determine this.

COMMENT. Whether or not a transcranial operation was indicated as a first procedure in this case is debatable. I would favor such an approach but grant freely that an orbital approach may have had equal merit. With the transcranial approach a vigorous effort could well have been made to remove the tumor, and this requires extensive removal of orbital roof, not a small one. Following such a procedure either a piece of mesh or a plate should be placed over the orbital roof defect. We have had the unfortunate experience of prolapse of frontal lobe tissue through such a defect when exenteration was performed subsequent to transcranial operation in which the orbital roof was partially removed. Then when the ophthalmic surgeon who enucleated the eye could not remove the tumor other than bit by bit, orbital exenteration was indicated.

Addendum. For additional information concerning orbital meningiomas in the young age group I contacted two useful sources of information, Dr. Algernon Reese's book[6] and Dr. Lorenz Zimmerman.

From the first source two cases are selected.

Case A. A boy was said to have had tuberculous meningitis. His left eye was blind and slightly proptosed. The optic nerve was pale and the disc was elevated. Nodules on the skin were known to be neurofibromas. The clinical diagnosis was glioma of the optic nerve. Through an orbital approach it was found that there was a meningioma involving the optic nerve sheaths. The observation made at the time of operation was unusual: tumor oozed from the optic nerve sheaths.

Case B. A 6-year-old girl was found at school to have a blind left eye. Visual acuity was 20/70 OD. A white mass, partially cystic, was seen to obscure the optic disc of the blind left eye. In the right fundus nasal to the nervehead there was a small, slightly elevated, white intraretinal mass. Through a Krönlein approach the left eyeball with the orbital optic nerve was removed. The pathologic diagnosis was neurofibromatosis involving the ciliary nerves and primary meningioma of the optic nerve sheaths.

From Dr. Zimmerman I received much help as regards primary orbital meningiomas in the group of cases under consideration. The first of his five cases is most interesting in that it exemplifies meningioma of the orbit having preceded evidence of neurofibromatosis involving the central nervous system, as in cases 3 and 4. Absence of follow-up information on his other cases is regrettable.

AFIP Acc. No. 94594. Dr. Zimmerman's note on this first case is as follows: "This was the case of a girl who was 8-years-old when her right eye was removed in 1943 because of a suspected intraocular tumor. There was no intraocular tumor, however, but a totally detached retina and changes that I believe are the result of old central retinal vein occlusion. The iris shows advanced rubeosis, ectropion uveae, and peripheral anterior synechiae. Present in the arachnoid around the optic nerve, observed both in cross sections and longitudinal section of the stump of the optic nerve attached to the globe, there is a psammomatous type of meningioma. The patient subsequently developed evidence of neurofibromatosis and is said to have died at age 30 as a result of cystitis and pyelitis 'presumably secondary to a neurofibroma of the spinal cord.' Previous to her death she had a craniotomy for cerebellopontine angle meningioma. Unfortunately, we have not been able to obtain sections from either the brain tumor or the spinal cord tumor. This case would seem to bear out your impression of the poor prognosis of meningioma in childhood and the case is of particular interest because the eye was enucleated before the child was recognized as having either a tumor of the optic nerve, a brain tumor, or neurofibromatosis."

AFIP Acc. No. 1226958. An 8-year-old girl had gradual loss of vision over a 2½-year period. Neurosurgical exploration showed no intracranial tumor, but a meningioma arising from the optic nerve sheaths occupied the posterior orbit.

AFIP Acc. No. 77664. A 14-year-old white boy was found to have a meningothelial tumor invading the orbital tissues. Information on this case is incomplete, but there was no evidence of recurrence for six years.

AFIP Acc. No. 43409. A 19-year-old Negro had a seven-year history of progressive exophthalmos. An exenteration of the orbit was performed. The tumor was a meningothelioma.

AFIP Acc. No. 1269808. An 11-year-old white boy had increasing proptosis for 1½ years. The tumor was found in the upper nasal quadrant of the orbit by a neurosurgeon. There are no follow-up reports.

Summary and conclusions regarding primary orbital meningiomas in youth

1. Evidence has been produced to support the conclusion that meningiomas primary within the orbit in children, while infrequent, cannot properly be considered rare. Possibly such tumors occur more often in children than in adults.

2. Delay in diagnosis characterizes such tumors.

3. Meningioma may be the correct diagnosis when glioma has been suspected. Glioma is automatically suspected when there is any evidence suggesting neurofibromatosis, notably café au lait spots. This accounts for misdiagnosis. This well might be kept in mind by those who consider radiation therapy, without benefit of biopsy or visualization, as indicated when orbital optic nerve glioma appears to be a proper diagnosis.

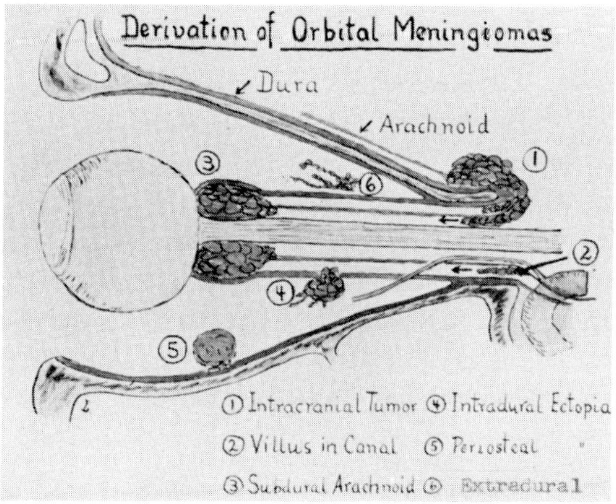

Fig. 9-14. Orbital optic nerve. This diagrammatic representation of the sites of orbital meningiomas does not include attainment of the orbit via the superior orbital fissure. Such tumors are characterized by extraocular palsies. *1,* Meningioma extends to within the orbit via the optic canal. *2,* An arachnoid villus from which a meningioma might obtain origin is shown. *3,* A meningioma has filled the subdural and subarachnoid spaces and surrounds the optic nerve as in case 2. Evidence has been produced to show that meningiomas within the dural sleeve cannot be removed without there being loss of vision in the eye. If growth proceeds in tumors that have become symptomatic, blindness is the ultimate result. *4,* A meningioma has developed from within the dura. It is ectopic. If such a tumor grows outside the dural sheath, its removal might at least temporarily provide improvement in vision. However, if growth proceeds within the sheath, blindness is the result. *5* and *6,* Meningiomas in these positions are ectopic. Vision well might improve when such a tumor is removed, but possible recurrence must be considered. (Courtesy Dr. Richard Lindenberg.)

4. Meningioma primary in the orbit in the young age group has a very bad prognosis as regards retention of vision in the affected eye. These tumors almost always have originated from within the dural sleeve. Possible exceptions to this generalization are considered subsequently.

5. The occurrence of meningiomas in members of the young age group who subsequently developed central neurofibromatosis is remarkable (see cases 3 and 4 and the first case cited by Zimmerman). That meningiomas may develop in individuals who exhibit neurofibromatosis is not new information, but that this has been found in two of seven cases is noteworthy. Minimal evidence of neurofibromatosis when an orbital meningioma exists is reason for apprehension as regards the future (see case 2).

We now come to the problems that face the surgeon when a meningioma is present in the orbit of a child. Fig. 9-14 is a diagramatic representation of the various sites of orbital meningiomas.

6. It would be generally agreed that in the young age group symptomatic orbital meningiomas require surgical treatment. How extensive should this be?

It seems obvious from what has been said and from what is shown in Fig. 9-14 that total loss of vision in the affected eye rarely can be avoided. Meningiomas occasionally develop outside the dural sleeve, as recently observed by Dr. Thomas Acers, but this is the exception not the rule.* I believe apical orbital tumors are an indication for a transcranial approach, but many prefer an orbital approach when no abnormality of the optic canal is seen in tomograms, and admittedly they may be right. Certainly it seems reasonable that if loss of vision in the affected eye is considered unavoidable, what remains for the surgeon as an objective is to eliminate, in so far as possible, recurrence and spread. This means that in many cases orbital extenteration is indicated by the time the operation is performed. If the transcranial approach has been chosen, an effort should be made to remove the tumor in toto. A plate or mesh should be placed over the defect in the orbital roof. Depending on what has been found during the transcranial procedure, it may have become clear that orbital exenteration is also indicated. If so, it can be performed after ten days or two weeks. When the orbit is exenterated, there is often little or nothing gained in leaving the eye in situ and sometimes much to be gained by removing it; it may be necessary to include removal of the eyelids. I have indicated the ultimate in radical surgery for orbital meningioma and, on occasion, this is justifiable. There are cases in which less radical surgery may suffice, such as when the tumor obviously is grossly within the dural sleeve and suf-

---

*EDITOR'S NOTE. Karp and associates (Arch. Ophthalmol. **91**:24, 1974) believe meningiomas arising intraorbitally but *outside* the meningeal sheaths of the optic nerve to be extremely rare, and their origin difficult to document as being unequivocally outside the nerve sheaths (so-called "ectopic" meningiomas). J. S. G.

ficiently far forward that resection of tumor with the nerve may be readily performed. Each case must be treated on the basis of the surgeon's evaluations as how best to prevent recurrence and spread.

Meningiomas primary in region of the optic canal

Meningiomas primary in the region of the optic canal properly may be considered orbital tumors. They are considered separately here only because my experience with them has been restricted to adults.

In 1922 Dandy[9] described a case of bilateral meningioma involving the optic nerves from the posterior aspect of the optic canal and extending into the apex of each orbit. His preoperative reasoning suggested prechiasmal optic nerve involvement, and for this reason as well as the importance of the case, the 1922 paper merits reading or rereading. A girl, age 7 years, had a blind right eye and visual acuity of 8/200 OS when first examinations were made at the Johns Hopkins Hospital. There was bilateral restriction of ocular movements, and the sella was slightly enlarged. The optic discs showed pallor. There was a history of occasional vomiting. At operation a "dural endothelioma" was found encircling the optic nerves at their entrance into the cranial cavity. The tumors were 1½ cm in diameter; they extended to the posterior orbit. Around each tumor was a collection of cystic fluid making up a cyst; Dandy remarked that this was a feature of cerebellopontine tumors. Following removal of the tumors the visual acuity in the left eye improved to 20/200.

Craig and Gogela[10] stated that the Mayo Clinic experience included 17 cases of meningioma primary in the orbit and optic canal. In a 30-year-old woman they observed precisely what had been described by Dandy.

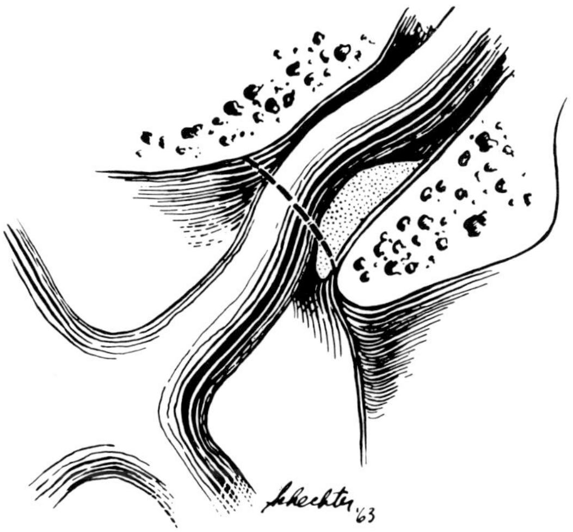

Fig. 9-15. Patient 8. Diagrammatic representation of site of meningioma.

Case 8. A white woman, age 51 years, complained of increasing impairment of vision in her right eye associated with headaches. Visual acuity was 20/200 OD, 20/15 OS. The right optic nerve was excessively pale. All technical examinations were unrewarding. One year after the tumor (Fig. 9-15) had been removed via a transcranial approach the vision of the right eye was perception of hand movements.

Case 9. A middle-aged woman described gradual loss of vision in the left eye. The optic nerve was pale. The field studies showed a central scotoma in the field of the affected eye. The patient disappeared and later committed suicide. At autopsy a small meningioma was found at the intracranial opening of the optic canal.

It seems unquestionable that tumors originating within the canal or its openings have essentially the same unhappy prognosis as a preponderant majority of meningiomas primary in the orbit. Possibly those that develop at the posterior opening of the canal have a slightly better prognosis on removal of the tumor than those situated within the canal.

Primary orbital meningiomas in adults

Primary orbital meningiomas are encountered from time to time in adults. It seems reasonable that an orbital origin is unusual but not rare.

Case 10. A 44-year-old white man complained of loss of vision in his right eye and persistent orbital pain (see Henderson[11]). The initial loss was said to have been rapid but then was gradually progressive for 18 months to hand movement perception. The only abnormal finding was an excessively pale optic disc in the right eye. All technical studies were unrevealing. Transcranial operation revealed adhesions about the right optic nerve. The optic canal was not unroofed. Within a year proptosis and ophthalmoplegia developed and the eye was blind. A repeat transcranial procedure was performed and a meningioma was removed from the apex of the orbit.

COMMENT. This case was previously reported as arachnoiditis providing gradual loss of vision.[12] Undoubtedly the arachnoiditis observed at the time of operation represented a reaction to what was then an occult, flat, meningioma at the apex of the orbit. When the arachnoiditis was discovered at operation, the neurosurgeon questioned the advisability of opening the canal. I was equally responsible for this not being done. The absence of proptosis and ophthalmoplegia seemed to indicate that it was unnecessary. Here again is an example of undue delay in diagnosis. In cases of progressive unilateral loss of vision where a transcranial procedure is indicated, and there are many such cases, it would seem wise to unroof the optic canal if arachnoiditis is suspected or if the intracranial nerve appears to be normal.

Case 11. B. T., a 55-year-old white woman, described progressive loss of vision in both eyes over a period of more than a year. There were no other complaints. Visual acuity was 20/100 OD, 20/50-1 OS. The optic discs were uniformly pale. The visual fields were markedly concentrically narrowed. All technical studies were unrevealing, except that in an arteriogram there was questionable elevation of the right anterior cerebral artery. Exploration of the chiasmal area revealed pronounced thickening of the arachnoid. The tissue was stripped away from the optic nerves, which looked normal. The tissue between the nerves seemed thicker than that about them. A biopsy was obtained but nothing further was done. The pathology report was *meningiosis,* a term some consider interchangeable with *primary diffuse sarcomatosis of the meninges* (Fig. 9-16).

COMMENT. Leaving terminology aside, it has seemed to us that this picture might properly be explained by a diffusely growing meningioma. It does not have the appearance of arachnoiditis. It cannot be stated with complete certainty that what was found at operation accounted for the loss of vision and visual field, but its seems unlikely that opening one or both orbits would have added to our knowledge. However, in recalling our ultimate finding in case 10, such an added undertaking might have produced something of interest.

Case 12. P. H. (409 501), a white woman 51 years old, described gradually increasing proptosis of the left eye over a period of eight years. In addition to a history of having had periods of vascular hypertension for several years, there was some loss of hearing in the left ear, thought to be middle ear deafness. Visual acuity was 20/20 OD,

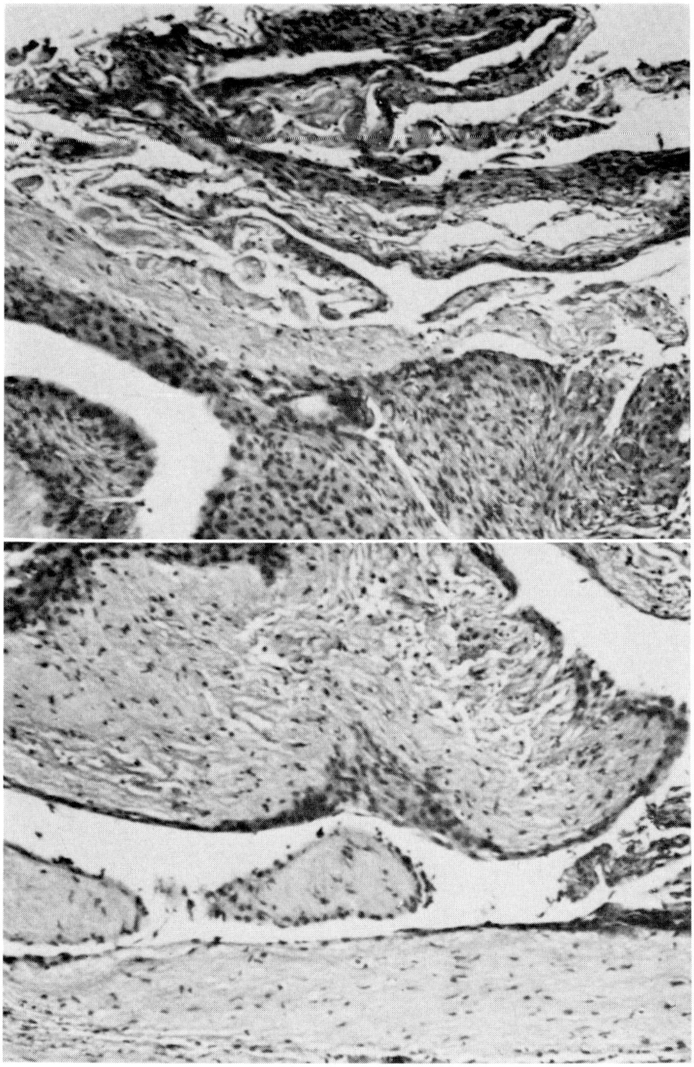

A

B

Fig. 9-16. Patient 11. **A,** Tissue removed from between optic nerves, showing arachnoid villi and cellular proliferation. Diagnosis from surgical pathology laboratory was meningiosis. The term *primary diffuse sarcomatosis of the meninges* has been used to describe such cases. **B,** Arachnoid villi. Evidence for tumor is somewhat less convincing than in **A.**

20/40 OS. There was edema of the disc of approximately 2 diopters. X-ray films and arteriogram were normal. There was a small nodular mass on the right leg shown to be a neurofibroma. A Krönlein operation was performed. The tumor was removed with much of the dura to the posterior aspect of the orbit. The tumor was a meningioma. The surgeon was not satisfied that all tumor tissue had been removed. A transcranial procedure showed no intracranial extension, but a small mass of tumor tissue was removed from the posterior orbit. We have no follow-up information.

COMMENT. This case exemplifies coincident orbital meningioma and neurofibromatosis in an adult. Which affection first provided evidence of its presence is not known. Unfortunately, the visual acuity of the left eye after operation was not recorded.

REFERENCES

1. Hayreh, S. S.: Arteries of the orbit in human being, Br. J. Surg. **50:**938-953, 1963.
2. Hayreh, S. S., and Dass, R.: The ophthalmic artery. I. Origin and intracranial course, Br. J. Ophthalmol. **46:**65-98, 1962a.
3. Hayreh, S. S., and Dass, R.: The ophthalmic artery. II. Intra-orbital course, Br. J. Ophthalmol. **46:**165-185, 1962b.
4. Walshe, F. M. R.: Head injuries as a factor in the etiology of intracranial meningioma, Lancet, **2:**993-996, 1961.
5. Russell, D. S., and Rubinstein, L. J.: Pathology of tumors of the nervous system, Baltimore, 1963, The Williams & Wilkins Company.
6. Reese, A. B.: Tumors of the eye, ed. 2, New York, 1963, Harper & Row, Publishers.
7. Mendiratta, S. S., Rosenblum, J. A., and Strobos, R. L.: Congenital meningioma, Neurology, **17:**914-918, 1967.
8. Ingalls, R. G.: Tumors of the orbit and allied pseudo tumors, Springfield, Ill., 1953, Charles C Thomas, Publisher.
9. Dandy, W. E.: Pre-chiasmal intracranial tumors of the optic nerves, Am. J. Ophthalmol. **5:**169-188, 1922.
10. Craig, W. M., and Gogela, L. J.: Meningioma of the optic foramen as a cause of slowly progressive blindness, J. Neurosurg. **7:**44-48, 1950.
11. Henderson, J. W.: Problem cases in neuro-ophthalmologic diagnosis, Am. J. Ophthalmol. **50:**1087-1097, 1960.
12. Little, H. L., Chambers, J. W., and Walsh, F. B.: Unilateral intracranial optic nerve involvement, Arch. Ophthalmol. **73:**331-337, 1965.

Chapter 10

Clinical approach to disorders of the third, fourth, and sixth cranial nerves

Ronald M. Burde
Joseph S. Karp

In any movement of one eye (duction), all six extraocular muscles play a role. To discuss the independent action of any individual extraocular muscle is strictly a hypothetical convenience,[1] although one that is quite useful clinically. For the most part, available reference texts base their concepts of extraocular muscle function on the writings of Duane,[2-4] who stated that the superior and inferior rectus muscles elevate and depress the eye in abduction, and the inferior and superior oblique muscles are the main elevator and depressor in adduction. Boeder, in 1961,[1] and then Jampel[5-8] have each challenged many of these concepts. The major differences are as follows:

1. The vertical recti are the main elevators and depressors in all positions of gaze (for example, in face of a superior oblique palsy it is still possible to depress the eye in the adducted position). The vertical recti contribute about 30% of the torsional force necessary to maintain the horizontal raphe parallel to the horizon in the primary position.

2. The main action of the obliques is a relative torsional movement that is constant for a given vertical position throughout the horizontal excursion range of the eye for a given strength of stimulation. However, the action of the oblique muscles can still best be isolated in adduction in the up- and downgaze positions as presented in the classic gaze diagram (Fig. 10-1).

Supported in part by grant EY-00016 from the National Eye Institute, Bethesda, Maryland.

3. Clinically, the horizontal recti play no primary role in vertical deviations.

Movements of both eyes together (conjugate movements) are termed *versions*. The accomplishment of a version requires simultaneous contraction of agonist muscles with appropriate inhibition of antagonists (Sherrington's law). The twelve extraocular muscles, six in each eye, have been grouped into six pairs working together in the six cardinal directions of gaze (Table 7). It has been stated that this grouping is a pairing with respect to the action of individual muscles in their fields of maximum action (yoke muscles). In light of our recent knowledge regarding the action of the vertical recti and obliques, the concept of yoke muscles must be modified from physiologic dogma to clinical pragmatism. Yoke muscles must be defined fuctionally as the pair of muscles in a particular field of gaze in which the function of one of the pair is most easily recognized clinically.

The coordinated movements of both eyes follow Hering's law.[9, 10] In all voluntary conjugate movements of the eyes equal and simultaneous innervation flows from the oculogyric centers (as yet theoretical "black boxes") to the muscles concerned with establishing the direction of gaze. This law does

Table 7. Yoke muscles of the eyes

Right eye	*Left eye*
Medial rectus	Lateral rectus
Lateral rectus	Medial rectus
Superior rectus	Inferior oblique
Inferior rectus	Superior oblique
Superior oblique	Inferior rectus
Inferior oblique	Superior rectus

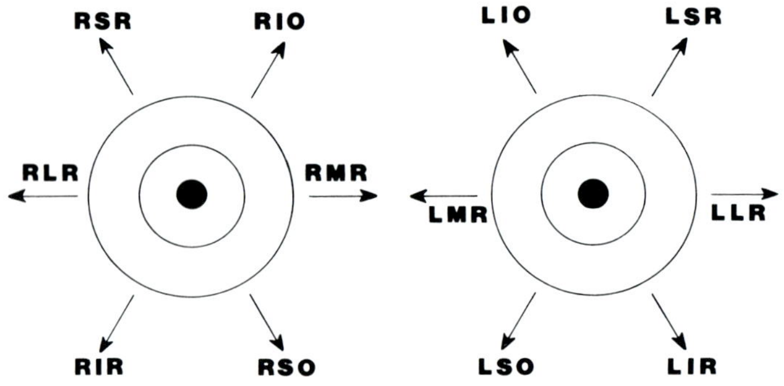

Fig. 10-1. Diagrammatic representation of direction of action of oculorotary muscles of each eye. View is from front. Arrows indicate direction of maximum action of each muscle. Parallel arrows running in same direction represent yoke muscles. (From Scobee, R. G.: The oculorotary muscles, St. Louis, 1952, The C. V. Mosby Co.)

not state that an equal amount of energy is sent to each muscle involved in a particular movement but does imply that the "amount of nervous energy" sent to the entire muscle unit of each eye is such that both eyes move conjugately. Thus, any condition that requires a relatively greater amount of energy to be expended in order to turn one eye in a given direction (for example, an eye with a paretic muscle) will correspondingly cause a greater amount of energy to be sent to the opposite eye, resulting in a larger excursion or deviation (Fig. 10-2). Therefore, a paresis of one of the extraocular muscles will produce a differential deviation depending upon which eye is fixating.

Paralytic strabismus is termed *noncomitant strabismus.* When the uninvolved eye is used for fixation, the usual case, the deviation measured is termed *primary deviation;* when the eye with the paretic muscle is used for fixation, the deviation measured is termed *secondary deviation.* Hering's law

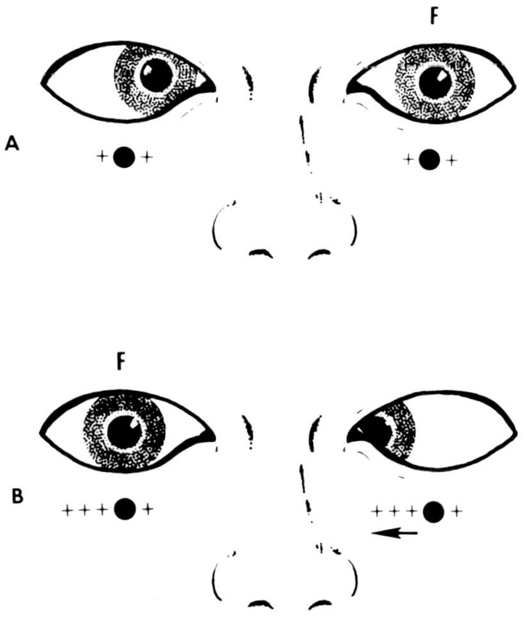

Fig. 10-2. A, Paretic right lateral rectus muscle, primary deviation. Left eye fixing *(F)* in straight-ahead gaze. Equal innervation to all four horizontal rectus muscles. Since right lateral rectus muscle cannot respond normally to input, designated by the "+" signs, right eye will be deviated medially by given amount, *X.* **B.** Paretic right lateral rectus muscle, secondary deviation. Right eye fixing *(F)* in straight-ahead position. Since greater input to the right lateral rectus muscle will be required to maintain right eye in straight-ahead position, greater innervation will be sent to yoke or left medial rectus muscle and result in a greater absolute deviation. (From Burde, R. M.: In Eliasson, S. G., et al., editors: Neurological pathophysiology, New York, 1974, Oxford University Press.)

dictates that secondary deviation is always greater than the primary deviation (Fig. 10-3). The deviation will also increase as the eyes are moved into the field of relative isolated action of the involved muscle or muscles. These changes in deviation with respect to both fixation and position are termed *noncomitancy*. With the passing of time the measured differential deviation becomes much less prominent or even nonexistent (spread of comitance).

Patients with nonparalytic deviations (basic esotropia or exotropia) are said to have a comitant deviation. An occasional neurologic patient may develop a comitant strabismus when a latent deviation, one compensated for by the fusion mechanism, is unmasked by a neurologic insult, such as a blow to the head or an ischemic attack.

Many neurologic deficits can develop insidiously, but the onset of diplopia, reflecting ocular motor dysfunction, is always acute; either the symptom is there or it is not, although it may be intermittent initially. Diplopia is one of the most annoying symptoms a patient can experience. The patient will subconsciously alter his head position to either bring his eyes into a field of single vision, into a position where the nose can act as an occluder, or into a position where the images are so widely apart that one can easily be ignored. Depending upon the age of the patient, a central adjustment may occur wherein one image is obliterated from conscious awareness (suppression).

In diplopia the image of regard falls on disparate retinal elements. When an individual with a normal ocular motor apparatus fixates on a given object

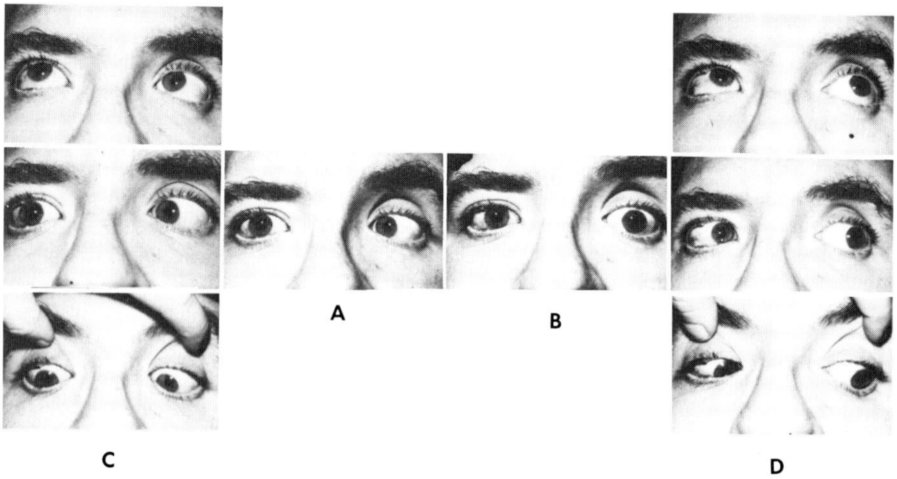

Fig. 10-3. Traumatic right sixth nerve palsy. **A,** Secondary deviation with paretic eye fixing. There is a marked increase in esotropia. **B,** Primary deviation with nonparetic eye fixing. **C** and **D,** Right and left gaze photographs emphasize weakness in field of action of right lateral rectus muscle.

in free space, that object is imaged on the fovea of each eye (Fig. 10-4). Each fovea has the innate property of implying the straight ahead or primary visual direction with respect to the individual (so-called egocentric localization). All other retinal receptors have a given visual direction with respect to the fovea. Those receptors in each eye that have the same visual direction are called corresponding retinal points. Within a given small area around the fovea the stimulation of slightly disparate points leads to the innate sensation of stereopsis.

With manifest deviations the image of regard falls on the fovea of the fixating eye and on nonfoveal points of the deviating eye. The fovea in the deviating eye is suppressed by a central mechanism, and the image of regard is projected in space along the line of visual direction that the stimulated points have with respect to the suppressed fovea. In a convergent strabismus, such as a sixth nerve paresis (Fig. 10-5), the image falls on the fovea of the fixating eye and on the nasal retina of the deviated eye. This image is projected temporally and appears on the same side of the real image as the deviated eye (uncrossed diplopia). Conversely, in divergent strabismus the object of regard is imaged on the temporal retina and projected nasally, appearing on the opposite side of the real object with respect to the deviated eye (crossed diplopia) (Fig. 10-6). If a deviated eye is hypertropic, or higher than the fixating eye, the object will fall on the superior retina and

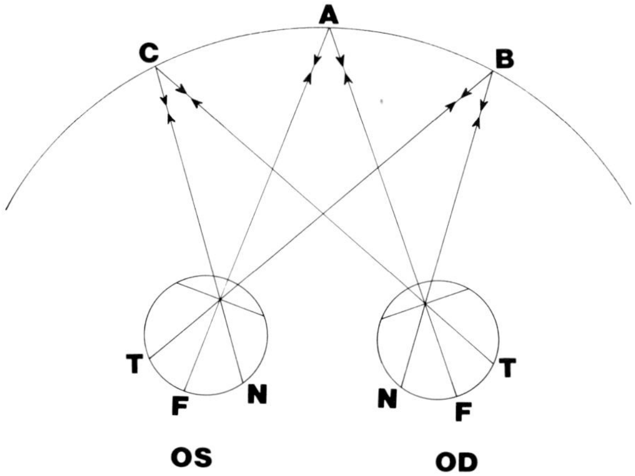

Fig. 10-4. *F*, Fovea; *A*, object in primary gaze; *B*, object in right field; *C*, object in left field; *T*, temporal retinal point; *N*, nasal retinal point. Image from object *A* falls on fovea of each eye and is seen straight ahead. Image from object *B* falls on nasal retina in right eye and temporal retina in left eye, which are corresponding retinal points, and is projected back to *B* in the right gaze field. Image from object *C* acts similarly vice versa. (From Roper-Hall, G., and Burde, R. M.: Clinical analysis of extraocular muscle paralysis. In Moses, R. A., editor: Adler's physiology of the eye, ed. 6, St. Louis, 1975, The C. V. Mosby Co.)

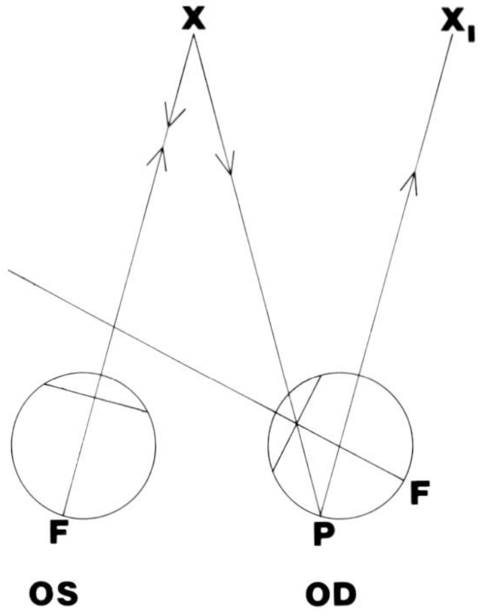

Fig. 10-5. *F,* Fovea; *X,* object; X_1, projected image of *X; P,* peripheral retinal point. Homonymous or uncrossed pathologic diplopia in a right esotropia. Image of *X* falling on fovea of left eye is projected straight ahead. Image of *X* falling on nasal retina of right eye is projected temporally, resulting in diplopic mental image, X_1, of object *X.* (From Roper-Hall, G., and Burde, R. M.: Clinical analysis of extraocular muscle paralysis. In Moses, R. A., editor: Adler's physiology of the eye, ed. 6, St. Louis, 1975, The C. V. Mosby Co.)

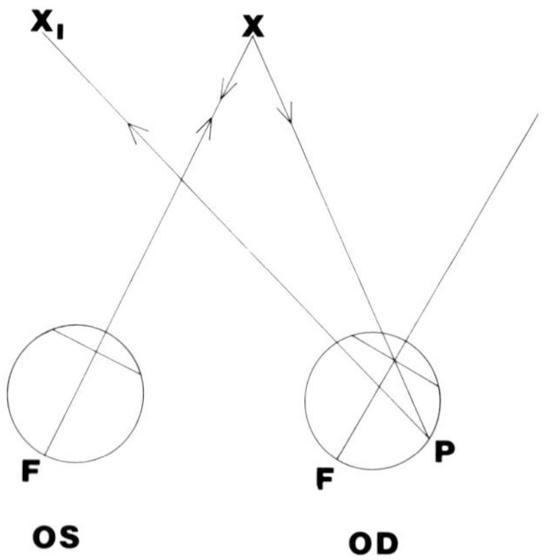

Fig. 10-6. *F,* Fovea; *X,* object; X_1, projected image of *X; P,* peripheral retinal point. Heteronymous or crossed pathologic diplopia in a right exotropia. Image of *X* falling on left fovea is projected straight ahead. Image of *X* falling on temporal retina of the right eye is projected nasally, resulting in X_1. (From Roper-Hall, G., and Burde, R. M.: Clinical analysis of extraocular muscle paralysis. In Moses, R. A., editor: Adler's physiology of the eye, ed. 6, St. Louis, 1975, The C. V. Mosby Co.)

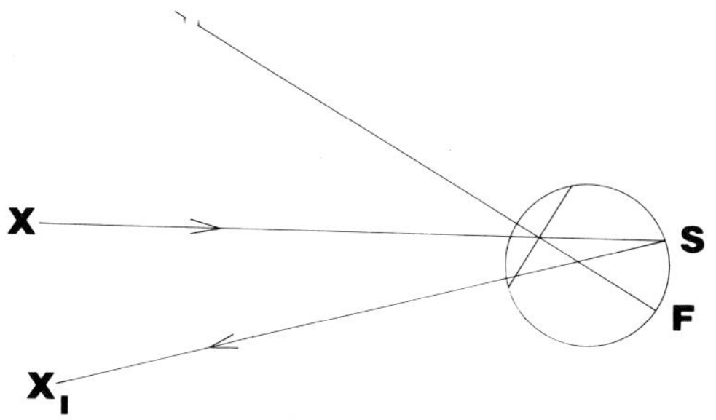

Fig. 10-7. *F,* Fovea; *X,* object in primary gaze; X_I, image of *X* projected below *X; S,* superior retinal point. Vertical diplopia in a right hypertropia. Image from object *X* falling on superior retina in right eye will be projected inferiorly below X, position where left eye (not shown) perceives image of object. (From Roper-Hall, G., and Burde, R. M.: Clinical analysis of extraocular muscle paralysis. In Moses, R. A., editor: Adler's physiology of the eye, ed. 6, St. Louis, 1975, The C. V. Mosby Co.)

Table 8. Limitation of elevation according to age*

Age brackets (years)	*Patients (N = 367)*	*Upward rotation (degrees)*
5-14	41	40.1
15-24	34	37.3
25-34	20	36.0
35-44	24	32.9
45-54	68	30.4
55-64	55	26.5
65-74	66	21.9
75-84	50	16.8
85-94	9	16.1

*From Chamberlain, W.: Am. J. Ophthalmol. **71:**343, 1971.

will be imaged below the real object; the opposite is true for a hypotropic eye (Fig. 10-7).

Under normal conditions the eye can move 45° to either side of, and 60° below and 40° above, the primary postion.[11] The ability to look up becomes increasingly limited with age (Table 8). Although total paralysis of any extraocular muscle is usually diagnosed easily, findings with partial pareses are often subtle, and diagnosis is frequently difficult.

EVALUATION

Evaluation of a patient with extraocular muscle paralysis obviously begins with a detailed history. A complete neuro-ophthalmologic and neurologic examination must be done in order to collect data relating to the company the extraocular paresis keeps, for this will often enable the clinician to specifically localize the site of the pathologic entity. The examiner should note the patient's head posture, since the patient will generally adopt a head position that will obviate the need for his eyes to move into the position of maximum function of the paretic muscle.

Evaluation of the ocular motor status is most accurately accomplished by an objective examination, using an occluder (paddle, finger, etc.) to perform a cover test. A qualitative or quantitative determination of the ocular deviation in seven positions of gaze should be made using an accommodative target both at near and at distance. In a cooperative patient, subjective testing of the ocular motor dysfunction by the use of confrontation diplopia fields may sometimes be the most useful method of isolating paretic muscles.

Guide to isolation of underacting muscles

Using a modification of Cogan's[11] rules for evaluating diplopia, the examiner first occludes one eye. If the diplopia is not relieved, the patient has monocular diplopia, a strictly ocular or perceptive problem. This simple step will often avoid hours of aggravation.

The second step is to place a red filter or a tongue blade with a red-green plastic filter combination before the patient's eyes to permit him to identify the images of the two eyes. In this way the diplopia can be described as horizontal, vertical, or a combination of both. If the diplopia is purely horizontal (the red and green image lie on the same horizontal plane with respect to the horizon) the involved muscle is one of four horizontal recti. If the diplopia is vertical the responsible muscle must be one of the vertical recti or one of the oblique muscles. It must be remembered that the lower image is always related to the higher, or *hypertropic,* eye. If the separation is oblique, then there is both a horizontal and vertical deviation; the horizontal component is ignored at first, for a vertical muscle paresis can dissociate the eyes allowing a latent eso- or exodeviation to become manifest.

Third, determination of the presence of a primary and secondary deviation should be attempted. The patient is instructed to look first at the red image, and using any frame of reference (for example, finger separation) is asked to judge how far the images are apart; then he is told to look at the green image and do the same. Thus he foveally fixates first with one eye, then with the other. The test position in which the deviation was largest is that situation in which the eye with the paretic muscle was used for fixation. If a differential deviation is present the paresis is limited to one eye. A circle may then be placed around each muscle in that eye in the appropriate schematic diagrams. For example, if the deviation is greatest with the right eye fixating, a circle is placed accordingly around either the vertically or horizontally acting muscles (Fig. 10-8).

Fourth, the patient is taken into right and left gaze. If the diplopia is horizontal this will isolate a lateral and medial rectus pair (one muscle from

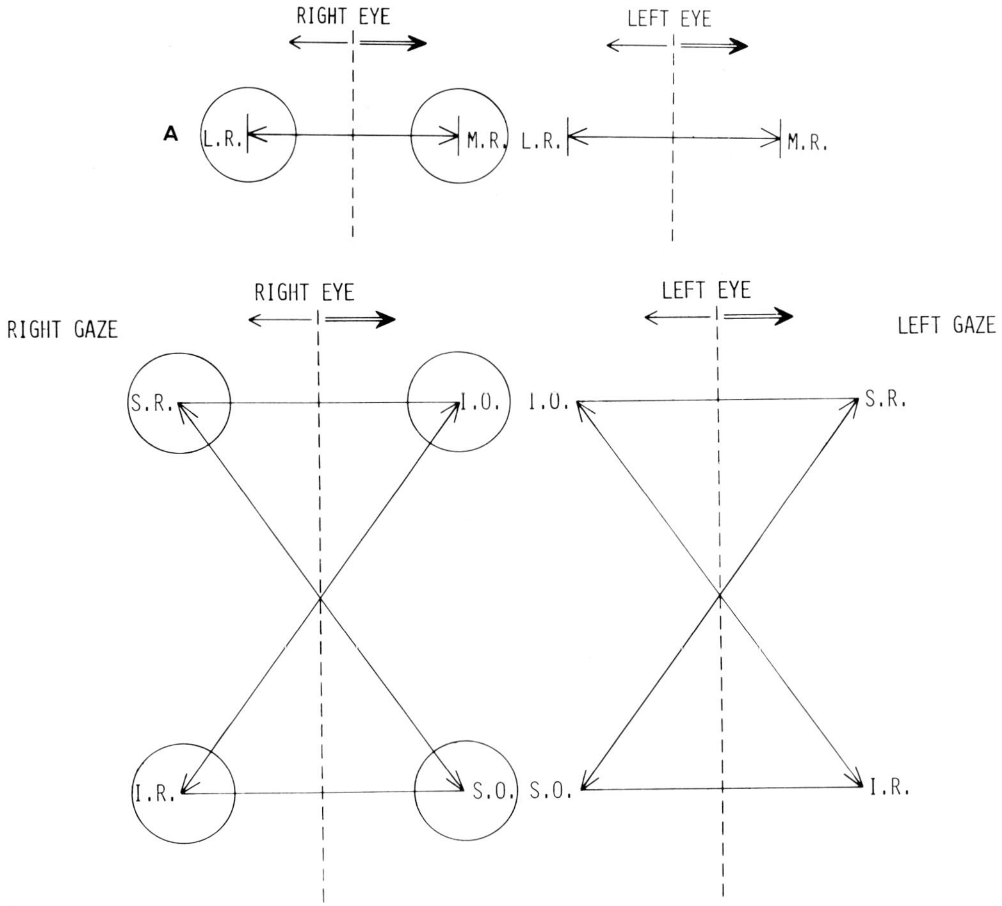

Fig. 10-8. A, Horizontal muscle isolation. *LR,* Lateral rectus; *MR,* medial rectus. **B,** Vertical muscle isolation. *SR,* Superior rectus; *IR,* inferior rectus; *SO,* superior oblique; *IO,* inferior oblique.

each eye). The separation will be greatest in the field of action of the paretic muscle. The diplopia is crossed if the medial rectus is paretic and uncrossed if the lateral rectus is involved. A circle may be placed around the two yoke muscles involved in the gaze positon in which the manifest deviation is greatest. The muscle with two circles around it is the paretic muscle (Fig. 10-9).

Isolation of the offending muscle in a vertical separation is determined by using a modification of the Parks three-step test.[12] First, a red glass is used to determine which eye is hypertropic. By the laws of projection the lower image will always be from the hypertropic eye. If one eye is higher than the other, either a weakness of the depressors on the side that is higher or a weakness of the elevators on the side is lower must be present. If, for example, the patient has a right hypertropia (when the red filter is over the

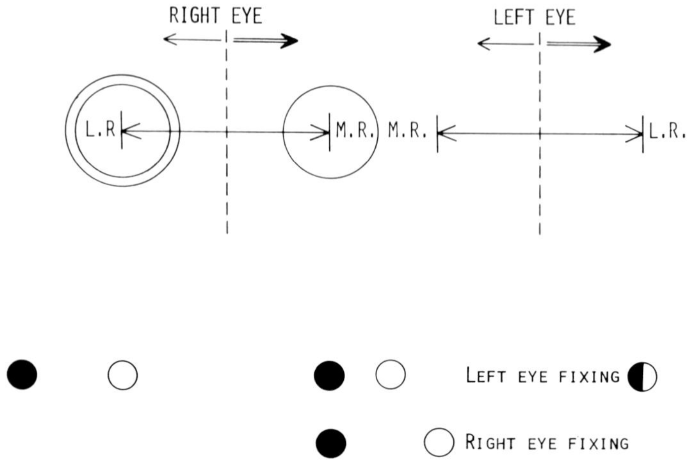

Fig. 10-9

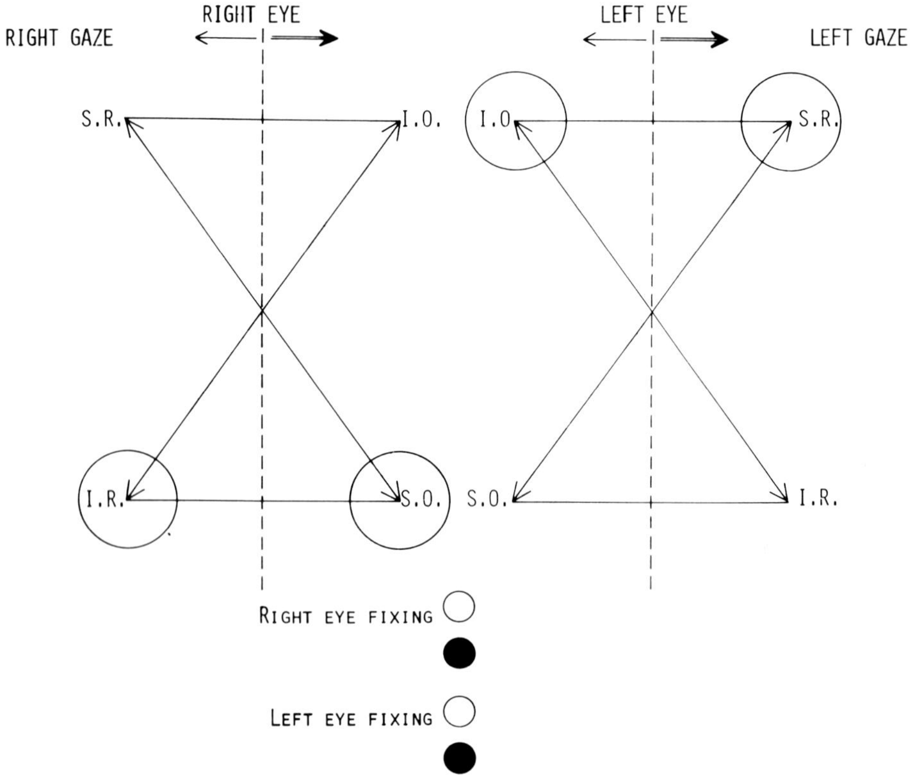

Fig. 10-10

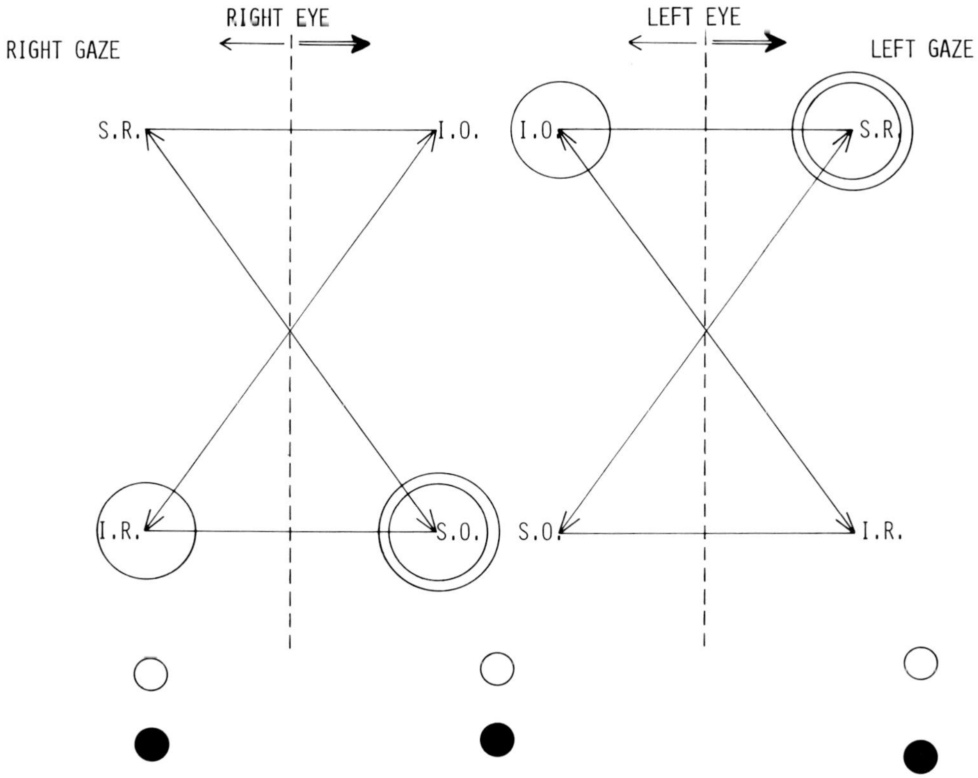

Fig. 10-11

right eye, the red image is lower), a circle is placed around the depressors of the right eye and the elevators of the left eye (Fig. 10-10).

The patient's eyes are then placed in right and left gaze, and the relative deviation is ascertained. If for example, the deviation is greatest in left gaze, a circle is put around the two muscles whose relative action is isolated in left gaze (Fig. 10-11). The degree of separation of images is then determined in up and down gaze to the left, and usually a differential deviation can be found. If the separation is greatest in down gaze the muscle that has its field of action in down gaze is circled; if it is greatest in up gaze the muscle with its field of action in up gaze is circled (Fig. 10-12). The muscle with three circles around it is the offending muscle.

The differential diagnosis between a superior rectus muscle palsy in one eye and a superior oblique muscle palsy in the other is often difficult.[12] The differential primary and secondary deviation, as well as the difference in deviation in up and down gaze, may be negligible secondary to changes involving the agonists, the yoke muscles, and their antagonists (for example, inhibitional palsy of the contralateral antagonist). The offending muscle may

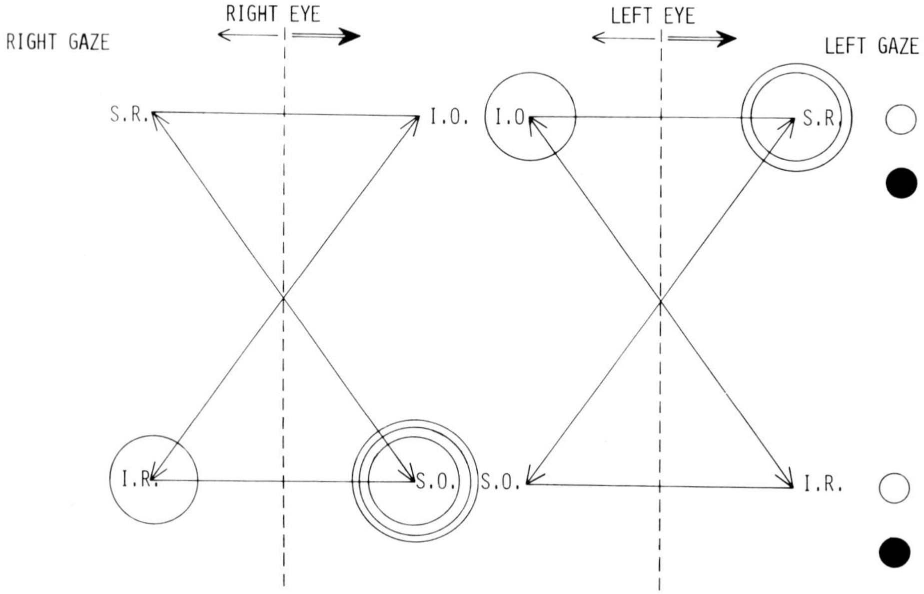

Fig. 10-12

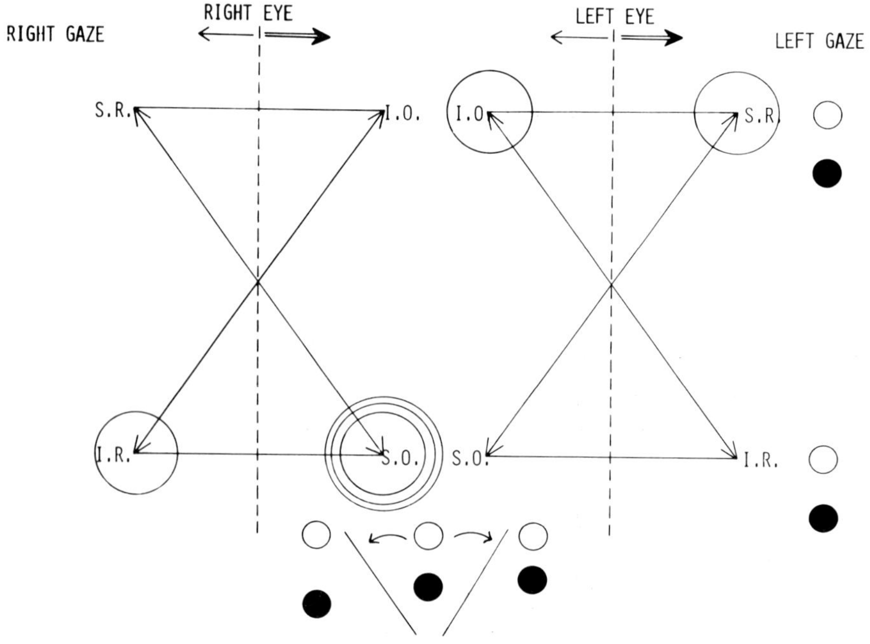

Fig. 10-13

then be isolated using the Bielschowsky head-tilt test. When the head is tilted to one side or the other there is an incycloduction of the eye ipsilateral to the head tilt and an excycloduction of the eye contralateral to the tilt. The neuronal arc originates in the vestibular apparatus. The intorters are the superior oblique and superior rectus muscles whose vertical actions balance each other when they act as intorting agonists. The inferior oblique muscle and inferior rectus muscle are the extorters, and their vertical actions likewise balance each other when acting as agonists. When the head is tilted toward the involved side in a superior oblique palsy, the superior rectus muscle will act unopposed and the vertical deviation will increase. When the head is tilted toward the opposite shoulder, the normal posture assumed by a patient with a superior oblique palsy, the involved eye will make a movement of excycloduction out of the field of the superior oblique muscle, and the deviation will decrease. If the superior rectus is the involved muscle, the head tilt will exaggerate the deviation when the head is tilted toward the involved side and the depressing action of the superior oblique on that side is unopposed. If the patient has a right hypertropia greatest in left gaze, a circle can be placed around the right superior oblique muscle if the vertical deviation is increased with head tilt to the right or around the left superior rectus muscle if the deviation is greatest with tilt to the left (Fig. 10-13).

Using the simple steps outlined—identifying the primary and secondary deviation, the hypertropic eye in vertical deviations, the increase in deviation first in right and left gaze, then in up and down lateral gaze, with the Bielschowsky head-tilt test when needed—isolation of a paretic muscle should become easier. If a vertical deviation is present that cannot be localized to a given muscle or muscles as outlined, the possibility of a skew deviation should be entertained, implying posterior fossa disease. Likewise, myasthenia gravis, which can on occasion masquerade as an isolated extraocular muscle palsy, can be ruled out by the use of a Tensilon or Prostigmin test.

Finally, before a sophisticated diagnostic investigation is undertaken, forced-duction testing should be performed. Inadequate anesthesia often makes this test difficult to perform and evaluate due to patient discomfort. After topical anesthesia, and before testing, a pledget of cotton soaked in 5% or 10% cocaine solution should be placed for 10 minutes on the conjunctiva over the insertion of the muscle to be grasped. The patient is then asked to look in the direction of gaze limitation; the insertion of the antagonist muscle is grasped, and an attempt is made to move the eye passively in the desired direction. Undue resistance to movement of the globe indicates an *intrinsic* pathologic condition in the orbit.

Another subjective but quantitative test for analyzing the degree and progression of extraocular muscle palsies is the plotting of diplopia fields with a Hess or Lees screen. In this test the patient is forced to fixate with one eye by the use of appropriate red and green filters while matching a measured set of points involving the nine positions of gaze with his other eye. The test is then repeated using the opposite eye to fixate. Interpretation of the chart requires looking for (1) the smallest field of action, (2) the largest deficit in that field of action, and (3) fields of overaction.

Since repeatable quantitation of a partial paresis is necessary to determine the progression of a given deficit, Feibel and Roper-Hall[13] have adapted the binocular single vision test to the almost universally available bowl perimeters. In this test the patient is seated at the perimeter with both eyes open, the head erect and centered, the chin and head rest adjusted so that the fixaion target is centered at eye level. The movable test target light is turned on (III_4e spot on the Goldmann and the 0,25 circle at Oo on the Tübinger). The patient is instructed to follow the light with his eyes. The test target is placed within the field of binocular single vision in order to make use of the patient's fusional amplitudes. The light is moved radially outward in all directions, and the patient is asked to report the onset of diplopia. The test quantitatively produces an outline of the area of binocular single vision (Fig. 10-14), can be performed in less than ten minutes, and serves as a quantitative determination of progression or regression of a given defect (Fig. 10-15).

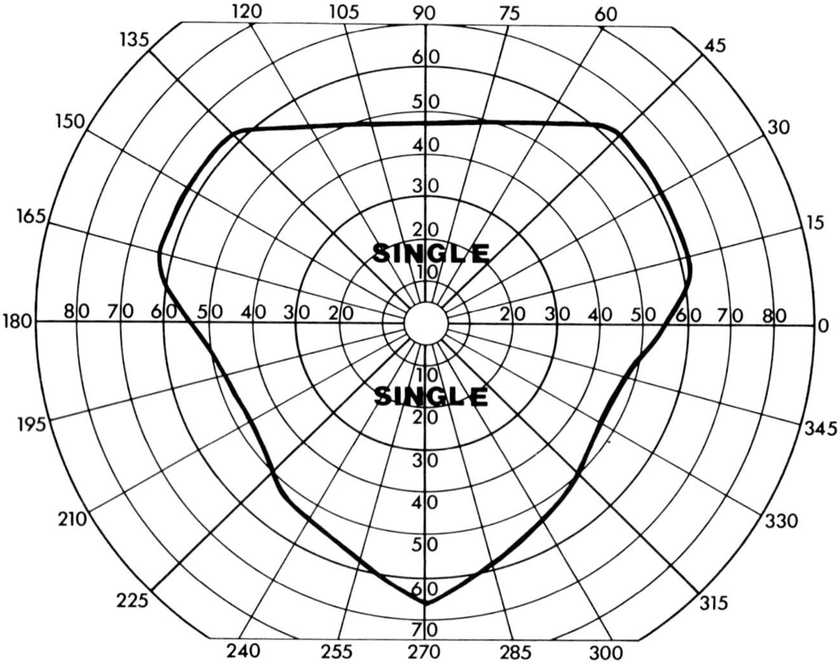

Fig. 10-14. Normal field of binocular single vision as demonstrated on Goldmann perimeter. (After technique of Feibel and Roper-Hall.)

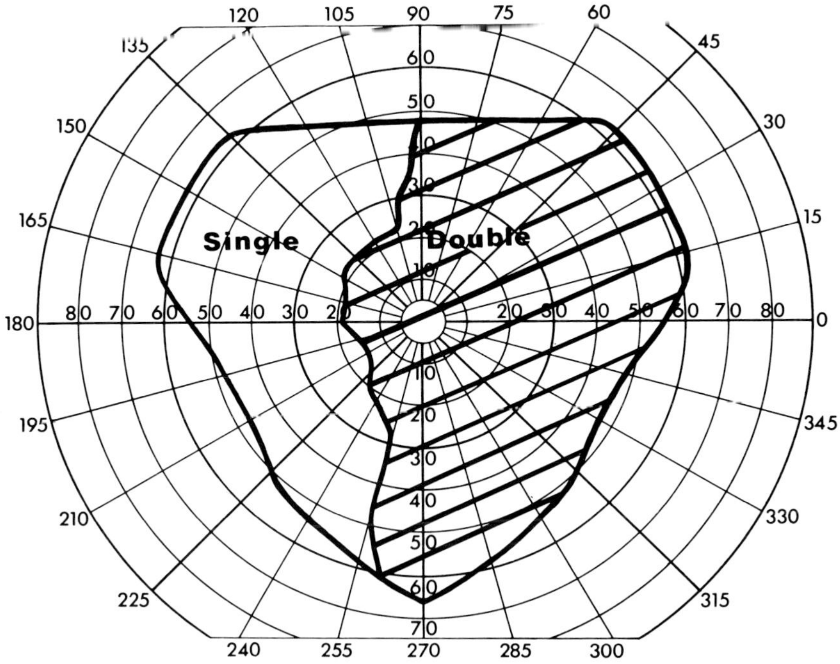

Fig. 10-15. Field of binocular single vision demonstrating progressive sixth nerve palsy. Lined section indicates area of double vision. (After Feibel and Roper-Hall.)

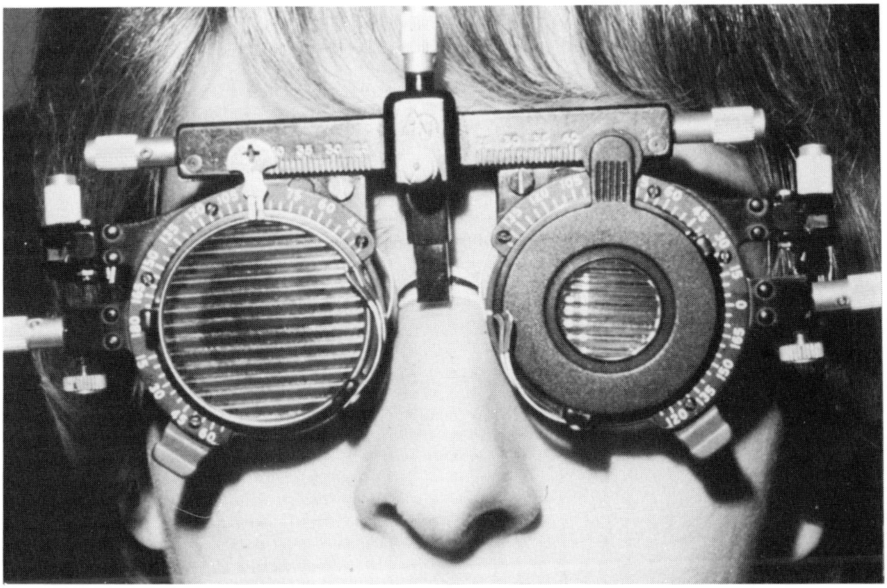

Fig. 10-16. Patient has bilateral fourth nerve palsies. Anterior cells have been turned by patient to set linear images perpendicular to horizon.

Torsional diplopia or disparity is best measured by using double maddox rods.[14] The rods are placed in the front cells of a trial frame with the bars of the rod parallel to the horizon on the 0°-180° axis along with the appropriate spherical distance correction in place in the back cell. The patient's head is placed in the erect position, and he is asked to look at a distant light spot. He is instructed to turn the cell control lever until the two linear images produced by the maddox rod are straight up and down (perpendicular to the horizon) (Fig. 10-16). The induced torsion secondary to the paresis is read in degrees from the cylinder axis marker on the trial frame. This test is invaluable in following the progression in a patient with bilateral superior oblique palsies (usually secondary to trauma).

PATHOLOGY

Oculomotor nerve

It is often more difficult to evaluate the oculomotor nerve than the trochlear or abducens nerve, because the third nerve innervates five extraocular muscles (including the levator) and the pupil. Complete paralysis of the third nerve leaves the pupil unreactive to direct or consensual light and the globe in an abducted and depressed position. If fourth nerve function is preserved, intorsion will result on attempted depression of the globe.

Like all cranial nerves the third nerve can be injured anywhere along its course from the brain stem to the muscles it innervates. Several series have been collected dealing with the pathology of the third nerve. Table 9 is a representative sample.[15-18] The four series represented are not exactly comparable. Rucker[15, 16] compiled all cases in a neurology practice with or without other neurologic signs but excluding palsies of the fourth and sixth nerves, whereas the patients collected by Green and co-workers[17] were from an ophthalmology hospital in an urban setting and had no other neurologic

Table 9. Comparison of causes of third nerve palsy

	Rucker[15] (*335 cases*)		*Rucker*[16] (*274 cases*)		*Green*[17] (*130 cases*)		*Goldstein*[18] (*61 cases*)	
	Number	*Percent*	*Number*	*Percent*	*Number*	*Percent*	*Number*	*Percent*
Aneurysm	64	19	50	18	38	30	11	18
Vascular disease (diabetes mellitus)	63	19	47	17	25	19	28	47
Trauma	51	15	34	13	14	11	5	8
Syphilis	6	2	0	0	12	9	0	0
Neoplasm	35	10.4	50	18	5	4	6	10
Undetermined	95	28	55	20	33	23	7	11
Miscellaneous	21	6	38	12	5	4	4	6

signs. The major concern in the series of Goldstein and Cogan[18] was pupillary sparing in third nerve palsies. Surprisingly, however, there are considerable similarities in the types of pathologic conditions recorded. In all series there is a high percentage of patients in whom the diagnosis was not determined even though sophisticated laboratory procedures were utilized. Likewise, posterior communicating and infraclinoid internal carotid aneurysms were also commonly encountered. These studies confirmed the general opinion that the pupil is almost always involved in third nerve palsies caused by aneurysms. Conversely, in all four series a few patients had documented aneurysms and normal pupillary reaction; thus normal pupils do not absolutely rule out this diagnosis.

In contrast, well over half of the patients with vascular causes of oculomotor palsy, including diabetes, had pupillary sparing. Dreyfus and associates[19] showed that the palsy resulted from an infarct of the nerve substance. It is hypothesized that the pupils are spared in those cases in which the superficial layers of the nerve escape ischemic insult. The general rule that palsies resulting from diabetic small vessel disease resolve within four months was supported in these series.

Trauma was a less frequent cause of third nerve palsy but was still common in all four series. The vast majority of trauma was blunt and frontal, but unfortunately the documentation of the exact location and extent of the injuries was poor. Third nerve palsy was caused by tumor approximately as often as by trauma. The authors reported involvment from supratentorial tumors by compression, and directly by metastatic and primary brainstem tumors. Pituitary tumors were by far the most frequent in Rucker's series,[15, 16] and metastatic tumors predominated in the series of Green and coworkers.[17]

Nine percent of Green's[17] patients had syphilis, while there were only six cases reported in the other three series combined. This discrepancy can be explained by the fact that Green's series was taken from a large urban hospital at a time when advanced syphilis was quite common. One would anticipate that this cause would be quite rare today since most cases of syphilis are probably diagnosed and treated, preventing progression to this stage.

Miscellaneous causes included a wide spectrum of neurologic and other diseases, including sinusitis, multiple sclerosis, migraine headache, postoperative complications, Hodgkin's disease, temporal arteritis, meningitis, and encephalitis. Although rare, these disorders take on added importance when third nerve palsies are evaluated on an age-related basis.

Fourth nerve palsy

The three largest series on isolated trochlear palsies are by Rucker[15, 16] and Burger and co-workers[20] (Table 10). Although Burger could not un-

Table 10. Comparison of causes of fourth nerve palsy

	Rucker[15] (*67 cases*)		*Rucker*[16] (*84 cases*)		*Burger*[20] (*33 cases*)	
	Number	*Percent*	*Number*	*Percent*	*Number*	*Percent*
Aneurysm	0	0	0	0	1	3
Vascular disease	24	36	13	15	6	18
Trauma	24	36	22	27	13	39
Neoplasm	3	4	7	8	7	21
Undetermined	9	13	29	33	2	6
Miscellaneous	7	10	13	15	3	9

cover the cause of fourth nerve palsy in only 6% of his series, we, along with Rucker, have found a large percentage of undiagnosed trochlear palsies that often improve spontaneously over a two- to six-month period. Of the known causes the most prevalent by far is trauma, usually severe and frontal in unilateral cases and vertex in nature in bilateral cases. Vascular disease, including diabetes, hypertension, and atherosclerosis, is the next most frequent, presumably causing ischemic injury to the nerve. Neoplasm was also common, and frequent sites included cerebellopontine angle, cerebellum, and metastases to the midbrain parenchyma. Miscellaneous causes included encephalitis, collagen disease, herpes zoster, and neonatal hypoxia. It is noteworthy that Rucker found no association of aneurysm with fourth nerve paresis and listed only one questionable case of demyelinating disease. Burger described one case of fourth nerve paresis secondary to ruptured posterior communicating aneurysm and one case of multiple sclerosis with isolated fourth nerve paresis. Walsh and Hoyt[21] list, in addition, migraine headache and sphenoid sinusitis as possible causes of fourth nerve paresis.

Sixth nerve paresis

Abducens palsies are by far the most common isolated extraocular nerve afflictions. In the three largest series[15, 16, 22] (Table 11) approximately one-fourth of the patients with isolated sixth nerve involvement were *undiagnosed*. Microvascular disease (diabetes and hypertension) and neoplasia were also frequently encountered. Contrary to common belief the vast majority of tumors responsible for sixth nerve paresis (both primary and metastatic) were present in the *posterior* fossa. Nasopharyngeal carcinoma was commonly implicated, but no pituitary tumors were listed.* The abducens

*EDITOR'S NOTE. See discussion of cranial nerve palsies with "pituitary apoplexy," Chapter 8. J. S. G.

Table 11. Comparison of causes of sixth nerve palsy

	Rucker[15] *(409 cases)*		*Rucker*[16] *(515 cases)*		*Schrader and Schlezinger*[22] *(104 cases)*	
	Number	*Percent*	*Number*	*Percent*	*Number*	*Percent*
Aneurysm	16	4	15	3	0	0
Vascular disease	57	14	46	9	38	37
Trauma	57	14	55	11	3	3
Neoplasm	82	20	159	31	7	7
Multiple sclerosis	15	4	36	7	13	13
Syphilis	7	2	0	0	10	10
Undetermined	129	32	112	21	25	24
Miscellaneous	46	11	92	18	8	8

nerve is proportionally less frequently affected in trauma and aneurysm than the oculomotor or trochlear nerves. Aneurysms that do cause sixth nerve palsy are usually located in the infraclinoid internal carotid.

Multiple sclerosis is more often a cause of sixth nerve palsy than of other isolated ocular motor palsy. In 7 of 13 cases of multiple sclerosis reported by Schrader and Schlezinger[22] sixth nerve paresis was the first manifestation. A total of 17 patients had syphilis in the three series reviewed. There was excellent response if therapy was begun less than ten weeks after the onset of symptoms.

Miscellaneous causes included sinusitis, Wernicke's disease, ophthalmoplegic migraine, meningitis, carotid cavernous fistula, spinal puncture, cerebral hematoma and hemorrhage, pseudotumor cerebri, postoperative complications, structural abnormalities, degenerative diseases, and isolated cases of numerous other entities.

AGE-RELATED INCIDENCE*

Once the extraocular muscle dysfunction has been localized to a given muscle or muscles, it is necessary to have formulated a rational scheme of diagnostic tests to establish the cause of the dysfunction. Isolated involvement of the nerves to the extraocular muscles begins at a similar age in the various ocular motor palsies. For this reason, age-related incidences will be considered together and obvious exceptions will be noted.

Birth to 20 years

By far the most common cause of extraocular muscle palsies in childhood is trauma. Since the trauma is usually severe, the cause is not in doubt.

*See Appendix, pp. 213-215.

A congenital cause is often overlooked. For example, unilateral ptosis is often a difficult diagnostic problem in a child if this cause is not considered. Likewise, Möbius syndrome presents with bilateral sixth nerve paresis secondary to abiogenesis of the sixth nuclei. Of added importance in children is meningitis and encephalitis. Any development of extraocular palsy with unexplained decrease in level of consciousness would compel the clinician to perform a complete neurologic evaluation. Likewise, suspected Hodgkin's disease, central nervous system leukemia, or tumor with or without multifocal involvement demands a full battery of diagnostic tests, including cerebrospinal fluid cytologic study. Although myasthenia gravis is not included in all series referred to in this chapter, on occasion it can present as isolated ocular motor palsy, especially as an isolated ptosis.

Knox and co-workers[23] have brought attention to the infrequent occurrence of isolated abducens palsy following acute viral illness in children that almost always resolves within ten weeks. Unlike more ominous possibilities, the postviral syndrome is benign, and invasive diagnostic procedures should be withheld when this diagnosis is strongly considered unless progression takes place. In cases where a prior history of sinusitis can be elicited, sinus x-ray films can help exclude this cause of ocular muscle palsy. In any child with apparent sixth nerve paresis, patching may uncover cross-fixating esotropia, which would obviate the necessity for involved evaluation. Finally, in all age groups an old photograph will often date the onset of the difficulty and document any progression.

Young adults

Many of the causes of unilateral ocular motor palsy occur in all age groups (trauma, malignancy, myasthenia gravis, sinusitis, etc.), but some causes become more frequent with age. Multiple sclerosis is a disease primarily of young adulthood. Any patient in this age group who develops a third or sixth nerve ocular muscle palsy, with a history of multifocal involvement at different times, requires a complete neurologic evaluation, including cerebrospinal fluid electrophoresis. Expanding aneurysms of the infraclinoid internal carotid or posterior communicating arteries can present with sudden onset of third nerve paresis, usually with the pupil involved, and more rarely, infraclinoid aneurysms can present with sudden onset of sixth nerve palsies. If neurologic investigation reveals xanthochromic cerebrospinal fluid, arteriography is usually diagnostic. Four vessel angiography is indicated because aneurysms are frequently multiple. Autoimmune disease, including systemic lupus erythematosus, can occasionally present with central nervous system complications, including ocular motor palsy. This diagnosis is suspected if there are other systemic manifestations and antinuclear antibody, lupus erythematosus preparations, sedimentation rate, and so on are positive. In young adults, as in other age groups, one must distinguish blepharoptosis, pseudoptosis, and Adie's syndrome (tonic pupil) from true oculomotor nerve palsy.

Older age group

By far the largest number of isolated palsies of the third, fourth, and sixth nerves occur in older adults. Although tumor, aneurysm, and trauma remain prevalent in the older age group, occlusive vascular disease becomes increasingly important in the differential diagnosis. Third nerve palsies caused by hypertension and diabetes tend to be of sudden onset, often spare the pupil, and may or may not be painful. A significant number of patients recover within four months. The sedimentation rate should be determined in any patient over 50 years old who develops an acute ocular motor palsy because fully 12% of patients with temporal arteritis present in this manner. In this age group it is especially important to keep microvascular disease in mind because these entities can be managed conservatively. Because of their significant morbidity in this age group arteriography and pneumoencephalography should be held in reserve unless progression can be documented.

REFERENCES

1. Boeder, P.: The co-operation of extraocular muscles, Am. J. Ophthalmol. **51:** 469, 1961.
2. Duane, A.: A new classification of the motor anomalies of the eye, Ann. Ophthalmol. Otolaryngol. **5:**969, 1896.
3. Duane, A.: The basic principles of diagnosis in motor anomalies of the eye, Arch. Ophthalmol. **48:**2, 1919.
4. Duane, A.: Anomalies of the ocular muscles, Arch. Ophthalmol. **11:**394, 1934.
5. Jampel, R. S.: Extraocular muscle action from brain stimulation in the macaque, Invest. Ophthalmol. **1:**565, 1962.
6. Jampel, R. S.: The action of the superior oblique muscle, Arch. Ophthalmol. **75:** 535, 1966.
7. Jampel, R. S.: The fundamental principle of the action of the oblique ocular muscles, Am. J. Ophthalmol. **69:**623, 1970.
8. Jampel, R. S., and Bloomgarden, C.: Individual extraocular muscle function from faradic stimulation of the oculomotor and trochlear nerves in the macaque, Invest. Ophthalmol. **2:**265, 1963.
9. Hering, E.: Die Lehre v. binokularen Sehen, Leipzig, 1868, Engelman.
10. Hering, E.: Dr. Raumsinn und die Bewegungen der Auges. In Hermann, L.: Handbuch der Physiologie, vol. 3, 1879. English translation by C. A. Radde, Baltimore, 1942, American Academy of Optometry.
11. Cogan, D. G.: Neurology of the ocular muscles, Springfield, Ill., 1956, Charles C Thomas, Publisher.
12. Parks, M.: Isolated cyclovertical muscle palsy, Arch. Ophthalmol. **60:**1027, 1958.
13. Feibel, R. M., and Roper-Hall, G.: Evaluation of the field of binocular single vision in incomitant strabismus, Am. J. Ophthalmol. In press.
14. von Noorden, G., and Maumenee, A. E.: Atlas of strabismus, ed. 2, St. Louis, 1967, The C. V. Mosby Co., p. 140.
15. Rucker, C. W.: Paralysis of the third, fourth, and sixth cranial nerves, Am. J. Ophthalmol. **46:**787, 1958.
16. Rucker, C. W.: The causes of paralysis of the third, fourth, and sixth cranial nerves, Am. J. Ophthalmol. **61:**353, 1966.
17. Green, W., Hackett, E., and Schlezinger, N.: Neuro-ophthalmologic evaluation of oculomotor nerve paralysis, Arch. Ophthalmol. **72:**154, 1964.
18. Goldstein, J., and Cogan, D.: Diabetic ophthalmoplegia with special reference to the pupil, Arch. Ophthalmol. **64:**592, 1960.

19. Dreyfus, P., Hakim, S., and Adams, R.: Diabetic ophthalmoplegia, Arch. Neurol. **77:**337, 1957.
20. Burger, L., Kalvin, N., and Smith, J. L.: Acquired lesions of the fourth cranial nerve, Brain **93:**567, 1970.
21. Walsh, F. B., and Hoyt, W. F.: Clinical neuro-ophthalmology, ed. 3, Baltimore, 1969, The Williams & Wilkins Company.
22. Schrader, E., and Schlezinger, N.: Neuro-ophthalmologic evaluation of abducens nerve paralysis, Arch. Ophthalmol. **63:**84, 1960.
23. Knox, D., Clark, D., and Schuster, F.: Benign VI nerve palsies in children, Pediatrics **40:**560, 1967.

Appendix

Outline of age-related approach to isolated fourth and sixth nerve palsies

Isolated fourth nerve paresis in children and adults

History	*Outpatient*	*Inpatient*
Bilateral		
Vertex or frontal blow Facial fractures		Usually seen as inpatient after motor vehicle accident
Unilateral		
Torticollis	Rule out ordinary torticollis by patching	
Trauma, oblique Frontal sinus surgery	Skull films	
Migraine or family history of migraine plus contraceptive pills	Fletchergram	
Herpes zoster	General medical examination Rule out neoplasia	
Evanescent diplopia	Tensilon testing	
Disseminated sclerosis	?	
Negative	General physical exam, neurologic exam Hemogram, heterophile, serum enzymes Skull films, including sinus films	
In addition over age 45 With or without head pain	Sedimentation rate Glucose tolerance test	
	If positive outpatient tests indicate If progression of paresis If development of additional signs and symptoms →	Complete evaluation

Apparently isolated sixth nerve paresis in children

History	*Outpatient*	*Inpatient*
Bilateral		
Present since birth or shortly thereafter	Rule out comitant strabismus Alternate patching Search for stigmata of congenital disease and birth trauma	
Acute onset		
Associated with trauma		Skull films including base views and orbital views
With other symptoms: pain, recurrent sinus or middle ear disease		(Consider battered child) Sinus films Towne's view
Headache with papilledema		Investigate causes of intracranial hypertension Drugs Heavy metals Systemic disease Central nervous system disease
Unilateral		
Present since birth or shortly thereafter	History or evidence of birth trauma Congenital defects (e.g., Duane's syndrome)	
Acute onset		
Associated with trauma	Evidence of orbital disease? Skull films with base views	If cannot be accomplished as an outpatient
Following "flu" syndrome, recurrent sinus or middle ear disease No pertinent history	Hemogram, heterophile, serum enzymes, skull views, Towne's view	Admit → Lumbar puncture?
Waxing and waning	Prostigmin test (I.M.)	
	If positive outpatient tests indicate If progression of paresis If development of additional signs and symptoms	→ Complete systemic screen Collagen vascular disease Granulomatous disease Infectious disease Neurological testings Lumbar puncture Brain scan Contrast studies

Apparently isolated sixth nerve paresis in adults

History	*Outpatient*	*Inpatient*
Bilateral		
Trauma	Approximate x-rays ? →	
Harbinger of increased intracranial pressure		Investigate cause of increased intracranial pressure
Syphilis	FTA-ABS (℞ penicillin)	
External pressure of living	Rule out spasm of the near reflex If divergence paralysis —Admit→	
Unilateral		
Trauma, significant or nonsignificant	X-ray skull, base views ? orbit	
Pain	Look for evidence of orbital inflammatory or neoplastic disease: forced ductions Investigate endocrine status, hemogram, skull films, Towne's view	
Evanescent diplopia	Tensilon test (+ Tonography) (+ EMG)	
Evidence of disseminated sclerosis	Lumbar puncture/protein electrophoresis/leukocyte migration inhibition ←→	?
Migraine (contraceptive pills)	Fletchergram for increased coagulability	
Negative	Similar to that in children: Careful physical examination Hemogram, heterophile, serum enzymes, protein electrophoresis, FTA-ABS, x-ray skull, Towne's view, polytomes of sphenoid sinus, chest x-ray	
In addition over age 45 Head pain	Careful physical examination STAT sedimentation rate Glucose tolerance With facial dysesthesia, nasopharyngeal examination	
	If positive outpatient tests indicate If progression of paresis If development of additional signs and symptons →	Complete evaluation

Chapter 11

Chronic progressive external ophthalmoplegia

Simmons Lessell

Chronic progressive external ophthalmoplegia (CPEO) is one of several names used to designate an uncommon disorder of ocular motility. Patients with CPEO gradually lose the ability to elevate their eyelids and move their eyes. However, the smooth muscles of their irides and ciliary bodies continue to function normally. This type of ophthalmoplegia can occur in a variety of diseases. In some of them it constitutes the major, or only, clinical manifestation, but in others it may be a minor feature. Although physicians have recognized CPEO for over 100 years,[1] its pathogenesis is not understood, the significance of the electrophysiologic and histopathologic findings in the disorder is controversial, and there is no scientific basis for classification. Despite this situation, physicians must be in a position to utilize what *is* known about CPEO in order to help and understand people with the disorder.

SYMPTOMS AND SIGNS

Case 1. Fig. 11-1 shows the face of a patient with CPEO. Her facial characteristics are so typical of CPEO that they should immediately suggest the diagnosis. She is a 55-year-old, white, married, American-born woman of Portuguese descent who developed double vision at the age of 33 years. Shortly thereafter, the upper lids of both eyes began to droop. She claimed that there was progressive ptosis and limitation of eye movement until the age of 45 years. After that there was no progression. Her past medical history was otherwise negative. The only family history of relevance was that a sister, not available for examination, had developed strabismus in adult life. The patient was examined at age 48, at which time the photograph in Fig. 11-1 was taken. The patient tended to keep her head tilted back and kept her frontalis muscles contracted in order to compensate for severe bilateral ptosis. The maximum excursion of her upper eyelids was 4 mm on the right and 5 mm on the left. Her eyelids were very thin and the blood vessels within them stood out in relief. There was a poverty of facial expression, her lips were pursed, and her smile was transverse. Her facial muscles,

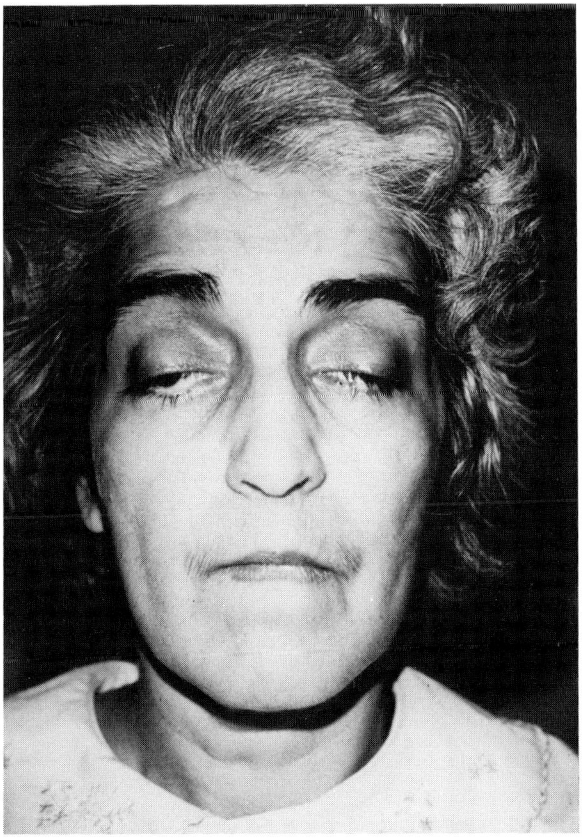

Fig. 11-1. Patient with chronic progressive external ophthalmoplegia.

including the orbicularis oculi, were weak. Her eyes were virtually fixed in partial abduction. She had no Bell's phenomenon, and reflex maneuvers did not improve the range of her ocular motions. There was no defect in pupillary motility or accommodation. Her vision was 20/30 in each eye. There was mottling of the retinal pigment epithelium in the region of the maculas of both eyes. The exposed portion of the left cornea was thin, but the cornea was not scarred, inflammed, or vascularized. There was mild, diffuse, symmetric weakness of the limbs, worse proximally, and the deep tendon reflexes were hypoactive. Barium swallow and pulmonary function studies were negative. Serum "muscle" enzymes were within normal limits. An intravenous injection of 10 mg of edrophonium chloride did not improve her ptosis or eye movements. Electromyography performed in limb muscles was interpreted as showing primary myopathic changes.

Case 2. Fig. 11-2 shows the face of another patient with CPEO. She suffers from a form of CPEO that involves the muscles of deglutition. She is a 72-year-old, white, married, Canadian-born woman of French descent. Her problem began at the age of 62 years, when, nearly simultaneously, she began to notice a slight drooping of the upper eyelids and difficulty in swallowing. Over the course of the ensuing years her symptoms slowly became worse. She denied any other medical problems. Her general physical examination was unremarkable, and her eye examination, apart from the eyelids, was

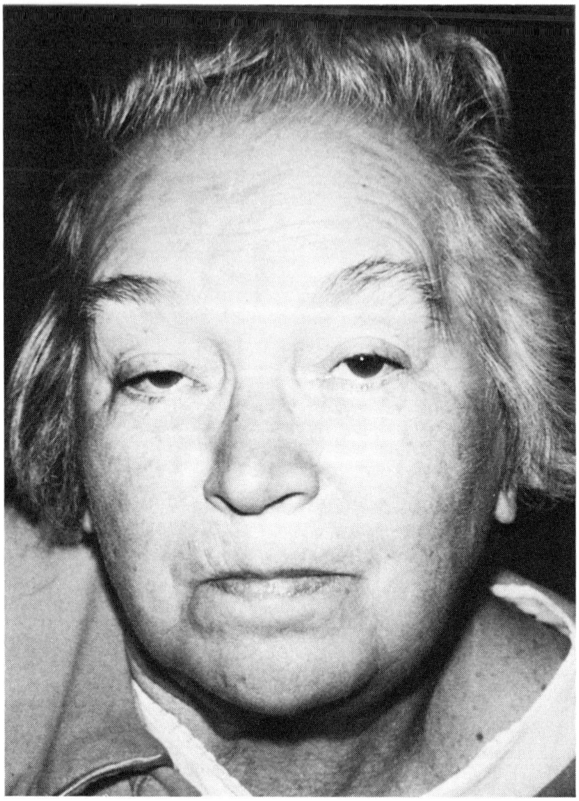

Fig. 11-2. Patient with chronic progressive external ophthalmoplegia.

also normal. There was no defect in pupillary function. She had moderately severe ptosis, which was associated with weakness of the orbicularis oculi muscles on both sides. She tended to keep her forehead furrowed in an attempt to overcome the ptosis. The eyelids were somewhat thin. There was no defect in eye movements. The neurologic examination showed very minimal weakness of the flexor muscles of the neck, the muscles of the face, and the proximal muscles of the arms. The deep tendon reflexes were considered normal. Her serum "muscle" enzymes were within normal limits. Electromyographic studies of her deltoid muscles showed "myopathic changes." Barium swallow showed weakness of pharyngeal muscles, with difficulty in initiating swallowing. None of her weakness was improved by an intravenous injection of 10 mg of edrophonium chloride.

Heredity

A positive family history has been obtained in about half of the reported cases of CPEO.[2] The frequency of a positive family history seems to be higher in the oculopharyngeal variant of CPEO than in other varieties of CPEO. Among the cases of oculopharyngeal muscular dystrophy found in people of French descent in Canada and New England, there is a striking pattern of autosomal dominant inheritance. This is beautifully documented in the reports of Barbeau[3] and Murphy and Drachman.[4] Barbeau has even traced the disorder back to early French settlers along the St. Lawrence River.

Several factors frustrate attempts to measure the hereditary tendency in a disease like CPEO. Illegitimacy, for example, can make a case that was actually dominantly inherited appear sporadic. Also, the relatively late onset of CPEO means that potentially affected siblings may have died before attaining the age of risk or may not otherwise be available for examination. Nevertheless, the physician should strive to obtain a complete and accurate family history. If there is involvement of relatives, it helps to rule out myasthenia gravis, the disease most difficult to distinguish from CPEO. Myasthenia gravis only rarely afflicts several members of a family. Another reason to obtain a family history is to provide a basis for genetic counseling of patients and their families. Finally, having the family history may help predict the patient's future course, since relatives who have had the disease for a longer period of time may have developed other manifestations.

Age of onset

In most instances the first symptoms of CPEO appear before the age of 30 years, but generally it is difficult to accurately determine the age of onset. The disease progresses so slowly that patients may not remember when it first began. Also, patients with CPEO are remarkably tolerant of their defect in eye movement and therefore may not acknowledge any infirmity in the early stages of their disorder. The age of onset is probably different for different variants of CPEO. In one variety of CPEO that is characterized by sporadic occurrence, small stature, cardiac conduction problems, and pigmentary retinopathy (the Kearns-Sayre syndrome[5, 6]), the onset tends to be early. On the other hand, the familial oculopharyngeal variant of CPEO tends to begin late.[3, 4, 7, 8]

I have chosen to eliminate from consideration cases of external ophthalmoplegia that are congenital.[9-11] This is because they are not ordinarily progressive and do not usually occur in kinships that include individuals with more conventional expressions of CPEO. However, there is evidence that CPEO can be congenital. First, there have been cases of congenital ophthalmoplegia in which postnatal progression occurred.[12] There have also been patients with congenital motor disorders ("flaccid" or "floppy" infants) who subsequently developed progressive ptosis or ophthalmoplegia or both. Centronuclear[13, 14] and myotubular[15] myopathy are congenital myopathies in which this has been described. I have seen one such case. That child had a nonprogressive congenital myopathy characterized by a flaccid quadriparesis. A muscle biopsy was said to show changes indicative of a primary disorder of muscle cells. At around 3 years of age the child's parents noted that he did not seem to move his eyes fully. This became progressively worse over the ensuing two years, so that by the time I saw him at age 5 years there was considerable restriction of his eye movements. Reflex maneuvers failed to improve his eye movements. There was no ptosis or facial weakness, and pupillary responses were normal.

Ptosis preceding ophthalmoplegia

In most patients with CPEO, the ptosis is evident before the ophthalmoplegia is recognized. However, there *have* been a few cases of ophthalmoplegia without ptosis.[16, 17] Also exceptional are the cases of CPEO in which the ptosis is recognized after the ophthalmoplegia.[18, 19]

There are, in addition, numerous cases of acquired bilateral ptosis, sometimes hereditary and of late onset, in which ophthalmoplegia and orbicularis oculi and other muscle weakness do not develop. It has been suggested that this type of ptosis can be due to a primary myopathy.[20] How acquired hereditary ptosis relates to CPEO is unclear, but since there are families with CPEO some of whose members have ptosis without ophthalmoplegia, one must conclude that ptosis can be a valid expression of CPEO even in the absence of ophthalmoplegia.[21]

Symmetry

Usually the ptosis and ophthalmoplegia are bilaterally symmetric. In some patients with CPEO the ophthalmoplegia is so symmetric that one is misled into believing that the patient has a supranuclear disorder of ocular motility.

There are some exceptions. Among these are cases in which the ptosis appears to be strictly unilateral[22, 23] and others in which there is a long interval between involvement of the first eye and of the second.[23-27] Also, in many cases of CPEO in the early stages one eye may be ptotic while the other remains normal.

Tolerance of ophthalmoplegia

Many physicians who have written about CPEO have commented upon the remarkable tolerance that patients with CPEO have to their ophthalmoplegia. As a result of this tolerance patients may not present themselves to doctors until late in the course of their illness, and then only at the urging of a friend or relative. Patients may fail to complain of diplopia even when they have obvious misalignment of their visual axes. Despite the lack of symptoms, one can demonstrate the diplopia by using a red lens or similar device. Tolerance of the diplopia usually cannot be explained by the symmetry of the ophthalmoplegia or the severity of the ptosis. In my own experience, patients are more likely to seek medical help because of their ptosis than because of their ophthalmoplegia.

Weakness of eye closure

Patients with CPEO who have severe ptosis usually have weak orbicularis oculi muscles. Unfortunately, patients vary in the degree to which they try to squeeze their eyes when requested to do so. Therefore, it is sometimes difficult to assess the strength of the orbicularis oculi muscles. Ophthalmologists generally neglect to examine the orbicularis oculi muscles in their routine examinations and so have a poor basis for making a clinical judgment of strength when confronted with cases like these. However, I think that orbicularis oculi weakness will usually be found if looked for in patients with CPEO.* The weakness of the orbicularis oculi muscles in cases of CPEO generally does not lead to exposure of the cornea *unless the patient has had lid surgery to correct the associated ptosis.*

In those rare instances in which patients develop CPEO as an expression of fascioscapulohumeral muscular dystrophy or myotonic dystrophy,[28] the orbicularis oculi weakness may be as striking as the ptosis. It may be *more* striking in such cases. There have been instances in which patients with myotonic dystrophy have sufficient impairment of closure of the eyes for exposure keratopathy to occur.

Remissions and diurnal variations

Patients with CPEO have a progressive disorder that may ultimately stabilize. They will enjoy neither diurnal improvement in their symptoms nor prolonged remissions, both of which may occur in myasthenia gravis. Abnormal fatigability has been noted in some cases of CPEO,[25] but that fatigability does not cause ptosis and ophthalmoplegia in the evening that disappear after rest. Patients with CPEO awaken with just as much ptosis and restriction of eye movements as when they retired the night before. In cases of ophthalmoplegia associated with Whipple's disease, fluctuation has occurred.[29] However, remissions are so exceptional in CPEO that a history of a remission should make the physician question the diagnosis.†

Thinned eyelids

If a patient with CPEO has severe ptosis for a long time, his upper eyelids are apt to become thin. The blood vessels of the upper lids may stand out in relief. One does not ordinarily find such thinning in normals or in cases of nonhereditary ptosis, although it has been seen in some cases of late-onset, hereditary ptosis.[20] Loss of bulk of the orbicularis oculi muscles is probably responsible for most of the thinning.

---

*EDITOR'S NOTE. Weakness of orbicularis oculi is also a common finding in patients with ocular myasthenia. J. S. G.

†EDITOR'S NOTE. Variability of ophthalmoplegia or ptosis, or both, is essentially pathognomonic of myasthenia. J. S. G.

Response of ptosis and ophthalmoplegia to anticholinesterase drugs

Anticholinesterase drugs such as edrophonium chloride and neostigmine do not improve the motility of the lids or eyes of patients with CPEO. Equivocal responses have been recorded in some patients with CPEO, and if one relies entirely on a patient's subjective responses, "positive" results may be obtained. However, if one defines a positive response to anticholinesterase agents as significant improvement determined by some objective method, one can assume that response to an anticholinesterase agent is evidence against the diagnosis of CPEO. There have been cases of CPEO, some of them familial, in which the patients have shown an unusual sensitivity to curare,[30-32] and one instance in which a patient was sensitive to succinylcholine.[33] While none of these patients seemed to have had myasthenia gravis, Rosenberg, Rowland, and their colleagues[34, 35] have questioned whether such patients who responded to curare can be safely classified as examples of CPEO.

One technique that has been used to aid in the diagnosis of myasthenia gravis is edrophonium chloride tonography.[36] In this test the intraocular pressure is monitored using an electronic tonometer in a fashion identical to that used to measure the facility of outflow of aqueous from the eye in patients suspected of having glaucoma. Edrophonium chloride is injected intravenously while the pressure is continuously recorded. Patients with myasthenia gravis have an abrupt rise in intraocular pressure when the drug is injected, followed by a gradual return to normal. Positive responses have been encountered in nonmyasthenic patients,[37] but not in cases of CPEO.

Smooth muscle functions of the eye

The only muscles of the eye that are ordinarily affected in CPEO are the striated muscles. The smooth muscles of the iris and ciliary body are not involved. Therefore, if a patient has evidence of pupillary paresis one should doubt the diagnosis of CPEO. However, CPEO may occur in the presence of neuromuscular disorders, some of which can have pupillary involvement as a feature.

Other findings

Table 12 lists some of the non–ocular motor findings that may occur in patients with CPEO. Table 13 lists some diseases in which CPEO may occur. Dr. Daniel Drachman[38] made a landmark contribution when he compiled lists like these to call attention to the phenomenon of "ophthalmoplegia plus." Rosenberg and colleagues,[34] and Jampel and associates[16] made similar contributions. My list is incomplete since I did not include several associations that have only been reported once. Their association with CPEO may have been by chance.

Dysphagia was alluded to earlier. It has been variously estimated that dysphagia afflicts between 3% and 50% of the patients with CPEO.[2, 39-41]

Table 12. Findings that may be associated with CPEO

Dysphonia	Corneal opacities
Dysphagia	Optic atrophy
Facial muscle weakness	Deafness
Neck muscle weakness	Atypical pigmentary retinopathy
Limb muscle weakness	Retinitis pigmentosa (classical)
Sphincter weakness	Proptosis
Lower motor neuron lesions	Cardiomyopathy
Ataxia	Cardiac conduction defects
Dystonia	Hypogonadism
Peripheral neuropathy	Early menopause
Corticospinal tract lesions	Small stature
Dementia	Delayed sexual maturation
Seizures	Curare sensitivity
EEG slowing	Succinylcholine sensitivity
Elevated CSF protein	

Table 13. Diseases in which CPEO may occur

Fazio-Londes disease	Werdnig-Hoffmann disease
Facioscapulohumeral dystrophy	Acanthocytosis
Myotonic dystrophy	Charcot-Marie-Tooth disease
Refsum's syndrome	Sanger-Brown's cerebellar ataxia
Primary systemic amyloidosis	Marie's cerebellar ataxia
Whipple's disease	Leigh's disease

The dysphagia occurs both in sporadic cases of CPEO and as a cardinal feature in a dominantly inherited variety. The latter, oculopharyngeal muscular dystrophy, characteristically begins late in life and tends to produce levator and orbicularis oculi weakness with little or no ophthalmoplegia.[3, 4, 40, 42, 43] The late Dr. Hermann Burian suggested that *palpebropharyngeal* might be a better name than *oculopharyngeal* since the muscles that move the eyes are frequently spared.[44] The pharynx is usually the level at which the problem in swallowing occurs.[40, 45] Weakness of the pharynx impairs the initiation of swallowing. As a result there may be regurgitation and aspiration. This makes the oculopharyngeal form of CPEO potentially fatal and is reflected in an undue representation of pneumonia among the causes of death in these patients.[39] Roberts and Bamforth[39] found small, nonperistaltic contractions throughout the body of the esophagus. Since the entire esophagus was involved, they suggested that there may be involvement of both the striated and smooth muscle of the esophagus in this disease. This has also been seen by others.[40, 46] Rarely, the laryngeal muscles and the tongue may also be involved.[39]

Pigmentary retinopathy is one of the more common associations of

CPEO.[5, 6, 16, 38] Only a few patients with CPEO have had typical retinitis pigmentosa,[5, 17] which consists of impaired night vision, contricted visual fields, bone corpuscular pigmentation of the retina, attenuated retinal blood vessels, waxy pallor of the optic discs, and depressed electroretinograms. Many of the patients with CPEO who have a retinopathy have one that does not look like classical retinitis pigmentosa.[48-52] In some, fine pigment may be dispersed over the fundus, deep to the retina, while the discs and blood vessels are generally normal. In other patients there may be pigmentation limited to the macula area or to the retinal periphery. Sometimes vision is subnormal or the fields are constricted. In rare instances an abnormal electroretinogram or subnormal visual acuity may be found in a patient with CPEO who has a normal fundus.[38] It should be noted that a form of pigmentary retinopathy is an essential feature of two of the diseases listed in Table 13, acanthocytosis[53] and Refsum's syndrome,[54] and macula pigmentation has been found in two others, myotonic dystrophy[55] and Leigh's disease.[56, 57]

Cardiac abnormalities are one of the most important associations of CPEO because they can threaten life.[5, 6, 38, 57, 58] In one variety of CPEO, the Kearns-Sayre syndrome conduction defects occur together with pigmentary retinopathy, small stature, and delayed sexual maturation. Stokes-Adams attacks can occur as a result of the conduction defect. Other cardiac abnormalities can occur in CPEO,[59] and one might expect that with time the same spectrum of cardiac abnormalities will be described in CPEO as has been described in the muscular dystrophies.[60, 61]

LOCALIZATION OF LESIONS—DIFFERENTIAL DIAGNOSIS

If a cooperative, nonaphasic patient does not move either eye when requested to do so, there are six possible levels in the ocular motor system at which a lesion could occur that would explain the problem. They are listed in Table 14.

Extensive lesions that bilaterally involve the pathways descending from the cerebral hemispheres to control gaze can produce immobile eyes. Such lesions occur, for example, in progressive supranuclear palsy (Steel-Richardson-Olzewski syndrome).[62-64] In that disease, the onset is in middle or late life and the progress of the ophthalmoplegia is slow. When the disease is fully established, the eyes appear to be immobile. Pupillary function is generally spared, as in CPEO. However, in supranuclear lesions the lower motor

Table 14. Possible sites of lesions causing ophthalmoplegia

Orbital tissues	Axons of cranial nerves
Muscle cells	Nuclei of cranial nerves
Motor end-plates	Descending gaze fibers (supranuclear)

neuron is intact, so that one can move the patient's eyes by using reflex methods. There are two ways to demonstrate this: (1) the doll head maneuver, the production of adversive eye movements by passively turning the patient's head, and (2) caloric stimulation of the semicircular canals. It should be easy to distinguish between CPEO and profound ophthalmoplegia due to gaze palsy, but it may be artificial to separate CPEO from gaze palsies of supranuclear origin. Jampel and co-workers[16] suggested that the ophthalmoplegia in a syndrome of CPEO they described might have been a result of supranuclear lesions. The progressive external ophthalmoplegia occasionally associated with Whipple's disease may also occur on a supranuclear basis.[65]

Bilateral infiltrative orbitopathies can produce slowly progressive, symmetric ophthalmoplegia. The commonest of these is the orbitopathy of Graves' disease. As in CPEO, the pupils are spared, but ptosis is usually absent and there may even be retraction of the upper eyelids. The lids are not thin, and the orbicularis oculi muscles are not weak in the infiltrative orbitopathies. Furthermore, exophthalmos and decreased orbital resiliency are frequently present in infiltrative orbitopathies. If one attempts to move the globes passively in these cases there is usually resistance (positive forced-duction test). This is due to the loss of elasticity of the involved muscle. The loss of elasticity of the extraocular muscles may also be reflected by a rise in intraocular pressure when the patient attempts to look into the field of action in which movement is limited. Patients with infiltrative orbitopathies may have diurnal variation in the severity of their diplopia, but unlike the myasthenic patients they are apt to have more diplopia in the morning than in the afternoon. The orbit probably becomes passively congested when the patient is recumbent. With the exception of very early cases, it should be easy to distinguish between CPEO and ophthalmoplegia due to infiltrative orbitopathies.

There is evidence in animals that CPEO can result from a defect at the level of the neuromuscular junction. There have been a series of investigations on a form of CPEO that occurs in mice with muscular dystrophy.[66-68] Although these mice fail to respond to anticholinesterase drugs, there is evidence of a structural defect at the myoneural junction. They have conglomerations of vacuoles within the muscle fibers in the regions adjacent to the nerve endings. The sarcoplasmic reticulum at those sites is also distended. In some instances the terminal axons were abnormal, with swelling and a paucity of synaptic vesicles. Abnormal terminal axons were found on some normal fibers.

The most prevalent disorder of the neuromuscular junction in man is myasthenia gravis. The cause of myasthenia is unknown, but studies have shown that patients with myasthenia gravis have deformed motor endplates in their limb muscles.[69-71] Recently, Farmbrough and associates[72] studied the number and distribution of acetylcholine receptors in the muscles of patients with myasthenia gravis. There was a reduction in the mean number of receptors per neuromuscular junction in the myasthenic as compared to normal patients. In about 15% of the cases of myasthenia gravis the clinical findings are limited to the eyes.[73] If they remain so limited for several years, nonocular muscles are apt never to be involved.[74] This is not invariable,[75] and Drachman[76] has indicated that a careful search frequently shows subtle involvement of other muscles in these patients. Like patients with CPEO, patients with myasthenia gravis may have progressive ptosis and ophthalmoplegia with sparing of the pupils. Weakness of the orbicularis oculi muscles and dysphagia may be present in both. To further complicate the issue, histopathologic and neurophysiologic evidence of atrophy and myopathy have been reported in patients with myasthenia gravis.[77, 78] Thus the symptoms and signs of myasthenia gravis so closely resemble those of CPEO that it may sometimes be difficult to distinguish between the two disorders. Nevertheless, patients with myasthenia gravis must be identified, because unlike patients with CPEO, they can be treated with drugs. Furthermore, myasthenia gravis is potentially fatal and is sometimes associated with thymic neoplasms and autoimmune diseases. Table 15 lists some features that may be helpful in distinguishing between myasthenia gravis and chronic progressive external ophthalmoplegia.

Lesions in the three other loci—cranial nerve nuclei, axons of the third, fourth, and sixth cranial nerves, and muscle cells of the extraocular muscles—each probably explain some cases of CPEO.

Nuclear abnormalities were described in postmortem studies of cases of CPEO reported in 1928[79] and 1943.[80] For a time thereafter all cases of CPEO were considered to be nuclear ophthalmoplegias. While this is not the current view and the nuclear basis of the ophthalmoplegia in those original cases is questioned, a case founded on histopathologic evidence can be made for the nuclei as the primary site of the lesion responsible for some cases of CPEO. Notable is the case reported by Daroff and coworkers[81] in which spongy changes were present in the nuclei of the nerves supplying the extraocular muscles. Another case with histopathologic evi-

Table 15. Comparison of CPEO and myasthenia gravis

	Myasthenia	*CPEO*
Diurnal variation in weakness	Typical	Atypical
Remissions	Sometimes	Rarely if ever
Symmetry	Atypical	Typical
Atrophy of lids	Uncommon	Common
Response to edrophonium chloride	Typical	Rarely if ever

dence of a nuclear lesion was reported by Brion and De Recondo.[82] Also, in the progressive bulbar paralysis of childhood (Fazio-Londe's disease) progressive ophthalmoplegia may occur with ptosis and facial muscle weakness.[83] There have also been a few cases of hereditary neurogenic muscular atrophy (Werdnig-Hoffmann type as well as adult type) with ophthalmoplegia.

It should be noted that the neuropathologic record would suggest that the nuclei of the third, fourth, and sixth cranial nerves tend to escape damage in most degenerative disorders of the central nervous system. Even in a disorder such as amyotrophic lateral sclerosis, in which motor neurons are destroyed up and down the neuraxis, these cranial nerves nuclei are almost invariably spared. In some diseases, such as the Parkinson-dementia complex of Guam,[84] and Werdnig-Hoffmann disease,[85-87] there are lesions in these nuclei in patients who have no clinical evidence of a defect in eye movement.

Occasionally one reads that multiple sclerosis has been considered in the differential diagnosis of patients with chronic progressive external ophthalmoplegia. This seems unreasonable to me. While multiple sclerosis produces lesions of the brain stem that cause nystagmus, internuclear ophthalmoplegia, and sometimes gaze palsies, it does not cause an unremitting, chronically progressive, lower motor neuron type of paralysis of multiple extraocular muscles. Intrinsic tumors of the brain stem would be a more reasonable consideration in the differential diagnosis. Some brain stem gliomas are relatively benign and grow slowly, so that the impairment of eye movements is slowly progressive. That papilledema tends to occur late if at all in patients with brain stem gliomas might further contribute to difficulty in diagnosis. Furthermore, bilateral facial diplegia and dysphagia can occur both with CPEO and with intrinsic brain stem gliomas. One would assume that growth of the neoplasm ultimately would produce symptoms and signs that would shed doubt on the diagnosis of chronic progressive external ophthalmoplegia.

At least in theory, the axons of the third, fourth and sixth cranial nerves are other possible primary sites for lesions that could cause CPEO. The sparing of pupillary function in CPEO is sometimes cited as evidence against this possibility. However, pupillary function *can* be spared in oculomotor nerve paralysis as shown by lesions of the oculomotor nerve caused by diabetes mellitus. It should be pointed out, however, that there is no histopathologic evidence to prove that any case of CPEO was actually due to a lesion that primarily involved the axons of third, fourth, or sixth cranial nerves. It is also highly unlikely that the opportunity would arise to permit autopsy of a case of CPEO so early in the course of the illness that the lesions would still be limited to the axons.

The available evidence suggests that most cases of CPEO are due to a primary disease of muscle cells. In 1951 Kiloh and Nevin[2] reviewed a large number of cases of CPEO and concluded that the clinical and histopathologic evidence favored the view that CPEO was due to a myopathy. Briefly, the evidence for a myopathic cause of CPO is as follows:

1. Electromyograms of the extraocular muscles generally show a "myopathic" pattern.[22, 23] In most cases of CPEO, abnormal limb and facial muscles have also shown a "myopathic" pattern.

2. Nerves that have been found in biopsy specimens of extraocular muscles from cases of CPEO have appeared normal.[2, 88]

3. The extraocular muscles from cases of CPEO show a lesion that is thought to indicate a primary disease of muscle cells.[2] Nearly all limb muscles that have been biopsied and found abnormal in cases of CPEO have shown a myopathic pattern of damage.

4. Sparing of the smooth muscle function of the iris and ciliary body is considered evidence against a neural lesion.

5. In most cases in which the nuclei of the third, fourth, and sixth cranial nerves have been examined in the brain stem, they have been found to be normal.[12, 25, 89-91]

6. The lack of response to anticholinesterase medications and the absence of "myasthenic" responses on electrophysiologic testing are thought to make an end-plate lesion unlikely in CPEO.

I have already mentioned that there is reason to doubt that some of this evidence is conclusive. In an eloquent essay in the *Archives of Ophthalmology,* Dr. Robert Daroff[92] has marshalled the arguments for and against myopathy being the basis of CPEO. Rosenberg and colleagues,[34] Stephens and co-workers,[90] and Drachman[38] have also dealt with this issue. I will not recount all their arguments, but they force one to conclude that the question of the primary site of the lesion in CPEO has not been answered by the data presently available. Electromyography and histopathologic examination do not allow one to distinguish with certainty between myopathy and chronic denervation of ocular muscles. The electromyographic changes that are so useful in identifying the cause of limb muscle weakness do not apply readily to the ocular muscles.[93] The electromyograph thus has limited usefullness in evaluating ophthalmoplegia. Normal tracings have even been found in cases of profound ophthalmoplegia![94] The limitations of histopathologic examination have been proved decisively by the observations of Dr. David Drachman and his associates. They found that chronically denervated limb muscles in patients who had had poliomyelitis showed a myopathic picture.[95] More pointed was the observation that experimentally denervated ocular muscles also present the appearance of a myopathy.[96] One should also be aware that in the nonocular muscular dystrophies, a neurogenic cause is considered possible.[97-100]

ABNORMAL MITOCHONDRIA IN CPEO

An intriguing finding in the limb and eye muscles of many patients with CPEO is deformity of mitochondria.[24, 33, 101-105] Abnormal mitochondria have also been found in the eye muscles of dystrophic mice.[68] Dr. William Olson and his colleagues[102] described a series of cases with abnormal mitochondria. The changes in limb muscles consisted of "clusters of normal and abnormal mitochondria and excessive lipid droplets." They did not examine the extraocular muscles, but other investigators have found similar mitochondrial changes in the eye muscles of patients with CPEO. Histochemical studies have shown that the abnormal-appearing mitochondria not only have retained their enzyme activity but may have an excess of it. In recent reports, mitochondrial deformities were also present in the cerebellum[103] and skin[104] of patients with CPEO. Interestingly, the several electron microscopic studies of the hereditary oculopharyngeal variety of CPEO have not shown the same mitochondrial deformities.[45, 106] The ultrastructural features apparently so common in cases of CPEO are not found in myasthenia gravis or the more prevalent forms of muscular dystrophy such as myotonic dystrophy, and limb girdle and fascioscapulohumeral muscular dystrophy. It is too early to say what the structural and chemical abnormalities in mitochondria that have been found in the muscle cells in CPEO mean. Similar changes have been found in muscles and other tissues in a variety of other disorders.[107-110]

MANAGEMENT

I think the following steps should be carried out whenever a diagnosis of CPEO is considered.

1. Complete medical history of patient and family. Attempt to obtain photographs of the patient and his relatives. Sometimes a series of photographs will document the rate of progression of the patient's illness and reveal age of onset. Urge the patient to contact siblings, especially those not seen for a long time. The value of the family history lies not only in helping to distinguish CPEO, which is often familial, from disorders like myasthenia gravis, that are rarely familial, but also in helping to predict complications that might occur in the index case.

2. Complete ocular evaluation. One should attempt to establish the patient's visual function in terms of both visual fields and acuity. The fundus should be examined carefully after the pupils have been dilated in an attempt to recognize the presence of any pigmentary changes. If these are found or if there are symptoms suggesting retinal dysfunction, tests of dark adaptation and electroretinography should be performed. The cornea should be carefully evaluated for evidence of lesions that may have resulted from exposure of the cornea. The range of motion of the globes and eyelids should be measured and recorded by the best available means. Photographs provide an excellent record. Determine if the range of eye movements can be increased by reflex means. Particularly attend to the position of the globes when the eyes are gently closed as in sleep. Is the cornea exposed? Look for the presence of a Bell phenomenon. Estimate the strength of closure of the lids. Look to see whether the lids are abnormally thinned. Also look for evidence of fatigability of eye movements and lid movements in order to help recognize evidences of myasthenia gravis.

3. Complete neurologic examination. Many patients who deny difficulties with nonocular muscles will be found to have it when examined. Occasionally the ophthalmologist will be surprised to learn from the neurologist that the eye movement disorder is part of a generaized neuromuscular disease that requires management in its own right.

4. Electrocardiogram. An electrocardiogram should be obtained because of the occurrence of cardiac lesions in patients with CPEO. Look particularly for defects in cardiac conduction.

5. Fluoroscopy with barium swallow. The patient's pharyngeal and esophageal functions can be evaluated with fluoroscopy with a barium swallow. Patients who complain of difficulty in swallowing should be referred for more refined testing.

6. Electromyogram of limb muscles and measurement of nerve conduction times. An electromyogram of the limb muscles and measurement of nerve conduction times will help to define the nature of the muscle weakness, rule out myasthenia gravis, and to determine if there are lesions in the peripheral nerve.

7. Muscle biopsy. The extraocular muscles would be of interest, but there is limited justification for biopsying them. Biopsy of limb muscles has a high yield in cases of CPEO even when the muscles in question are not known to be weak. The site chosen for biopsy should be distant from the site of any previous electromyographic studies; the electromyography needle can produce structural changes. The biopsy should be obtained in close collaboration with the individual who will examine it. One should be prepared to study the material histochemically and electromicroscopically. It is important to carefully plan and orchestrate the biopsy so that the material can be appropriately stretched, fixed, and examined.

8. Edrophonium chloride test. No matter what evidence one has to suggest that the patient does not have myasthenia, one still should perform an edrophonium chloride test. Edrophonium chloride tonography might also be included.* While there may be such an entity as anticholinesterase-negative, curare-positive myasthenia gravis,[35] I am not convinced that curare testing should be done in questionable cases of CPEO. A therapeutic trial of

---

*EDITOR'S NOTE. See also paper by Spector and associates (p. 270) reporting effect of edrophonium and optokinetic nystagmography. J. S. G.

steroids might be tried, since ocular myasthenia may be responsive to ACTH or corticosteroids even if anticholinesterase drugs are not helpful.[111-114] So far I have no personal experience with such trials.

A recent publication has indicated that there may be specific findings on electro-oculography in CPEO.[115] The patient who was studied had a "consistent, repeatable, unique pattern of reduced saccadic velocity bilaterally in both the horizontal and vertical directions." Saccadic eye movements are slow in myasthenia gravis but are reversed by edrophonium chloride. Therefore, electro-oculography in the vertical and horizontal directions in both eyes combined with edrophonium chloride testing may be an important adjunct in the diagnosis of patients with CPEO.

9. *Level of serum "muscle" enzymes.* I am uncertain whether it is valuable to examine the level of "muscle" enzymes in the serum of these patients, but such evaluation probably should be done. One would expect elevation of certain enzymes to favor a diagnosis of primary muscle disease rather than a neurogenic disorder or myasthenia gravis. In most series of cases of CPEO in which the ocular findings were dominant, the enzymes have been normal. An occasional patient with significant involvement of limb muscles has had elevated serum enzymes. Koerner and Schlote[49] made an interesting observation concerning the serum enzymes in their cases of CPEO associated with pigmentary retinopathy. Four of their six patients had elevation of the serum levels of one or more "muscle" enzymes (creatine phosphokinase, aldolase, and lactate dehydrogenase) at rest. In three of the four, exercise tended to elevate the levels of one or more of the enzymes. This observation demands that others seek to confirm it.

Other specific tests for patients with CPEO would depend upon the patient's complaints and findings on the various examinations.

TREATMENT

Three problems that occur in patients with CPEO are amenable to treatment: ptosis, dysphagia, and heart block.

The management of the ptosis in patients with CPEO is difficult, because these patients frequently have deficient upward movement of the eyes and deficient closure of the eyelids. If the ptosis is treated too vigorously, the patient may be unable to protect his corneas. In deciding about ptosis surgery in cases with good mobility of the eyes, I think one must take into account the duration of the patient's illness and how the illness has behaved in affected relatives. In end-stage CPEO one can gauge what the potential for exposure keratopathy is, but early in the course of the illness one may not be able to predict what will happen. The patient may appear to have isolated ptosis with mild ophthalmoplegia but years later may entirely lose Bell's phenomenon, and his orbicularis oculi muscles may become weak. Thus a ptosis operation that is done early in life and seems ideal at the time may later seem to have been radical surgery when the patient's disease has progressed. In many cases one should avoid operating altogether. This does not mean that the ptosis cannot be treated. I have seen patients, managed by others, in whom a mechanical ptosis crutch has succeeded in maintaining satisfactory lid elevation. My own experience with lid crutches has been unsatisfactory, but crutches are worth trying. I have had much more success using tape. A transparent form of tape is used, and I find that patients can maintain satisfactory elevation of the lid without risk of exposure. Several patients have been using tape for years without any problems. The patients in whom lid surgery has been most effective in my experience have been those with the familial form of oculopharyngeal muscular dystrophy. These patients had a good range of eye movements and therefore have managed to protect their corneas from my levator resections. The subject of surgery for the ptosis in this particular disorder has been authoritatively discussed by Dr. Carl Johnson and Dr. Toichiro Kuwabara in a recent issue of the *American Journal of Ophthalmology*.[45] *Exercise great caution in selecting both the patients for ptosis surgery and the technique to be used.*

The dysphagia that occurs in some patients with CPEO is often amenable to surgery.[116] If the dysphagia is contributed to by failure of the cricopharyngeal muscle to relax, which can be demonstrated radiographically, relief may be obtained by myotomy of the inferior constrictor muscle.

Cardiac conduction effects in CPEO can be not only troublesome but fatal. Heart block can be prevented by the implantation of a demand pacemaker. It should be recognized that the cardiac problems that occur in some patients with CPEO might not be amenable to pacemaker therapy.

CONCLUSION

CPEO is important not because it is common but because it may occur in association with a variety of other neurologic and systemic abnormalities, because it may indicate the presence of a heredofamilial disorder, and because it may be amenable, at least in part, to therapy. In the preceding presentation I have described typical examples of CPEO and reviewed typical findings in CPEO. I have also described some atypical presentations and complications. It seems that CPEO can result from lesions at several levels in the ocular motor system and is not necessarily a myopathy. The limitations of the available techniques for distinguishing between neuropathy and myopathy contribute to the problem of understanding the pathogenesis of individual cases of CPEO. The observation of unusual ultrastructural abnormalities in many cases of CPEO is interesting but at the moment does not help one classify cases of CPEO or understand the cellular events that lead to the limitation of eye and lid movements. Hopefully, continuing investigation of CPEO will lead to therapy that can reverse or retard the development of ophthalmoplegia and ptosis.

REFERENCES

1. von Graefe, A.: Verhandlungen arztlicher Gesellschaften, Klin. Wochenschr. **5:**125-127, 1868.
2. Kiloh, L. G., and Nevin, S.: Progressive dystrophy of the external ocular muscles (ocular myopathy), Brain **74:**115-143, 1951.
3. Barbeau, A.: The syndome of hereditary late onset ptosis and dysphagia in French Canada. In Kuhn, E., editor: Progressive Muskeldystrophie, Myotonie, Myasthenie, Berlin, 1966, Springer Verlag.
4. Murphy, S. F., and Drachman, D. B.: The oculopharyngeal syndrome, J.A.M.A. **203:**1003-1008, 1968.
5. Kearns, T. P., and Sayre, G. P.: Retinitis pigmentosa external ophthalmoplegia and complete heart block, Arch. Ophthalmol. **60:**280-289, 1958.
6. Kearns, T. P.: External ophthalmoplegia, pigmentary degeneration of the retina and cardiomyopathy: a newly recognized syndrome, Trans. Am. Ophthalmol. Soc. **63:**559-625, 1965.
7. Szobor, A.: Data on the oculopharyngeal syndrome. A clinicopathological study, Eur. Neurol. **9:**242-259, 1973.
8. Lewis, I.: Oculopharyngeal muscular dystrophy. A family study. In Brunette, J. R., and Barbeau, A., editors: Progress in neuro-ophthalmology, Amsterdam, 1969, Excerpta Medica Foundation.
9. Laughlin, R. C.: Congenital fibrosis of extraocular muscles, Am. J. Ophthalmol. **41:**432-438, 1956.
10. Flieringa, H. T.: Familiare Ptosis congenital kombiniert mit anderen angeborenen beweglichkeits Defekten der Bulbusmuskulatur, Z. Augenheilkd. **52:** 1, 1924.
11. Jonkers, G. H.: Familial ptosis congenita combined with other congenital defects of motility of the ocular musculature, Ophthalmologica **120:**372-374, 1950.
12. Cogan, D. G.: Pathology of abiotrophic ophthalmoplegia externa, Johns Hopkins Med. J. **3:**42-56, 1962.
13. Bethleen, J., et al.: Centronuclear myopathy, Eur. Neurol. **1:**325-333, 1968.
14. Sher, J. H.: Familial centronuclear myopathy, Neurology (Minneap.) **17:** 727-742, 1967.
15. Spiro, A. J., et al.: Myotubular myopathy, Arch. Neurol. **14:**1-4, 1966.
16. Jampel, R. S., et al.: Ophthalmoplegia and retinal degeneration associated with spinocerebellar ataxia, Arch. Ophthalmol. **66:**247-258, 1961.
17. Heller, W.: Ueber Zw klinisch verschiedene Falle von chronischer progressiver Ophthalmoplegie, Z. Augenheilkd. **64:**136-142, 1928.
18. Jocas, M.: Rec. Ophtalmol. **15:**141-148, 1893. Cited by Kiloh, L. G., and Nevin, S.[2]
19. Hanke, V.: Neurol. Zentralbl. **14:**121, 1895. Cited by Kiloh, L. G., and Nevin, S.[2]
20. Fuchs, E.: Ueber isolirte doppelseitige Ptosis, Albrecht von Graefes Arch. Klin. Ophthalmol. **36:**234-259, 1890.
21. Fiorenza, I.: Contributo alla conoscenza dell' oftalmoplegia nucleare a tipo familiare, Pediatria (Napoli) **29:**200, 1921.
22. Magora, A., and Zauberman, H.: Ocular myopathy, Arch. Neurol. **20:**1-7, 1969.
23. Teasdale, R. D., and Sears, M. L.: Ocular myopathy: clinical and electromyographic considerations, Arch. Neurol. **2:**281-292, 1960.
24. Zintz, R., and Villiger, W.: Elektronenmikroskopische Befunde bei 3 Fallen von chronisch progressiver okularer Muskeldystrophie, Ophthalmologica **153:**439-459, 1967.
25. Beckett, R. S., and Netsky, M. G.: Familial ocular myopathy and external ophthalmoplegia, Arch. Neurol. **69:**64-72, 1953.
26. Fagin, I. D.: Chronic ophthalmoplegia externa: classification of causes. Report of case, Am. J. Ophthalmol. **25:**968-973, 1942.
27. Atland, W.: Arch. Ophthalmol. **38:**296, 1909. Cited by Kiloh, L. G., and Nevin, S.[2]
28. Lessell, S., et al.: Ophthalmoplegia in myotonic dystrophy, Am. J. Ophthalmol. **71:**1231-1236, 1971.
29. Badenoch, J., et al.: Encephalopathy in a case of Whipple's disease, J. Neurol. Neurosurg. Psychiatry **26:**203-210, 1963.
30. Mathew, N. T., et al.: Familial ocular myopathy with curare sensitivity, Arch. Neurol. **22:**68-74, 1972.

31. Ross, R. T.: Ocular myopathy sensitive to curare, Brain **86:**67-74, 1963.
32. Jacob, J. C., and Varkey, G.: Curare sensitivity in ocular myopathy, Can. Anaesth. Soc. J. **13:**449-453, 1966.
33. Lessell, S., et al.: Myopathy and succinylcholine sensitivity, Am. J. Ophthalmol. **68:**789-796, 1969.
34. Rosenberg, R. N., et al.: Progressive ophthalmoplegia. Report of cases, Arch. Neurol. **19:**362-376, 1968.
35. Rowland, L. P., et al.: Myasthenic syndromes, J. Nerv. Ment. Dis. **38:**548-600, 1958.
36. Glaser, J. S., et al.: The edrophonium tonogram test in myasthenia gravis, Arch. Ophthalmol. **76:**368-373, 1966.
37. Wray, S. H., and Pavan-Langston, D.: A reevaluation of edrophonium chloride (Tensilon) tonography in the diagnosis of myasthenia gravis, Neurology (Minneap.) **21:**586-593, 1971.
38. Drachman, D. A.: Ophthalmoplegia plus. The neurodegenerative disorders associated with progressive external ophthalmoplegia, Arch. Neurol. **18:**654-674, 1968.
39. Roberts, A. H., and Bamforth, J.: The pharynx and esophagus in ocular muscle dystrophy, Neurology (Minneap.) **18:** 645-652, 1968.
40. Bray, G. M., et al.: Ocular myopathy with dysphagia, Neurology (Minneap.) **18:**678-684, 1965.
41. Walton, J. N.: Some clinical and genetic aspects of muscular dystrophies. In Paul, W. M., et al., editors: Muscle, New York, 1965, Pergamon Press, Inc.
42. Taylor, E. W.: Progressive vagus-glossopharyngeal paralysis with ptosis. A contribution to the group of family diseases, J. Nerv. Ment. Dis. **42:**129-139, 1915.
43. Victor, M., et al.: Oculopharyngeal muscle dystrophy, N. Engl. J. Med. **267:**1269-1272, 1962.
44. Cogan, D., et al.: Classification of primary ocular myopathies. A panel. In Brunette, J. R., and Barbeau, A., editors: Progress in neuro-ophthalmology, Amsterdam, 1969, Excerpta Medica Foundation.
45. Johnson, C. C., and Kuwabara, T.: Oculopharyngeal muscular dystrophy, Am. J. Ophthalmol. **77:**872-879, 1974.
46. Lewis, L.: Late-onset muscle dystrophy: oculopharyngoesophageal variety, Can. Med. Assoc. J. **95:**146-150, 1966.
47. Erdbrink, W. L.: Ocular myopathy associated with retinitis pigmentosa, Arch. Ophthalmol. **57:**335-338, 1957.
48. Woordenburg, P. J., et al.: Genetics and ophthalmology, vol. 1, Springfield, Ill., 1961, Charles C Thomas Publisher, p. 438.
49. Koerner, F., and Schlote, W.: Chronic progressive external ophthalmoplegia associated with retinitis pigmentary changes and evidence in favor of ocular myopathy, Arch. Ophthalmol. **88:**155-166, 1972.
50. Thorson, J. C., and Bell, W. E.: Progressive dystrophic external ophthalmoplegia with abiotrophic fundus changes, Arch. Ophthalmol. **62:**833-838, 1959.
51. Walsh, F.: Clinical Neuro-ophthalmology, ed. 2, Baltimore, 1957, The Williams & Wilkins Company, pp. 644-646.
52. Chamlin, M., and Billet, E.: Ophthalmoplegia and pigmentary degeneration of the retina, Arch. Ophthalmol. **43:**217-223, 1950.
53. Kornzweig, A. L., and Bassen, F. A.: Retinitis pigmentosa, acanthrocytosis and heredodegenerative neuromuscular disease, Arch. Ophthalmol. **58:**183-187, 1957.
54. Refsum, S.: Heredopathia atactica polyneuritoformes, J. Nerv. Ment. Dis. **116:** 1046-1050, 1952.
55. Burian, H. M., and Burns, C. A.: Ocular changes in myotonic dystrophy, Am. J. Ophthalmol. **63:**22-34, 1967.
56. Cogan, D. G.: Personal communication.
57. Crosby, T. W., and Chou, S. M.: "Ragged-red" fibers in Leigh's disease, Neurology (Minneap.) **24:**49-54, 1974.
58. Lind, I., and Prame, G.: Chronic progressive external ophthalmoplegia and muscular dystrophy, Acta Ophthalmol. (Kbh.) **41:**497-507, 1963.
59. Shy, G. M., et al.: A generalized disorder of nervous system, skeletal muscle and heart resembling Refsum's disease with Hurler's syndrome. I. Clinical pathologic and biochemical characteristics, Am. J. Med. **42:**163-168, 1967.
60. James, T. N.: Observations on cardiovascular involvement, including cardiac conduction system in progressive mus-

cular dystrophy, Am. Heart J. **63**:18 56, 1962.
61. Perloff, J. K., et al.: The cardiomyopathy of progressive muscular dystrophy, Circulation **33**:625-648, 1966.
62. Steele, J. C., et al.: Progressive supranuclear palsy. A heterogeneous degeneration involving the brain stem, basal ganglia and cerebellum with vertical gaze and pseudobulbar palsy, nuchal dystonia and dementia, Arch. Neurol. **10**:333-359, 1964.
63. Behrman, S., et al.: Progressive supranuclear palsy. Clinicopathological study of four cases, Brain **92**:663-678, 1969.
64. Dix, M. R., et al.: Progressive supranuclear palsy (the Steele-Richardson-Olszewski syndrome), J. Neurol. Sci. **13**: 237-256, 1971.
65. Lampert, P., et al.: Encephalopathy in Whipple's disease, Neurology (Minneap.) **12**:65-71, 1962.
66. Pachter, B. R., Davidowitz, J., and Breinin, G. M.: Morphological changes associated with the myoneural junction in extraocular muscle of the dystrophic mouse, Acta Neuropathol. (Berl.) **24**:214-221, 1973.
67. Pachter, B. R., Davidowitz, J., and Breinin, G. M.: A phase-electron microscopic study of extraocular muscle dystrophy in the mouse, Invest. Ophthalmol. **11**:715-722, 1972.
68. Pachter, B. R.: A light and electron microscope study in serial section of dystrophic extraocular muscle fibers, Invest. Ophthalmol. **12**:917-923, 1973.
69. Woolf, A. L.: Morphology of the myasthenic neuromuscular junction, Ann. N. Y. Acad. Sci. **135**:35-59, 1966.
70. Coers, C., and Desmedt, J. E.: Abnormal end-plates in myasthenic muscle, Lancet **2**:1124, 1958.
71. Coers, C., and Woolf, A. L.: Innervation of muscle, Oxford, 1959, Blackwell Scientific Publications, Ltd.
72. Farmbrough, D. M., et al.: Neuromuscular junction in myasthenia gravis: decreased acetylcholine receptors, Science **182**:293-295, 1973.
73. Rowland, L. P., et al.: Myasthenic syndromes, J. Nerv. Ment. Dis. **38**:548-600, 1958.
74. Ferguson, F. R.: A critical review of the clinical features of myasthenia gravis, Proc. R. Soc. Med. **55**:49-52, 1962.
75. Turner, J. W. A.: Myasthenia gravis, Proc. R. Soc. Med. **67**:763-769, 1974.
76. Drachman, D. A.: Discussion of paper by Smith, J. L., Trans. Am. Acad. Ophthalmol. Otolaryngol. **78**: 797-798, 1974.
77. Oosterhuis, H., and Bethlen, J.: Neurogenic muscle involvement in myasthenia gravis, J. Neurol. Neurosurg. Psychiatry **36**:244-254, 1973.
78. Rowland, L. P.: Myasthenic myopathy and thymoma, Neurology (Minneap.) **23**:282-288, 1973.
79. Langden, N. M., and Cadwalader, W. B.: Chronic progressive external ophthalmoplegia, Brain **51**:321-333, 1928.
80. Jedlowski, P.: Sulla oftalmpliegia externa nucleare cronica progressiva, Riv. Oto-neuro-oftal. **20**:203, 1943.
81. Daroff, R. B., et al.: Spongiform encephalopathy with chronic progressive ophthalmoplegia (central ophthalmoplegia mimicking ocular myopathy), Neurology (Minneap.) **16**:161-169, 1966.
82. Brion, S., and De Recondo, J. D.: Ophthalmoplegie nucleaire progressive et heredo-degenerescence spino-cerebelleus. Etude d'un cas anatomo-clinique, Rev. Neurol. (Paris) **116**:383-400, 1967.
83. Gomez, M. R.: Progressive bulbar paralysis in childhood (Fazio-Londe's disease), Arch. Neurol. **6**:317-323, 1962.
84. Lovelance, R. E., et al.: The Kugelberg-Welander syndrome, Trans. Am. Neurol. Assoc. **91**:286-288, 1966.
85. Brandt, S.: Werdnig-Hoffmann's infantile progressive muscular atrophy Copenhagen, 1950, Ejnar Munksgaards Forlag.
86. Thieffry, S., et al.: Quarante cas de maladie de Werdnig-Hoffmann avec onze exambns anatomiques, Rev. Neurol. (Paris) **93**:621-644, 1955.
87. Byers, R. K., and Bankec, B. Q.: Infantile muscular atrophy, Arch. Neurol. **5**:140-164, 1961.
88. Molbert, E., and Doden, W.: Chronisch-progressive Okulare Muskeldystrophie im elektronmikroskopischen Bilde, Ber. Dtsch. Ophthalmol. Ges. **62**:392-397, 1959.
89. Schwarz, G. A., and Liu, C.: Chronic

progressive external ophthalmoplegia, Arch. Neurol. **71:**31-53, 1954.

90. Stephens, J., et al.: On familial ataxia, neural amyotrophy, and their association with progressive external ophthalmoplegia, Brain **81:**556-566, 1958.
91. Stojanow, V. W., and Janisch, W.: Die okulare Muskeldystrophie, Psychiatr. Neurol. Med. Psychol. (Leipz.) **14:**130-134, 1962.
92. Daroff, R. B.: Chronic progressive external ophthalmoplegia. A critical review, Arch. Ophthalmol. **82:**845-850, 1969.
93. Breinin, G.: The electrophysiology of extraocular muscle, Toronto, 1962, University of Toronto Press.
94. Papst, W.: Die okulare Muskeldystrophie, Klin. Monatsbl. Augenheilkd. **132:** 691-707, 1958.
95. Drachman, D. A., et al.: Myopathic changes in chronically denervated muscle, Arch. Neurol. **16:**14-24, 1967.
96. Drachman, D. A., et al.: Experimental denervation of ocular muscles. A critique of the concept of "ocular myopathy," Arch. Neurol. **21:**170-183, 1969.
97. McComas, A. J., et al.: Multiple muscle analysis of motor units in muscular dystrophy, Arch. Neurol. **30:**249-251, 1974.
98. McComas, A. J., et al.: An electrophysiological study of Duchenne dystrophy, J. Neurol. Neurosurg. Psychiatry **34:**461-468, 1971.
99. McComas, A. J., et al.: Electrophysiological study of dystrophia myotonica, J. Neurol. Neurosurg. Psychiatry **34:**132-139, 1971.
100. Sica, R. E. P., and McComas, A. J.: An electrophysiological investigation of limb girdle and facioscapulohumeral dystrophy, J. Neurol. Neurosurg. Psychiatry **34:**469-474, 1971.
101. Morgan-Hughes, J. A., and Mair, W. G. P.: Atypical muscle mitochondria in oculoskeletal myopathy, Brain **96:** 215-224, 1973.
102. Olson, W., et al.: Oculocraniosomatic neuromuscular disease with "ragged-red" fibers, Arch. Neurol. **26:**193-211, 1972.
103. Schneck, L., et al.: Ophthalmoplegia plus with morphological and chemical studies of cerebellar and muscle tissue, J. Neurol. Sci. **19:**37-44, 1973.
104. Karpati, G., et al.: The Kearns-Shy syndrome. A multisystem disease with mitochondrial abnormality demonstrated in skeletal muscle and skin, J. Neurol. Sci. **19:**133-151, 1973.
105. Crosby, T. W., and Chou, S. M.: "Ragged-red" fibers in Leigh's disease, Neurology (Minneap.) **24:**49-54, 1974.
106. Rebeiz, J. J., et al.: Oculopharyngeal dystrophy—a presenescent myopathy. In Brunette, J. R., and Barbeau, A., editors: Progress in neuro-ophthalmology, Amsterdam, 1969, Excerpta Medica Foundation.
107. Radnot, M.: Mitochondrial crystals in muscles of a patient with spastic entropion, Am. J. Ophthalmol. **75:**713-719, 1973.
108. Shafiq, S. A., et al.: Giant mitochondria in human muscles with inclusions, Arch. Neurol. **17:**666-671, 1967.
109. DeRecondo, J., et al.: Etude ali microscope electronique des lesions musculaires d'atrophie neurogene par atteinte de la corne anterieure, Rev. Neurol. (Paris) **114:**169, 1966.
110. Schaff, Z., et al.: On the ultrastructure of Gilbert's disease, Morphol. Igazsagugyi Orv. Sz. **10:**17, 1972.
111. Fischer, K. C., and Schwartzman, R. J.: Oral corticosteroids in the treatment of ocular myasthenia gravis, Neurology (Minneap.) **24:**795-798, 1974.
112. Gibberd, F. B., et al.: Treatment of ocular myasthenia with corticotropin, J. Neurol. Neurosurg. Psychiatry **34:**11-13, 1971.
113. Cape, C. A.: Ocular response to corticotropin in myasthenia gravis, Arch. Ophthalmol. **90:**292-293, 1973.
114. Warmolts, J. R., and Engel, W. K.: Benefit from alternate-day prednisone in myasthenia gravis, N. Engl. J. Med. **286:**17-20, 1969.
115. Metz, H. S., and Meshel, L.: Ocular saccades in progressive external ophthalmoplegia, Am. J. Ophthalmol. **6:**623-628, 1974.
116. Montgomery, W. W., and Lynch, J. P.: Oculopharyngeal muscular dystrophy treated by inferior constrictor myotomy, Trans. Am. Acad. Ophthalmol. Otolaryngol. **75:**986-993, 1971.

Chapter 12

Assessment of pupillary abnormalities

John A. McCrary, III

The purpose of this chapter is to acquaint practicing ophthalmologists, neurologists, and neurosurgeons with disorders that may affect pupillary function. The use of the pupil as a diagnostic tool for localization of neurologic lesions is of undisputed value. This chapter deals first with the current understanding of the normal neuroanatomy and neuropharmacology of pupillary function. Following this is a short description of normal pupillary physiology, then a section on clinical testing. The final section deals with common clinical abnormalities of the pupil. It is not the purpose of the chapter to describe every known disorder of the pupil. In the interest of brevity, those disorders of questionable importance, those rarely seen, and those previously described that frankly do not exist will not be discussed.

NORMAL PUPILLARY NEUROANATOMY AND NEUROPHARMACOLOGY

Parasympathetic influence on pupil

The amount of parasympathetic outflow to the pupil is the main factor governing its size. The activity of this system is primarily a function of the quantity of light input into the afferent side of the pupillomotor arc, which governs the output of the efferent pupillomotor pathway. A number of factors may modify the output of the parasympathetic connections to the pupil.

The afferent neural relay for the pupillary response to light begins with the afferent relay for vision at the photoreceptor layer of the retina. This pathway proceeds inward by synaptic connections through the bipolar and ganglion cell layers of the retina. The axons of the ganglion cell layer, which constitute the nerve fiber layer of the retina, continue centripetally toward the scleral canal, eventually forming the optic nerve. They advance toward the optic chiasm where the pathways decussate. Slightly more than half of the visual afferents pass from each eye into the opposite optic tract (retinal representation for visual field temporal to fixation) while the remainder continue more or less directly posteriorly toward the ipsilateral optic tract (retinal representation for visual field nasal to fixation). Thus the afferents for the pupil and the afferents for vision follow the same basic route in the retina, optic nerve, chiasm, and optic tract. Whether or not there are two separate systems for vision and for pupillary function is still debated. In all probability, the afferents for the pupillomotor system are simple axonic branches coming from the visual afferents in the extreme posterior optic tract. These pupil afferents enter the brain stem through the brachium of the superior colliculus and subsequently make their way into the pretectal region of the diencephalic brain stem. At this point a synaptic connection exists in the pretectal nucleus. An intercalated neuron passes from this nucleus around either side of the sylvian aqueduct forming a second decussation. The intercalated neurons achieve their final synaptic destination in the Edinger-Westphal nucleus. At this point the afferent side of the arc is completed (Fig. 12-1).

The efferent parasympathetic pupillomotor pathway begins at the Edinger-Westphal nucleus. Preganglionic parasympathetic fibers arise from the Edinger-Westphal nucleus, a midline structure located just rostral to the third nerve nuclei in the mesencephalic brain stem. These parasympathetic motoneurons pass ventrally through the brain stem in association with the fasicular components of each third cranial nerve. They exit the ventral stem located superiorly and superficially in the root of the third nerve. These fibers gradually rotate downward and medially as they pass forward toward the superior orbital fissure. When viewed from behind, the pathways rotate counterclockwise in the right third nerve, and clockwise in the left third nerve. Ultimately these pathways descend into the inferior division of the third nerve as it divides near the superior orbital fissure. They continue forward into the orbit through the inferior division and ultimately gain access to the ciliary ganglion through the short (motor) root. Within the ganglion, synaptic connections are made with postganglionic parasympathetic fibers that pass forward into the globe as the short ciliary nerves. These parasympathetics terminate in the pupillary sphincter or the ciliary body (Fig. 12-1). The majority, approximately 90%, are devoted to accommodation, whereas 5% are directed toward the iris sphincter. These terminals secrete acetylcholine to bring about pupil constriction by increasing the activity of the iris sphincter. Damage to the ciliary ganglion or the postganglionic parasympathetic pathways results in denervation supersensitivity to weak cholinergic solutions.

Near synkinesis. The anterior portion of the occipital cortex appears to be the primary locus for the initiation of the near synkinesis, which consists of accommodation, convergence and constriction of the pupil. The subcortical

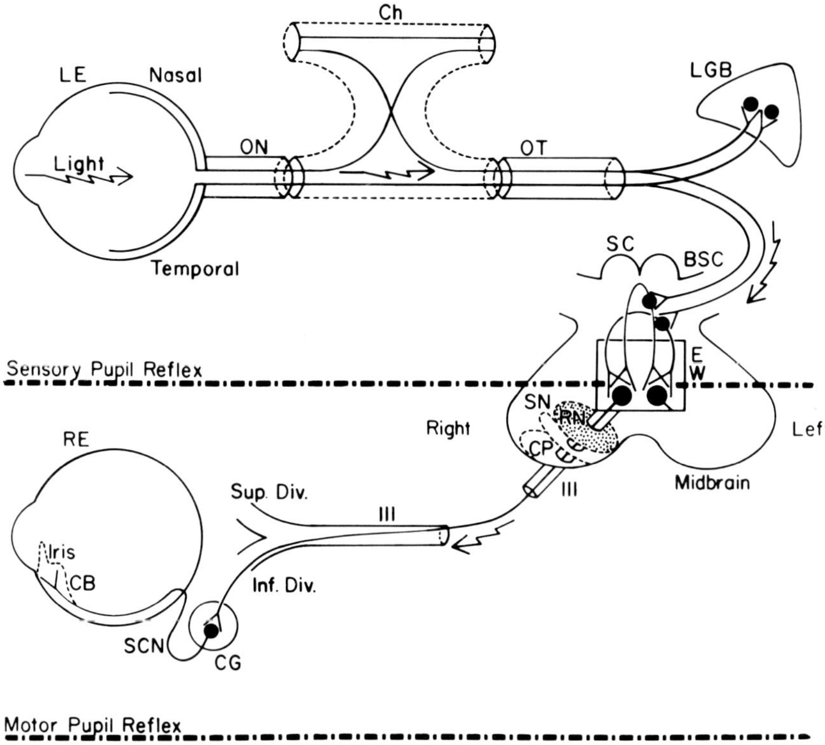

Fig. 12-1. Diagrammatic representation of neural pathway for pupillary light reflex. Sensory portion (top) includes optic nerve *(ON)*, chiasm *(Ch)*, optic tract *(OT)*, lateral geniculate body *(LGB)*, brachium of the superior colliculus *(BSC)*, and superior colliculus *(SC)*. At beginning of motor arc (bottom) is Edinger-Westphal nucleus *(EW)*, followed by substantia nigra *(SN)*, red nucleus *(RN)*, cerebral peduncle *(CP)*, oculomotor nerve *(III)*, ciliary ganglion *(CG)*, and short ciliary nerves *(SCN)*.

pathway from the occipital associational cortex passes downward through corticotectal connections into the pretectum of the brain stem. After synapsis, the pathways are routed into the tegmental portion of the mesencephalic brain stem; ultimately these neural elements synapse in the Edinger-Westphal nucleus and the nuclei of each oculomotor nerve to mediate miosis, accommodation and convergence. These neurons enter the Edinger-Westphal nucleus and third nerve nuclei from a ventral route as compared to the pathways that are concerned with the pupillary response to light. This would explain anatomically the ability of the pupils to constrict during the near synkinesis while being unable to respond to stimulation from a bright light.

Inhibitory pathway to Edinger-Westphal nucleus. A group of polysynaptic corticomesencephalic and spinal reticulomesencephalic neurons modify the activity of the Edinger-Westphal nucleus. The activity of these pathways is extremely important in governing the resting pupillary size in ambient light. A decrease in the level of cortical activity with subsequent loss of inhibition of the Edinger-Westphal nucleus allows the parasympathetic pupillomotor fibers to increase their output. This results in a small pupil diameter in each eye, most commonly seen in sleep. Similarly, decreased inhibitory activity from the spinal cord level mediated by the reticular formation achieves the same result. Increased inhibition of the Edinger-Westphal nucleus through either of these pathways produces a larger pupil size.

Sympathetic influence on pupil

The effect of activity of the sympathetic autonomic nervous system on pupillary size is less important than that of parasympathetic activity. The sympathetic pathway has its origin in the posterior hypothalamus. The first-neuron sympathetic axons then proceed caudally through the brain stem. At each succeeding level (mesencephalic, pontine, and medullary) the pathways diverge laterally. Subsequently they adopt a superficial location in the cervical spinal cord just beneath the dentate ligaments. These pathways continue downward in the cervical cord to the C_8-T_2 level. At this juncture they turn inward to synapse with the second-neuron cell bodies in the intermediolateral gray substance (ciliospinal center of Budge). This ends the first-neuron sympathetic pathway. The second neuron passes out of the spinal cord through the white rami and then enters the cervical sympathetic chain. These constituents ascend through the inferior, middle, and superior cervical ganglia. Those sympathetic components earmarked for the orbit undergo a final synaptic connection in the superior cervical ganglion. The third-order neurons pass from the superior cervical ganglion into the carotid sympathetic plexus. They enter the cranial vault through the foramen lacerum closely investing the internal carotid artery. These fine fibers continue upward into the cavernous sinus. Upon leaving the cavernous sinus they project anteriorly to enter the orbit through various routes. Some fibers enter the orbit with the ophthalmic division of the fifth cranial nerve, and they ultimately pass into the nasociliary branch of the ophthalmic division. Utilizing the long ciliary nerves, they achieve the pupillary dilator muscle. At this point they secrete norepinephrine as the chemical product of the terminal boutons. Other sympathetics enter the globe through the sympathetic root of the ciliary ganglion; they come through the superior orbital fissure, pass without synapsis through the ciliary ganglion, and enter the globe with the short ciliary nerves to provide vasomotor control of blood vessels within the globe.

Increased activity of the sympathetic nervous system due to stimulation through pain, fear, or other modalities will produce a rapid dilatation of the pupils through stimulation of this three-neuron arc to the dilator muscle of the iris. The pathways of the sympathetic nervous system that innervate vasomotor control and sweating for the face are essentially all confined to the distribution of the external carotid circulation. Only the central portion of the forehead is supplied by sympathetic neurons that follow the internal carotid branches.

NORMAL PUPILLARY PHYSIOLOGY

Direct light reflex. In the normal individual, the pupil constricts rapidly and extensively when subjected to suprathreshold light stimulation. This response generally has a latency period of approximately 0.25 seconds, although the latency may be increased as the strength of the stimulus is reduced. The gradation of the direct light reflex is essentially a linear function of the intensity of the light stimulus and the degree of dark adaptation. Placing a very bright light before the eye of an individual who has remained in a darkened room for several minutes will evoke a rapid, extensive constriction of the pupil.

Consensual (indirect) light reflex. The response of the pupil in the eye opposite to the stimulus source is usually identical to that of the directly stimulated eye. This behavior of the pupil in the nonstimulated eye is known as the consensual, or indirect, light reflex. Because of the decussation of visual afferents previously described, the reaction of the pupil in the consensually stimulated eye is a carbon copy of that elicited in the directly stimulated eye. The rate of constriction, the latency period, and the extent of constriction are equivalent in all respects. Normally the speed of redilatation after removal of the light source from the stimulated eye is the same in both eyes. This latter response is known as the darkness reflex.

Near reflex (synkinesis). When an effort is made to direct visual attention on an object near the face, the pupils promptly constrict. Although accommodation, convergence, and miosis occur simultaneously in the near synkinesis, each can be generated independently under special test circumstances. The triad of ocular signs associated with observation of an object near the face is not a true reflex but a synkinesis. The near synkinesis is produced by using the patient's finger as the near stimulus. An adequate near synkinesis can be generated even in an individual with bilateral blindness using this method. The tactile sensory stimulation obtained by using the patient's finger as the target for fixation allows the generation of an adequate near synkinesis. In the normal individual the near synkinesis does not generate the extensive constriction of the pupil seen with light stimulation. This point is important in considering the entity known as light-near dissociation. To evaluate the constriction of the pupil to a near stimulus one must indirectly illuminate the patient's eyes sufficiently to make observations of the pupillary contraction.

Pupillary unrest. When the pupils of a normal individual are observed under steady illumination, small, nonrhythmic oscillations are visible. The amplitude of excursion is usually 0.5 mm. These movements should not be confused with hippus. Pupillary unrest may be blocked in the normal individual by psychosensory stimulation. It may be increased with fatigue.

Hippus. Large rhythmic oscillations of the pupils of 1.0 mm or more in a patient with depressed alertness is called hippus. Though hippus is described in many normal individuals with decreased alertness,[1] it is seen in a number of pathologic states causing diffuse brain damage, such as hypoxia, cerebral contusion, metabolic encephalopathy, and toxic states. Although considered here under the category of normal pupillary physiology, hippus obviously does occur in certain pathologic conditions.*

Psychosensory reflex. Increased levels of alertness may be produced by a number of means. Pinching the skin of the neck (ciliospinal reflex), stimulation with sound, or other methods may be utilized to elevate the patient's level of central nervous system activity. When this happens, neural discharges through the sympathetic trunks cause rapid bilateral dilatation of the pupils. This normal reflex may be fatigued with repeated stimulation.

Fatigue effect. The diameter of the pupils decreases and oscillation increases as an individual fatigues. A generalized decrease in the level of central nervous system activity tends to produce such an effect. The relationship of the fatigue effect to pupillary unrest and hippus can be readily appreciated. Increased stimulation by the psychosensory reflex may block the fatigue effect temporarily. Widely dilated pupils that oscillate slightly or not at all under steady illumination result from such stimulation.

Humoral effects. The pupil of a normal individual may dilate as a result of an outpouring of adrenergic amines. These adrenergic substances may be derived from the heart and great vessels and also from the adrenal stores. The effect of these circulating amines on the pupil takes several seconds to develop, as opposed to the almost instantaneous responses that occur with psychosensory stimulation. Slower dilation of the pupil may also arise from the effect of increased activity of the polysynaptic pathways through the reticular activating system inhibiting the Edinger-Westphal nucleus. Both of these mechanisms are influential in governing the overall size and function of the pupil.

Size. The normal pupil ranges from 2 to 6 mm in diameter, averaging about 3.5 mm. In infants the iris dilator muscle is not well developed and the pupil therefore is small.† The pupils in infants dilate poorly under the effect of mydriatic and cycloplegic agents. The pupil size gradually increases in childhood and youth. Maximum sizes are reached during youth. After the age of 30 years the average pupillary diameter begins to decrease very slowly. In the elderly, pupil diameters are quite similar to those in earliest

---

*EDITOR'S NOTE. For most clinicians, "pupillary unrest" and hippus are equivalent and nonpathologic. J. S. G.

†EDITOR'S NOTE. In addition, in the infant diminished activity of the brain-stem reticular activating system reduces inhibition of pretectal pupilloconstrictor center, with resultant miosis. J. S. G.

life. The pupil becomes less responsive to light with age. The pupil diameter is not significantly related to either sex or iris color, although older reports in the literature have suggested such relationships. The average size is greater in the myopic individual than in the hyperopic individual.[2] Anisocoria is common in normal individuals. Some appreciable difference in pupillary size is seen in 17% to 20% of normal persons; a difference of 1.0 mm or more occurs in 4% to 5% of the population.*

CLINICAL TESTING

Accurate evaluation of the pupils requires time and perseverance on the part of the examiner. In evaluating the pupils, one should attempt to standardize room lighting as much as possible, especially when measuring pupil responses to light and near in the same individual on several occasions. It is advisable to have a standardized pattern for illumination of the examination room when the pupils are tested. When the pupils are examined at the bedside, one has to reduce room lighting to obtain maximum pupillary responses to light stimulation. It is important that a bright light be used for pupil stimulation. For the ophthalmologist the best light source is the indirect ophthalmoscope turned to the 7.5-volt setting. Disposable penlights generate a very bright light but have a short life span. These should be changed frequently if used for pupil testing. Before the response of the pupil to light is evaluated, the patient should fixate on some specific distant object. With a comatose individual this obviously is impossible. Obtunded individuals may or may not be capable of distant fixation. After the patient fixates on the distant object, the examiner should measure or estimate the size of each pupil. Measuring the size of the pupil is preferable. The measurement, of course, should be recorded. After each pupil has been measured, the direct light response should be checked on at least three successive trials. The responses are surveyed and graded on a scale of 0 to 4+. This is an arbitrary scale but is far superior to the "PERLA" classification, which is meaningless. One may also grade the consensual response. This is somewhat more difficult; the oblique illumination of the nonstimulated eye must be sufficient to allow the response of the indirectly reacting pupil to be seen.

Following direct light testing, one should develop the habit of testing for a Marcus Gunn pupillary sign.[3, 4] The examiner presents a bright light source before the better eye. He notes the speed and extent of pupil constriction and then moves the light rapidly across the nose to stimulate the defective eye. If a Marcus Gunn sign is present, the pupil of the defective eye will dilate slightly or extensively depending on the severity of the sensory defect. In the normal individual when no significant difference between conduction velocity in retina or optic nerve exists between the two eyes, swinging light quickly from the right eye to the left eye and back to the right eye again yields an

*EDITOR'S NOTE. Anisocoria may vary during a 24-hour period. This "central" anisocoria defies explanation. J. S. G.

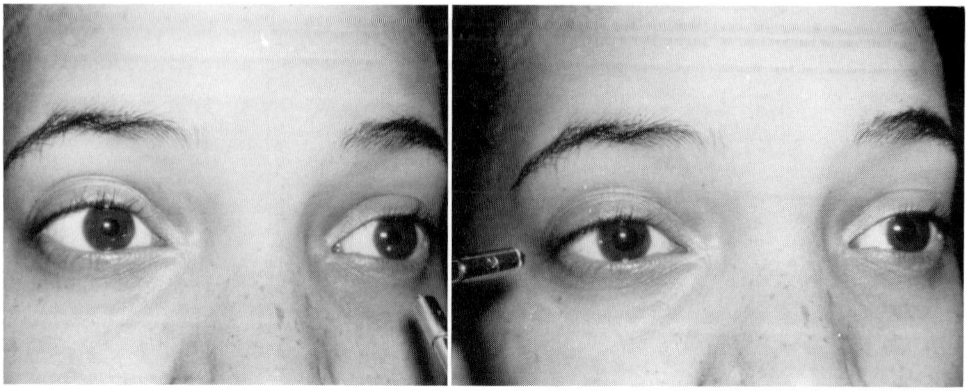

Fig. 12-2. Patient has afferent pupil defect on right due to optic neuritis. If light is moved from left eye to right eye, pupils dilate rather than constrict. When light is moved from right eye to left eye, both pupils constrict immediately. Thus, patient has Marcus Gunn pupillary sign on right.

immediate constriction of the pupil as soon as the light strikes each eye alternately. With a Marcus Gunn pupil, however, when the light strikes the affected eye there is no crisp constriction of the pupil. Instead the pupil fails to constrict. In fact, the pupil dilates slightly under the influence of the light (Fig. 12-2). When the light is then returned to the better eye, the pupil immediately shows a constrictive motion. The presence of a Marcus Gunn pupil is therefore proof that a conduction defect exists in one eye. It localizes the defect anterior to the chiasm. Obviously, when the pupil of the eye with sensory loss dilates under light stimulation, the opposite pupil does the same. Thus, there is a consensual and a direct Marcus Gunn sign.

Pupil measurements and the responses to testing for direct and consensual light reflex, near reflex, and presence of a Marcus Gunn pupil may be recorded very simply as follows:

R.E.	4.0 mm	3+	4+	(2+ Marcus Gunn)
L.E.	4.0 mm	4+	4+	

I generally do not record the consensual light response unless there is a specific need to do so, as when looking for evidence of residual visual function in an eye that is blind according to the patient's history. In this circumstance, a consensual reponse in the unaffected eye when the "blind eye" is stimulated indicates the presence of some residual visual function in the "blind eye."

CLINICAL PUPILLARY ABNORMALITIES

Afferent pupillary defects

In general, pure afferent pupillary defects do not produce anisocoria. This has been repeatedly documented by pupillographic investigation. Any anisocoria associated with sensory loss in one or both eyes must be due either to a preexisting inequality in pupillary size or to some involvement of sympathetic or parasympathetic motor supply to the pupil. Afferent defects are associated with abnormalities in the visual acuity or visual field of the affected eye. When the defect is unilateral, the patient will show one of three types of pupillary abnormalities: the amaurotic pupil, unilateral light-near dissociation of the pupil, or the Marcus Gunn pupil. With marked bilateral afferent defects, the patient generally shows bilateral light-near dissociation.

The amaurotic pupil, the pupil of a blind eye, has certain stereotyped characteristics that set it apart from other sensory pupillary abnormalities. For example, when the blind eye is stimulated, one does not see a direct or a consensual pupillary response. When the uninvolved eye is stimulated, one can see a good direct and a good consensual response. Also the patient shows equal and adequate constriction of both pupils to the near synkinesis. It is imperative that careful testing for residual consensual response in the unaffected eye be carried out before deciding that the defective eye is blind. This can be done best by placing one hand vertically over the bridge of the patient's nose to prevent extraneous light input into the unaffected eye. The affected eye is stimulated with the indirect ophthalmoscope light at maximum intensity. A consensual response is looked for. This observation may require an assistant. Some oblique illumination must be used for the pupil reaction to be seen. If no consensual response can be elicited, the eye is truly blind. Although one may accept the fact that from a psychic viewpoint the patient may be "blind" when a consensual response can be elicited, one should be extremely careful in accepting the affected eye as being physiologically blind. This is particularly important when considering surgical removal of a traumatized eye. The presence of residual consensual pupillary response in the unaffected eye indicates that some visual function may still remain. There is reason for caution in considering enucleation in such a case.

Unilateral light-near dissociation

When a conduction defect of the optic nerve or retina of one eye is not sufficiently serious to produce blindness, the responsiveness of the pupil to direct light stimulation will often decrease markedly, whereas the pupil will constrict better on near fixation. This is light-near dissociation. It may occur monocularly in a patient in whom neural conduction is seriously impaired by extensive retinal or optic nerve damage. Like the Marcus Gunn pupil, light-near dissociation is not seen when monocular visual decrease is due to uncorrected refractive error, irregular astigmatism, lenticular abnormalities such as lenticonus or cataract, or opacification of the vitreous body. The detection of unilateral light-near dissociation in an eye with opaque media indicates that the patient has a significant problem with either the retina or the optic nerve in that eye. The cause cannot be known until further diagnostic studies are carried out, but one can predict that the patient's visual outcome will be less than would be expected normally if a lens extraction is undertaken.

Marcus Gunn pupil (afferent pupillary defect/swinging flashlight sign)

In patients who have even less severe involvement of the retina or the optic nerve, the only evidence for a conduction deficiency may be the Marcus Gunn pupil. Involvement of the optic nerve or retina may not be severe enough to produce a slowing of the direct pupillary response to light or the findings consistent with the amaurotic pupil, but there may be a significant sensory defect involving one eye. When both eyes have a sensory defect, the eye with an afferent pupillary sign has the more severe impairment. There is no such entity as a bilateral Marcus Gunn pupil. Retinal disease sufficient to produce an afferent pupillary defect is usually rather extensive. On rare occasions, large destructive lesions of the macula alone can produce an afferent pupillary abnormality. The Marcus Gunn pupil is most helpful in recognizing optic nerve disease when vision is fairly good. A Marcus Gunn pupil may be the only objective evidence that a patient with visual complaints and 20/20 visual acuity actually has a lesion involving the optic nerve. It is one of the key diagnostic findings in the 20% of patients with optic neuritis who have reasonably good visual acuity. Optic nerve disease sufficient to produce a visual field defect or a defect in visual acuity or both will rarely if ever fail to show a Marcus Gunn pupil unless some other pupillary abnormality masks its presence. Involvement of the parasympathetic pathways to the pupil may obscure a Marcus Gunn phenomenon.

In a patient with a motor pupil defect in one eye and an associated conduction defect, one can observe the consensual pupil response when the light is moved from the better eye to the affected eye and back again. If, on moving the light from the better eye to the affected eye, the pupil in the better eye fails to show a prompt constriction or dilates as light floods the eye with the motor pupil defect, then the motor-defect eye has an afferent conduction defect as well. Some have used the term *inverse Marcus Gunn pupillary sign* for this phenomenon, but I object to this terminology. The term *consensual,* or *indirect, Marcus Gunn pupillary sign* could be used. A more acceptable term might be *consensual afferent pupillary defect.*

With subtle afferent pupillary abnormalities, it may be necessary to alternate the light between the better eye and the affected eye several times. It may take five minutes of careful pupil testing in order to bring out a really subtle Marcus Gunn defect. The time spent on careful testing of the subtleties of conduction pupillary defects is well worth the investment. I have personally seen several patients who were thought to have functional loss of the visual acuity or visual field in one eye but had a Marcus Gunn pupil on careful examination. It is obvious that such a person has organic, not functional, visual loss. The importance of this sign cannot be overemphasized. The Marcus Gunn pupil is generally associated with defective visual acuity or visual field or both. There may be a normal direct response to light but a Marcus Gunn pupil can still be seen.

Bilateral light-near dissociation

Bilateral dissociation of the light and near response occurs in several conditions. It may be present in bilateral retinal disease or bilateral damage to the optic nerve. It is also seen as a common feature of involvement of the chiasm. In this circumstance it is often called tabes pituitaria, since pituitary adenomas are a common cause of chiasmal compression, bitemporal visual field defects, and slowing of the light response of the pupils. Light-near dissociation may also be present in lesions affecting the optic tract. It is commonly present in disease of the mesencephalic brain stem wherein the afferent pathways for the light reflex are compromised. One of the common causes for light-near dissociation due to tectal compression is pinealoma (Fig. 12-3).[5]

A

B

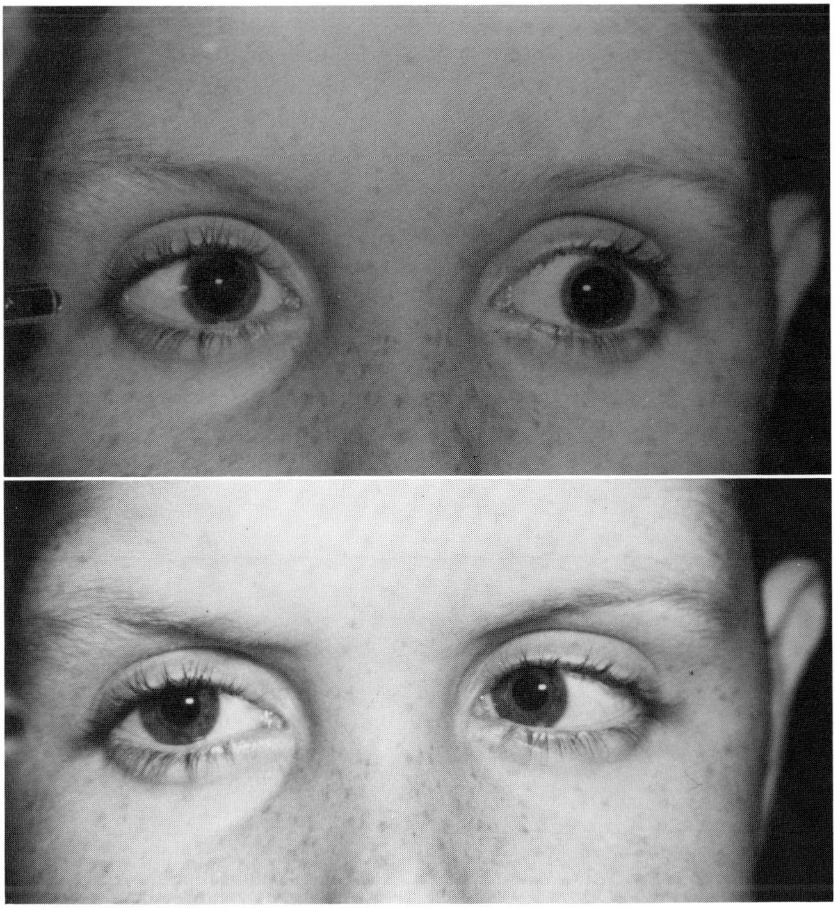

Fig. 12-3. Bilateral light-near dissociation of pupils due to pinealoma in 13-year-old boy. **A,** Bilateral dilated pupils and markedly defective constriction on exposure to bright light. **B,** Excellent constriction of pupils to near synkinesis.

It may be seen with large cerebellar neoplasms that press upward against the tectal plate. Intrinsic brain stem disease such as glioma, vascular malformation, and vascular occlusive or embolic disease in elderly individuals may lead to light-near dissociation. It may occur as a posttraumatic phenomenon in some individuals.*

Mixed pupillary defects

The category of mixed pupillary defects incorporates the defects that may compromise pupillary function on either the sensory or the motor side of the parasympathetic pupillary arc. The two leading causes for light-near dissociation in this category include neurosyphilis and diabetes mellitus. Optic nerve disease is, of course, commonly associated with neurosyphilis. Optic atrophy is especially common with tabes dorsalis. The most common pupillary abnormality in neurosyphilis is light-near dissociation, which is often accompanied by anisocoria. Diabetes mellitus may occasionally evoke light-near dissociation if the patient has had the disease for several years.† Light-near dissociation results from involvement of both the retina and optic nerve with hemorrhagic or neovascular changes as well as vascular occlusive disease affecting the optic nerve. Direct effects on the iris are also important. Light-near dissociation is also said to occur in the early development of and late recovery from Hutchinson's pupil (see below) and from the effect of cycloplegic or mydriatic preparations.

Another classic example of a defect resulting from mixed sensory and motor damage is the Argyll Robertson pupil. This pupillary defect has the following features:

1. Moderately good vision in the affected eye
2. Small diameter
3. No light response
4. Some constriction of the pupil to the near synkinesis
5. Poor dilatation with mydriatics
6. Usually bilateral

The Argyll Robertson pupil is, of course, the most well-known sign of central nervous system syphilis. It is classically seen in approximately 13% of patients with tabes dorsalis and approximately 8% of those with general paresis. Over 70% of the patients with neurosyphilis, however, have some abnormality of pupillary function, most commonly light-near dissociation. The exact location for the defect producing light-near dissociation, such that there is essentially a total loss of light responsiveness of the pupil in one or

---

*EDITOR'S NOTE. Unlike the pupils in neurosyphilis, which are *small* and show light-near dissociation, tumors involving the upper midbrain (e.g., pinealoma) produce *mid-dilated* (about 5 mm) pupils. J. S. G.

†EDITOR'S NOTE. These pupils are usually *large* and sluggishly reactive in patients who have had juvenile onset diabetes for many years. J. S. G.

both eyes but retention of the near response, has been classically thought to be the mesencephalic brain stem. The brain stem in the region of the afferent input to the Edinger-Westphal nucleus has been suggested over the years as the primary locus for small lesions producing the Argyll Robertson pupil. This would preferentially spare the pathways necessary for evoking pupil constriction by the near synkinesis.

Syphilis of the central nervous system is a multifocal disorder. Its effects range far and wide and include direct effects on the eye. This suggests that the Argyll Robertson pupil is not a result of a small lesion in the mesencephalic brain stem but of multifocal disease. Therefore, I think the Argyll Robertson pupil is best classified as a defect of the mixed type.

Efferent pupillary defect

Efferent pupillary defects may be classified as pure parasympathetic defects or pure sympathetic defects.

In the pure parasympathetic defect, the involved pupil is larger than the normal pupil and therefore the patient has an acquired anisocoria. The anisocoria is more profound in the light than in the dark, and the patient has no abnormality of the visual field or visual acuity of the affected eye, aside from the defect produced by involvement of accommodation and thus defective near vision.

The patient with a sympathetic defect shows anisocoria that is more profound in the dark than in the light. In this case the smaller pupil is defective. The patient has no defect in visual acuity or visual field; he may have an increased range of accommodation and actually have better than normal accommodative amplitude in the involved eye.

Benign anisocoria should be distinguished from the anisocoria produced by parasympathetic or sympathetic defects. Benign anisocoria may be classified into two general types, congenital anisocoria and fatigue anisocoria. Congenital anisocoria is very common. Such anisocoria is generally rather subtle. It remains about the same in the light and the dark; in other words, the same relative difference in pupil size exists in light and dark. It is important to look at old photographs of the patient in order to determine whether the anisocoria is recently acquired or long-standing. Fatigue aniscoria increases as fatigue deepens. Marked stimulation, either psychosensory or through the use of amphetamines, causes a return toward isocoria. Anisocoria returns when the patient becomes fatigued.

Parasympathetic efferent defects. A classification of common parasympathetic efferent defects includes the following:

1. Cycloplegic drops
2. Hutchinson's sign
3. Adie's pupil
4. Tonic pupil

5. Misdirection of third cranial nerve
6. Traumatic mydriasis
7. Acute glaucoma

CYCLOPLEGIC DROPS. A dilated and fixed pupil in a patient who has not sustained ocular trauma and complains only of the sudden onset of blurred vision and difficulty with reading is the prototype for the effect of cycloplegics on the eye. This is extremely common in the hospital among nurses required to instill cycloplegic medications into the eyes of patients under their care. These individuals may inadvertently contaminate themselves with their fingers, which have been in contact with the solution. This will lead to a rapid dilatation of the pupil with loss of varying amounts of accommodation depending on the amount and type of medication introduced into the eye. A similar problem occurs in the mothers of children who are being treated with cycloplegic agents for esotropia in preparation for a cycloplegic refraction.

The most rapid way to differentiate cycloplegic effect, from a neurologic cause of a dilated and fixed pupil, is to use the pilocarpine test advocated by Thompson and co-workers.[6] In this test one uses 0.5% to 2% pilocarpine. If the patient has had a cycloplegic drop instilled, the pilocarpine will fail to cause the pupil to constrict because the acetylcholine receptor sites are blocked. This test is particularly important as a diagnostic tool when the patient has had atropine instilled. If one suspects that cycloplegic instillation is the cause for iridoplegia but cannot elicit an adequate history of exposure, then one must wait for the cycloplegic effect to abate. In the case of atropine, this may take a week or longer.*

HUTCHINSON'S SIGN. The dilated and fixed pupil that occurs with increased intracranial pressure and herniation of the uncus of the temporal lobe over the tentorial margin is the hallmark of shifting intracranial contents with compression of the third cranial nerve. Compression of the upper medial aspect of the third nerve against the dorsum sellae occurs as the uncus continues to be pushed medially by a space-taking lesion such as a subdural hematotma. Compression of the third nerve in this manner involves the parasympathetic pathways to the pupil before other impairment of third nerve function occurs. Because of their superficial location, the parasympathetics for pupil and accommodative function in the third nerve are the first to be compromised by compression effect. It is not uncommon to see a contralateral hemiparesis develop with a "blown pupil." On some occasions, the patient may have the hemiparesis ipsilateral to the dilated and fixed pupil, which is known to the neurologist and neurosurgeon as the

---

*EDITOR'S NOTE. Pharmacologic accidents (atropine, belladonna-alkaloids, etc.) tend to produce a larger pupil (6 mm and greater) than do oculomotor palsies. A large light-fixed pupil in the presence of normal ocular motility, and an otherwise intact patient, should be considered a *pharmacologic* accident. J. S. G.

Kernohan's notch syndrome. In this condition the third cranial nerve ipsilateral to the lesion is compressed, and shifting of intracranial contents produces contralateral compression of the corticospinal pathways at the midbrain level. The patient therefore develops a third nerve palsy ipsilateral to the lesion as well as an ipsilateral hemiparesis due to compression of contralateral corticospinal pathways. As the Hutchinson's pupil develops with increased shifting of cerebral contents, the ocular motor function of the third nerve may become compromised. A prompt reduction of intracranial pressure by appropriate surgical means, such as localization and drainage of a subdural hematoma, will result in a return of ocular motor and pupillary function. Bilateral dilated and fixed pupils in a patient with increased intracranial pressure indicates that the patient is developing a tentorial pressure cone with obstruction of vascular supply into the mesencephalic brain stem. This is an ominous sign. The survival rate in patients who develop bilateral dilated and fixed pupils and demonstrate decerebrate posturing is poor despite adequate and prompt neurosurgical intervention.

ADIE'S PUPIL. Adie's tonic pupil[7] indicates a specific diagnostic classification. This classification should not be used to describe all tonic pupils. The pupillary abnormality arises from damage to the postganglionic parasympathetics or the parasympathetic ganglion cells in the ciliary ganglion. Although the disorder has been reported after viral infections, such as herpes zoster, varicella, and mumps, usually no cause can be established. Specific diagnostic criteria for this classification include the following:

1. Unilaterality in 80% of the cases
2. Affected pupil usually large
3. Direct light reflex almost or completely abolished
4. Pupil dilates slowly in dark
5. Pupil contracts slowly if at all when exposed to bright light
6. Miosis occurs during accommodation and may exceed that of the normal pupil in some circumstances
7. Pupil dilates slowly when accommodation stops (tonic redilatation—an important diagnostic sign)
8. Pupil dilates normally with mydriatic agents
9. Most common in women 20 to 40 years old
10. Patient must be neurologically intact except for loss of knee or ankle jerks or both
11. Prompt miosis after instillation of 2.5% Mecholyl or $\frac{1}{16}$% pilocarpine

Weak cholinergic solutions produce marked constriction of the pupil in the affected eye but no significant constriction of the pupil in the normal eye. This chemical test is used to complete the diagnostic evaluation of Adie's tonic pupil. A positive Mecholyl test may also be seen in other forms of tonic pupil disorders. It may be present with Argyll Robertson pupil and the pupillary defects associated with myotonic dystrophy and amyloidosis. The postdenervation supersensitivity that produces a positive Mecholyl test remains unchanged throughout life. Adie's tonic pupil rarely occurs in males.

TONIC PUPIL. Other causes for the tonic pupil defect include the polyneuropathy of diabetes mellitus and alcohol abuse, syphilis, trauma to the eye or orbit, orbital inflammatory disease, retrobulbar alcohol injection, and even metastatic choroidal neoplasms. Obviously the latter are an exceptionally rare cause of tonic pupil. The term Adie's tonic pupil should not be used to describe these disorders. It is incumbent upon the ophthalmologist, neurologist, and neurosurgeon to exclude these possible causes when dealing with a tonic pupil that does not fit the diagnostic criteria usually applied to Adie's tonic pupil. One should specifically search the history for evidence of previous alcohol abuse, significant ocular trauma, or diabetes mellitus. Appropriate testing for diabetes mellitus and syphilis may be necessary. A glucose tolerance test and FTA-ABS test should be part of the routine work-up for these other types of tonic pupils. The most common missed diagnosis is the syphilitic tonic pupil.* A tonic pupil defect has been reported in some patients with pineal tumors. The majority of these individuals do not have a tonic pupil, however, but they often demonstrate marked light-near dissociation.

MISDIRECTION OF THIRD CRANIAL NERVE. When a patient has experienced severe impairment of third nerve function, recovery of function may lead to misdirection-in-regeneration of the third nerve. This may be complete or partial but almost every patient who experiences a total third nerve palsy shows some evidence of misdirection-in-regeneration within a few weeks or months following the insult. The classic findings in misdirection-in-regeneration of the third nerve include horizontal gaze-lid dyskinesia (the involved eyelid retracts as the eye is adducted, and becomes ptotic as the eye is abducted), limitation of vertical gaze, adduction upon attempted vertical gaze, monocular optokinetic responses, pseudo-Graefe's sign (retraction of the upper lid with attempted down gaze), and pseudo–Argyll Robertson pupil. The affected pupil is generally much larger than the normal one. It tends to constrict somewhat on attempted adduction, exhibits some dilatation on abduction, shows a very poor or complete lack of responsiveness to light, and often constricts somewhat during the near synkinesis.

TRAUMATIC MYDRIASIS. Individuals who have had significant blunt trauma to the eye develop a traumatic mydriasis with great regularity. Prior to the mydriasis, the pupil may be smaller than normal. Then the pupil dilates and becomes essentially fixed to light and near. After sufficient

---

*EDITOR'S NOTE. Most tonic pupils are of unknown cause and benign. Syphilis is *not* generally thought to produce this characteristic syndrome, and to confront the patient with such clinical speculations may prove deleterious. J. S. G.

time has passed, a tonic quality may surface. In 50% of the patients with posttraumatic mydriasis, there is a permanent dilatation of the pupil. There may be some irregularity to the pupil outline if a disinsertion of the iris root or sphincter tear has occurred. With disinsertion of the iris root, one will see a peripheral defect in the iris, seen better with transillumination than with direct lighting of the iris surface. Other associated abnormalities include angle recession with the late onset of a monocular glaucoma, dislocation of the crystalline lens, and retinal edema concentrated at the macular region (Berlin's edema). Similar changes in pupil function may also result from penetrating injury to the eye.

ACUTE GLAUCOMA. Patients who have sustained a sudden rise in intraocular pressure with an attack of acute narrow-angle glaucoma exhibit a middilated pupil fixed to light and near, one of the diagnostic features of acute glaucoma. Experimental elevation of intraocular pressure above the diastolic pressure within the eye adversely affects the ability of the pupil sphincter to constrict, even after instillation of large amounts of pilocarpine. It has been suggested that there is a preferential resistance of the iris dilator to the effect of increased intraocular pressure.[8] The sphincter, on the other hand, is extremely sensitive to elevation of pressure. The use of an adrenergic blocking agent such as thymoxamine to selectively block iris dilator function theoretically might be practical in treating an attack of narrow-angle glaucoma.

The pupil will begin to constrict in response to cholinergic agents once the intraocular pressure has been reduced below the diastolic pressure of the intraocular vascular supply. Vigorous treatment with Diamox, osmotic diuretics, and even retrobulbar injection of a local anesthetic may be necessary in order to control the attack and reduce pressure sufficiently to allow pilocarpine to become effective.

Lesions of the sympathetic pathway. Oculosympathetic paresis (Horner's syndrome) is a relatively common disorder. Many disease entities may lead to a defect in sympathetic neural innervation of the eye. The lesion can affect any portion of the three-neuron pathway that comprises the route for sympathetic input to the eye.

The miosis in patients having sympathetic lesions is rather minimal (Fig. 12-4, *A*). Sympathetic denervation is often overlooked because of the minimal change in pupillary diameter. It is not uncommon to see only a 0.5-mm decrease in the diameter of the pupil, even with the most devastating sympathetic lesions. The ptosis is usually inextensive, often only 1.0 mm; it can easily escape detection unless specifically searched for. Enophthalmos is regarded as one of the classic signs of Horner's syndrome, but this is a relative enophthalmos due to the ptosis. The eye only appears to be retroplaced in the orbit. Exophthalmometry indicates that there is no true enophthalmos. Anhidrosis, another of the classic features of

A

B

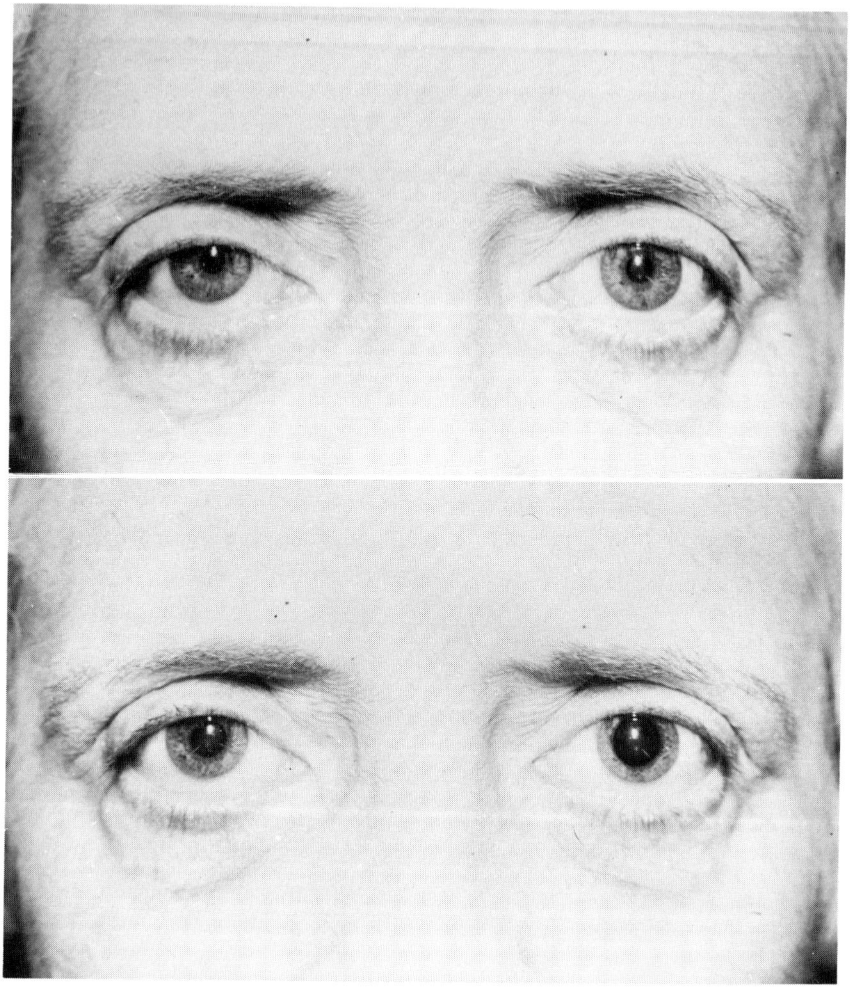

Fig. 12-4. A, Patient has oculosympathetic paresis on right. Note minimal amount of ptosis and slight miosis of affected eye. **B,** Same patient after instillation of two drops of 4% cocaine. Normal left pupil is widely dilated while right pupil is only modestly dilated. Patient has positive cocaine test on right, which is clearly consistent with diagnosis of Horner's syndrome.

Horner's syndrome, is extremely variable in extent. Generally, it is found only when the lesion is located proximal to the takeoff of the external carotid artery from the common carotid, because the pathways for vasomotor control and sweating for the face follow the external carotid, except those destined for innervation of the central portion of the forehead. Other less important features of Horner's syndrome include transient flushing of the face, increase in skin temperature, decrease in intraocular pressure, and, if sympathetic damage occurs before the age of 2 years, heterochromia iridis. The pale iris is ipsilateral to the lesion. Although the pupil is small in diameter when there are lesions of the sympathetic pathway, it has an intact response to light and to near. There is loss of psychosensory dilatation of the pupil as one would expect.

Horner's syndrome is clinically apparent whenever the first, second, or third neuron is involved. The miosis seems to be more profound as the lesions become more peripheral (closer to the eye). Denervation supersensitivity results from third-neuron lesions. Weak adrenergic solutions have been suggested as a useful means of diagnosis of a third-neuron Horner's syndrome. Recent evidence indicates that such testing may not be as useful as was previously believed.[9] The diagnosis of Horner's syndrome is best established by being suspicious that it may be present and by looking for subtle ptosis and miosis. Lesions in the sympathetic neural chain are best localized by the neurologic company they keep. Careful study of the regional neuroanatomy of the sympathetic pathway is most helpful in establishing localization. Also helpful in this regard are 4% cocaine (Fig. 12-4, *B*) and 1% Paredrine.[9]

REFERENCES

1. Yoss, R. E., Moyer, N. J., and Hollenhorst, R. W.: Hippus and other spontaneous rhythmic pupillary waves, Am. J. Ophthalmol. **70:**935-941, 1970.
2. Borgmann, H.: Grundlagen fur eine klinsche Pupillographic. IV. Abhangigkeit der Pupillenweite und der Lichtreaktion von Geschlecht, Irisfarbe und Refraktion, Albrecht von Graefes Arch. Klin. Ophthalmol. **185:**11-21, 1972.
3. Gunn, R. M.: Retro-ocular neuritis of the optic nerve, Lancet **4:**412, 1904.
4. Thompson, H. S.: Afferent pupillary defects, Am. J. Ophthalmol. **62:**860-873, 1966.
5. Seybold, M. E., et al.: Pupillary abnormalities associated with tumors of the pineal region, Neurology (Minneap.) **21:** 232-237, 1971.
6. Thompson, H. S., et al.: The fixed dilated pupil. Sudden iridoplegia or mydriatric drops? A simple diagnostic test, Arch. Ophthalmol. **86:**21-27, 1971.
7. Hedges, T. R.: The tonic pupil, Arch. Ophthalmol. **80:**21-25, 1968.
8. Rutkowski, P. C., and Thompson, H. S.: Mydriasis and increased intraocular pressure. I. Pupillographic studies, Arch. Ophthalmol. **87:**21-24, 1972.
9. Thompson, H. S., and Menscher, J. H.: Adrenergic mydriasis in Horner's syndrome. Hydroxyamphetamine test for the diagnosis of postganglionic defects, Am. J. Ophthalmol. **72:**472-480, 1971.

Chapter 13

Short papers

Familial paralysis of horizontal gaze

A syndrome associated with pendular nystagmus and progressive scoliosis

James A. Sharpe
J. L. Silversides

Paralysis of all conjugate horizontal eye movements is usually acquired from lesions in the pons. It can be a congenital disorder, either sporadic[1, 2] or familial,[1, 3] that is either isolated, or associated with facial palsy in Möbius syndrome.[4, 5]

This paper describes paralysis of lateral gaze, pendular nystagmus, and progressive scoliosis in a family. Convergence during attempted lateral gaze and acquired spastic facial contraction with facial myokymia are inconstant manifestations of this familial syndrome of horizontal gaze paralysis.

CLINICAL DATA

Family study

Four siblings with paralysis of horizontal gaze and their family were examined by us in Kingston, Jamaica in 1971 and 1973. The family was Chinese of Hakka extraction. The pedigree is shown in Fig. 1. Consanguinity could not be detected. The parents believed that all the children had had full eye movements in early childhood. In 1974, two of the affected patients (Fig. 13-1: III-3, III-4) and three of their brothers (III-6, III-8, III-9) emigrated to Toronto where they attended the Neuro-ophthalmology Clinic, Toronto Western Hospital.

A Jamaican physician first documented gaze paralysis in one brother (III-3) whom he examined for scoliosis in early adolescence. Examination of the other children showed scoliosis and horizontal gaze palsy in two

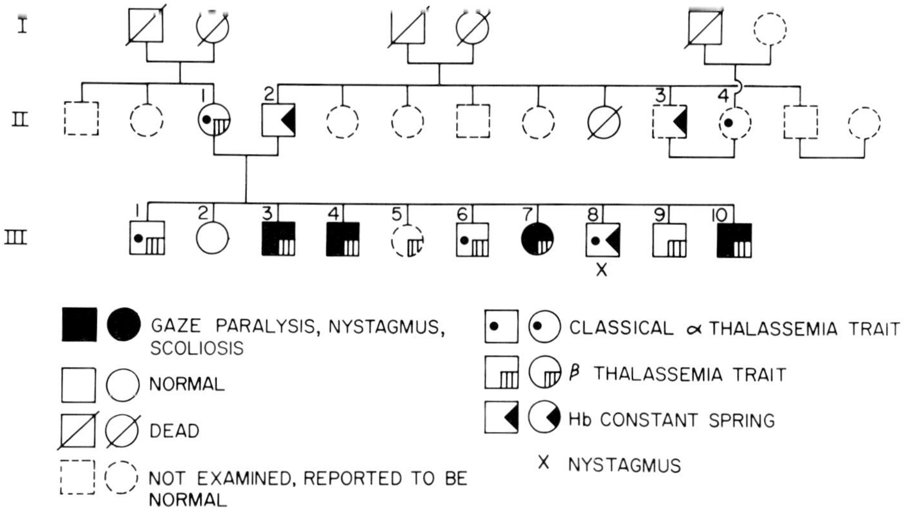

Fig. 13-1. Pedigree of family.

(III-4, III-7). The same physician reported that the youngest child (III-10) had full eye movement when first examined at the age of 2 years. By his fourth year, this boy had early scoliosis and partial limitation of lateral gaze. In 1973, when he was 14 years old, his horizontal eye movements were paralyzed. We found pendular nystagmus in all four of the propositi and in one brother (III-8) who did not have gaze paralysis or scoliosis. All but one sibling (III-5) had myopia. Only three (III-3, III-6, III-10) had myopia greater than 5 diopters. Their parents were not myopic.

Milner, Clegg, and Weatherall[6] identified genetically independent disorders of hemoglobin synthesis in this family. One brother (III-8), his father (II-2), and an uncle (II-3) and six of his children not shown in Fig. 13-1 had an abnormal elongated alpha-chain structure, termed hemoglobin Constant Spring after the name of the road in Kingston where the family lived. Other family members including the propositi had alpha-thalassemia-1 trait or beta-thalassemia trait. Inheritance of both an alpha-thalassemia-1 trait and hemoglobin Constant Spring produced clinical manifestations of hemoglobin H disease in one brother (III-8) and two cousins, previously reported in detail.[6] The abnormal hemoglobins assorted independently. It was apparent that the hematologic abnormalities were unconnected with the neuro-ophthalmic disorder reported here.

The propositi

Case 1. A 30-year-old man (III-3) developed progressive scoliosis of the thoracic spine after the age of 10 years, requiring spinal fusion at age 13. His mother stated that his gestation and birth had been normal and that eye movements had been full in early childhood. A physician had detected absence of lateral gaze in early adolescence, and the patient had realized that he turned his head to look to either side. He never experienced illusionary movement of the environment. He had worn glasses for myopia since the age of 11 years. For three years prior to our examination in Jamaica in 1973, he had had a tight pulling sensation of his face, mainly about the left side of the mouth. For about two years, he had been aware of involuntary flickering movements of his face. The patient was admitted to the neurology service of the Toronto Western Hospital in November 1974.

General physical examination showed severe thoracic scoliosis, convex to the left (Fig. 13-2). Neurologic examination revealed normal intellectual function. Muscle tone, strength, and coordination were normal. Tendon reflexes were active, the jaw jerk was brisk, and the patient had unsustained clonus of both ankles. Superficial reflexes were normal, and plantar reflexes were flexor. There were no sensory deficits.

NEURO-OPHTHALMIC FINDINGS. The visual acuity in each eye was 20/80 with correction of –15.5 S +1.25 cx 90° OD and –15.75 S OS. Near vision was Jaeger 2 bilaterally. Color vision and the visual fields were normal. His pupils were 5 mm in diameter and briskly reactive to light and near stimuli. The cornea and ocular media were normal on slit lamp examination. Fundoscopy showed myopic crescents at the

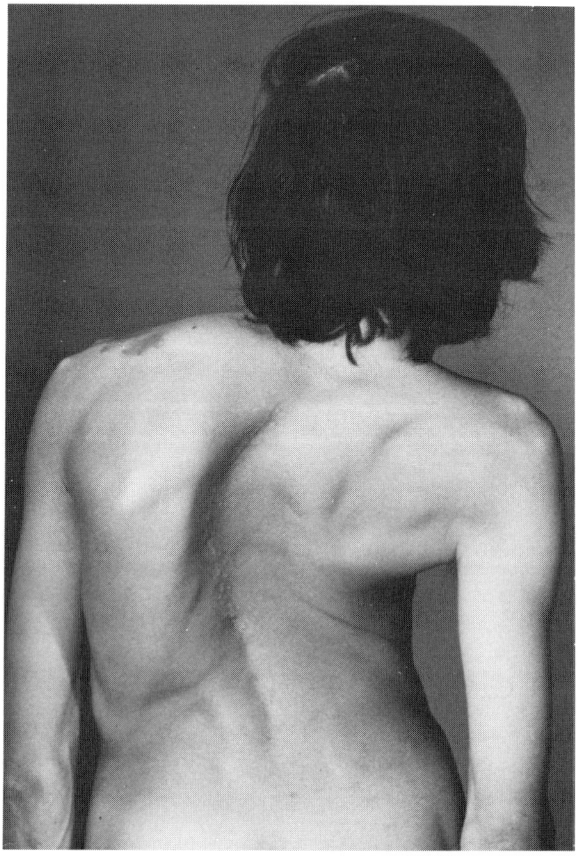

Fig. 13-2. Case 1. Scoliosis at age 30 years was progressive from early adolescence.

discs and enhanced visibility of choroidal vessels. The maculae and peripheral retinas were normal.

Lateral gaze was absent. Vertical pursuit was saccadic, but upward and downward excursion of the eyes was full. Caloric and rotational vestibular stimulation and oculocephalic maneuvers did not overcome the paralysis of lateral gaze. Full lateral excursion of each eye was accomplished only by forced duction. The patient had horizontal pendular nystagmus of very low amplitude in all positions of vertical gaze. The oscillations were not always obvious on inspection of the eyes, but fundoscopy showed them to be continuous. Small amplitude head oscillations occurred during maximal visual effort. The patient had a right exotropia of 15° at near and an alternate suppression pattern when tested with fusion targets. Convergence was normal, and it damped the nystagmus.

The patient's facial muscles were contracted, with deepening of the nasiolabial folds, retraction of the angle of the mouth, and inconstant narrowing of the palpebral fissures. The intensity of facial contraction was variable but consistently more evident on the left side (Fig. 13-3). Small vermiform movements occurred randomly over both sides of the face and platysma and less frequent larger flickering movements undulated over the brow and lower face. These involuntary movements did not involve specific groups of facial muscles nor did they produce an organized pattern

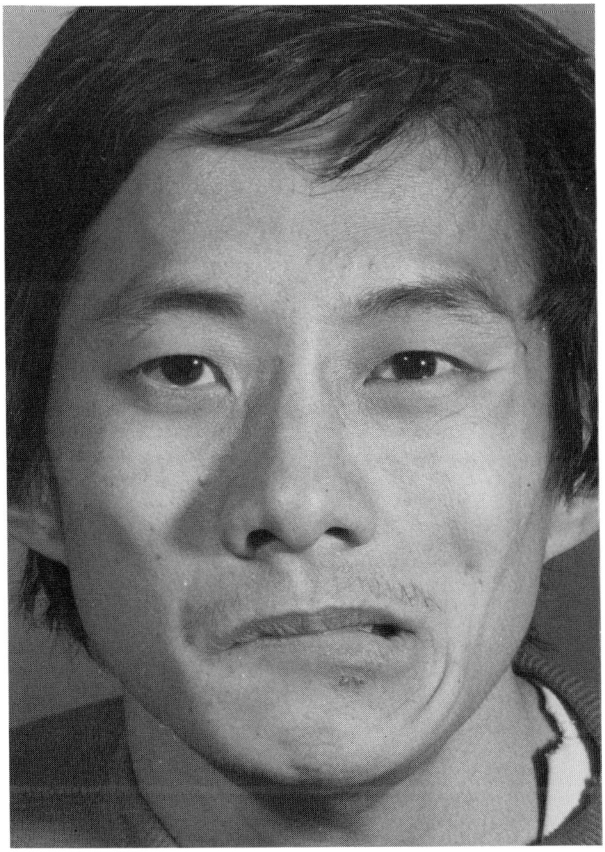

Fig. 13-3. Case 1. Facial contraction with the patient at rest, showing retraction of angle of mouth on the left side with mild narrowing of palpebral fissure.

of facial movement. Voluntary and emotional movements were full without weakness, abnormal synkinesis, or associated movements. Salivation, lacrimation, and taste were normal. There was no ptosis. Hearing and cranial nerves V, IX, X, XI, and XII were normal.

LABORATORY INVESTIGATIONS. Skull x-ray films were normal, without evidence of basilar impression. X-ray films of the spine showed extensive rotary scoliosis extending from the sixth cervical level to the upper lumbar vertebrae. No underlying abnormalities of the vertebrae were present. Pneumoencephalography and computerized axial tomography showed normal brain stem and cerebellar size and contour. An electroencephalogram was normal. Audiograms showed no impairment of hearing. The cerebrospinal fluid had 2 white cells per milliliter and a protein concentration of 14 mg/100 ml. An electrocardiogram was normal. The following values were also obtained: hemoglobin, 12.4 g/100 ml; reticulocytes, 0.6%; white blood cell count, 6300/ml, with a normal differential count. Platelets were normal. Peripheral blood films showed erythrocyte microcytosis, hypochromia, and bizarre poikilocytes. Hemoglobin electrophoresis showed only Hb A and increased Hb A_2 and Hb F consistent with beta-thalassemia trait. The VDRL test was negative. Levels of serum enzymes, calcium, and phosphorous were normal, as were results of urinalysis and urinary amino acid chromatography.

The results of electromyography and nerve conduction studies, described in a separate report, are summarized here. Stimulation of the facial nerves showed normal latencies and muscle action potentials. Needle electrode examination of the facial muscles showed no evidence of denervation. During attempted relaxation, continuous muscle potentials were present on both sides of his face. This continuous activity was more prominent in the left lower facial muscles. Superimposed on this background activity were intermittent bursts of repetitive muscle potentials. These periodic bursts were asynchronous in right and left facial muscles. Voluntary and mimetic facial movements were full, but the number of motor units active during maximal effort was reduced. All motor unit potentials were of normal amplitude and duration.

Case 2. A 28-year-old man (III-4) was not aware of impairment of lateral gaze until 12 years old, but his siblings noticed impaired eye movements after his eighth year; he had to turn his head to look to the side. At the time of our examinations in 1971 and 1973, lateral eye movements were absent. One year later, the patient crossed his eyes when lateral gaze was tested with his head fixed. However, he habitually preferred to turn his head. He never had facial twitching. He wore glasses for myopia since the age of 12. He denied oscillopsia. Curvature of the spine began when he was 10 years old and progressed despite insertion of a Harrington rod at age 23.

General physical examination in November 1974 showed severe thoracic scoliosis convex to the right. Results of neurologic examination were normal apart from the cranial nerve findings. The patient exhibited slowness in starting volitional and emotional movements of his face, particularly on the right side. Once initiated, facial movement and strength were full. No spontaneous movements or abnormal synkinesis of the face were present.

NEURO-OPHTHALMIC FINDINGS. Distance visual acuity was 20/40 with −2.5 spherical correction in each eye, and near acuity was Jaeger 1. Color vision and the visual fields were normal. Fundoscopy showed only myopic crescents of the discs.

The patient showed paralysis of lateral gaze. Attempted fixation to either side produced convergence, pupillary constriction, and accommodation instead of conjugate lateral eye movements (Fig. 13-4). Ocular retraction did not accompany this substituted convergence. Cold caloric irrigation of either ear and oculocephalic maneuvers did not overcome the lateral gaze palsy. Full abduction was achieved by forced ductions under topical anesthesia. Upward and downward gaze was full, but vertical pursuit was saccadic. Convergence amplitudes were normal. The patient had conjugate horizontal oscillations of the eyes in all positions of vertical gaze. Head oscillations occurred during intense efforts to fixate. Convergence in forward and attempted lateral gaze stopped the nystagmus. Optokinetic stimulation to either side produced convergence without nystagmus. Vertical optokinetic responses were reduced.

LABORATORY INVESTIGATIONS. Skull x-ray films were normal. X-ray films of the spine

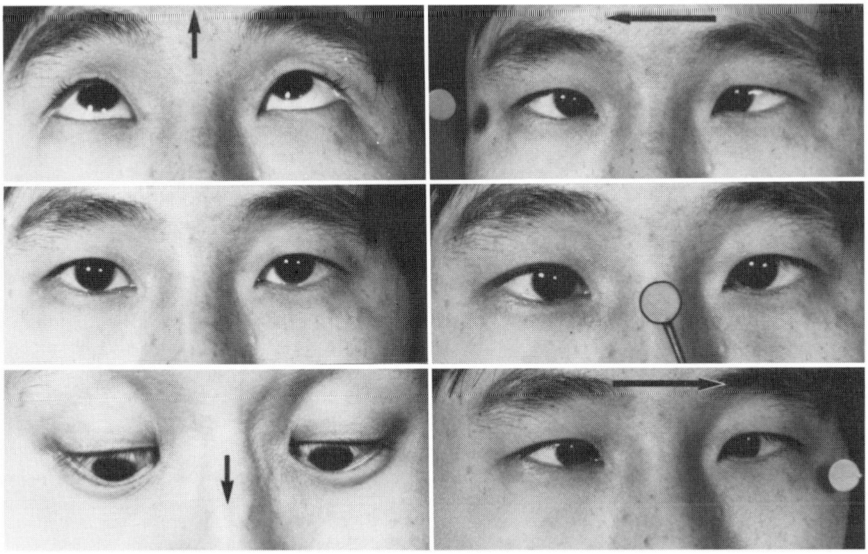

Fig. 13-4. Case 2. **A** and **C,** Upward and downward gaze are full. **E,** Convergence is normal. **D** and **F,** Attempted lateral gaze to right and left, showing substituted convergence.

showed scoliosis with curvature extending from the fifth cervical to the first lumbar vertebra and a Harrington rod between T_3 and L_1. No defects of vertebral structure were present. Audiograms and an electrocardiogram were normal. Hemoglobin level was 12.2 g/100 ml; white blood cell count was 8000/ml. Platelets were normal. Peripheral blood films showed hypochromia, bizarre poikilocytes, and target cells. Hemoglobin electrophoresis showed a pattern of beta-thalassemia trait identical to that in case 1. Results of chromosomal analysis of peripheral white cells by trypsin banding was normal.

Case 3. In this 23-year-old woman (III-7) scoliosis began after the age of 8 years. She had paralysis of lateral gaze that was complete when examined in Jamaica in 1973. Its precise duration could not be determined. Her parents thought that her eye movements were full in early childhood. General physical examination showed severe thoracic scoliosis. Her intellect was normal. The corrected visual acuity was 20/20 in each eye. Pupillary reactions were normal. The visual fields were full and the fundi were normal apart from myopic crescents at the discs. Lateral gaze was absent. Vertical excursions and convergence were normal. The patient had horizontal pendular nystagmus of low amplitude in all positions of vertical fixation. The left nasiolabial fold was flat but facial movements were normal, without contraction or myokymia. Results of neurologic examination were otherwise normal.

Case 4. The youngest child (III-10), age 14 years, developed mild scoliosis in his fourth year. A physician reported normal lateral eye movements at age 2 and some impairment of lateral gaze at age 4. Examination in 1971 and 1973 showed severe scoliosis convex to the left. Distance visual acuity was 20/60 in the right eye and 20/40 in the left eye with correction for high myopia. Near visual acuity was normal. The pupillary reactions were normal. The fundi showed myopic crescents with no other degenerative changes. Gaze was absent in both horizontal directions. Vertical gaze and convergence were full. Lateral eye movements were not elicited by doll's head maneuvers. The patient had low-amplitude horizontal pendular nystagmus in forward, upward, and downward gaze. Facial movements were normal and there were no other neurologic abnormalities.

• • •

A 22-year-old brother (III-8) had nystagmus, first detected in 1971. He did not have oscillopsia. Distance visual acuity was 20/25 in each eye with correction for myopic astigmatism, and near acuity was Jaeger 1. Gaze was full in all directions. Convergence was intact. His nystagmus was horizontal in all positions of fixation and pendular through a wide neutral zone. On extreme lateral gaze he had jerk nystagmus in the direction of deviation. The null region of best visual acuity and minimum nystagmus intensity was straight ahead. The nystagmus stopped during convergence. Optokinetic nystagmus was impaired in both lateral directions without visible inversion. Vertical optokinetic responses were normal. This patient did not have scoliosis, and results of neurologic examination were normal.

DISCUSSION

Paralysis of horizontal eye movements, nystagmus, and scoliosis in four members of this family were expressions of a genetic disease. Involvement of patients of both sexes and absence of these abnormalities in relatives for three antecedent generations indicated an autosomal recessive pattern of inheritance.

Lateral gaze paralysis was complete when we first examined these patients. Historical evidence suggested that the gaze paralysis was acquired and progressive,[6] but we did not observe the eye movements during early childhood. The ophthalmoplegia may have been present at birth and not detected until childhood or adolescence. The scoliosis and facial contraction were acquired and progressive and distinguish this syndrome from congenital nonprogressive paralysis of horizontal gaze[1-3] and Möbius syndrome.[4, 5]

Nine of the ten siblings were myopic. The myopia, like the disorders of hemoglobin synthesis, was genetically independent of the ocular motor and spinal abnormalities. The severity of myopia in our patients was not related to penetrance of gaze paralysis, nystagmus, or scoliosis.

All four of the propositi had scoliosis that progressed after childhood and adolescence. None had signs of segmental spinal neuromuscular involvement to specify a neurogenic mechanism. We have not identified a disturbance of connective tissue or bone metabolism responsible for the scoliosis. Familial studies of acquired scoliosis without recognized neuromuscular cause have implicated autosomal dominant or multifactorial inheritance.[7, 8] In this family, both the scoliosis and the ocular motor disorder were pleiotropic effects of autosomal recessive inheritance.

Facial myokymia and continuous contraction were progressive for three years in the oldest patient (case 1). The facial contraction was asymmetric, being consistently more evident on the left side. Facial myokymia and contraction are uncommon phenomena, typically observed in multiple sclerosis[9] and pontine neoplasms.[10-12] Pneumoencephalography and computerized axial tomography did not show a structural brain stem lesion in our patient. Electromyographic evidence has implicated a supranuclear disturbance of facial motor neuron innervation in myokymia and facial contraction.[10] Sethi and co-workers[12] reported facial myokymia from metastatic tumor in the pons sparing the facial nucleus and fascicle, thereby confirming its supranuclear origin. In our patient, electromyography showed spontaneous periodic muscle potentials on both sides of the face. These potentials persisted even when we could not see the myokymia. A background of continuous motor unit activity was the electromyographic correlate of the facial contraction. Normal strength and absence of fibrillation potentials suggested integrity of the facial nuclei and axons. Both this patient and one brother (case 2) developed slowness in starting volitional and emotional movements, but strength was normal. Slowness of initiation of facial movement and reduction of the interference pattern implied defective recruitment of motor neurons. O'Connor and associates[13] postulated that isolation of facial motor neurons caused continuous facial spasm. Degeneration of supranuclear inhibitory and excitatory fibers or interneurons in the pontine tegmentum may be responsible for facial contraction and myokymia in case 1.

The four propositi had horizontal pendular nystagmus* in all positions of vertical gaze. The nystagmus impaired distance visual acuity. Convergence damped the nystagmus and improved near acuity in each case. We could not establish the duration of nystagmus in these patients. Pendular nystagmus was the only neurologic disorder in one brother (III-8, Fig. 13-1), in whom we could observe eye movements through full excursions. The nystagmus did not exhibit binocular disparity of direction and amplitude or vertical components usually apparent in acquired pendular nystagmus from brain stem disease.[14] Neither this patient nor the propositi had oscillopsia. The oscillations were characteristic of congenital nystagmus. This patient was old enough to have developed the gaze palsy and scoliosis manifest in four of his siblings. We attribute their absence to delayed or reduced expressivity of the same pleiotropic genes that afflicted the propositi.

The paralysis of horizontal eye movements can be explained by bilateral involvement of the paramedian pontine reticular formation (PPRF) that mediates ipsilateral pursuit and saccadic eye movements.[15, 16] Failure of vestibular stimulation to move the eyes laterally signified disruption of the vestibuloocular reflex arc at the level of the caudal PPRF.[17, 18] We do not attribute the gaze paralysis to more widespread involvement of both medial longitudinal fasciculi and abducens nuclei since none of our patients had peripheral facial nerve palsy that regularly accompanies nuclear or fascicular paralysis of abduction. Convergence with pupillary constriction and accommodation was substituted for horizontal version in case 2. The patient used cross fixation to look to either side. Substitution of convergence can occur in congenital gaze paralysis,[1] or in gaze paralysis acquired from pontine le-

*EDITOR'S NOTE. Horizontal pendular nystagmus despite total horizontal gaze palsy is an enigma that defies explanation. J. S. G.

sions.[19, 20] Retraction of the nonfixating convergent eye, sometimes evident in the congenital form, was not present in case 2. Sparing of vertical gaze, pupillary constrictor reflex activity, upper lid function, and convergence assured normality of midbrain ocular motor function.

Neurologic system degenerations can produce predominant involvement of the brain stem reticular formation and supranuclear ophthalmoplegia.[21] Progressive supranuclear palsy[22] exemplifies such a disorder, with early paresis of vertical eye movements. The syndrome in our patients may be explained by degeneration in the pontine tegmentum. This familial disorder differs from all the neurodegenerative diseases associated with chronic progressive external ophthalmoplegia in which ocular movements are symmetrically impaired.[23, 24] The horizontal gaze paralysis, pendular nystagmus, and progressive facial contraction and scoliosis described here are distinctive features of a unique heredofamilial syndrome.

REFERENCES

1. Zweifach, P. H., Walton, D. S., and Brown, R. H.: Isolated congenital horizontal gaze paralysis, Arch. Ophthalmol. **81:**345-350, 1969.
2. Taumer, R., Schellenbeck, R., and Schmidt, D.: Kongenitale bilaterale horizontale Blickparese mit erhaltener Konvergenz, Albrecht von Graefes Arch. Klin. Ophthalmol. **187:**299-309, 1973.
3. Francois, J.: Congenital ophthalmoplegias. In Brunette, J. R., and Barbeau, A., editors: Progress in neuro-ophthalmology, vol. 2, Amsterdam, 1969, Excerpta Medica Foundation, pp. 387-421.
4. Van Allen, M. W., and Blodi, F. C.: Neurologic aspects of the Möbius syndrome, Neurology (Minneap.) **10:**249-259, 1960.
5. Danis, P.: Les paralysies oculo-faciales congenitales, Ophthalmologica **110:**113-137, 1945.
6. Milner, P. F., Clegg, J. B., and Weatherall, D. J.: Haemoglobin H diseases due to a unique haemoglobin variant with an elongated alpha chain, Lancet **1:**729-732, 1971.
7. Riseborough, E. J., and Wynne-Davies, R.: A genetic survey of ideopathic scoliosis in Boston, Massachusetts, J. Bone Joint Surg. (Am.) **55:**974-982, 1973.
8. Filho, N. A., and Thompson, M. W.: Genetic studies in scoliosis, J. Bone Joint Surg. (Am.) **53:**199, 1971.
9. Anderman, F., Cosgrove, J. B. R., Lloyd-Smith, D. L., Gloor, P., and McNaughton, F. L.: Facial myokymia in multiple sclerosis, Brain **84:**31-44, 1961.
10. Tenser, R. B., and Corbett, J. J.: Myokymia and facial contraction in brain stem glioma. An electromyographic study, Arch. Neurol. **30:**425-427, 1974.
11. Sogg, R. L., Hoyt, W. F., and Boldrey, E.: Spastic paretic facial contracture, Neurology (Minneap.) **13:**607-612, 1963.
12. Sethi, P. K., Smith, B. H., and Kalyanaraman, K.: Facial myokymia: a clinicopathological study, J. Neurol. Neurosurg. Psychiatry **37:**745-749, 1974.
13. O'Connor, P. J., Parry, C. B., and Davies, R.: Continuous muscle spasm in intramedullary tumors of the neuraxis, J. Neurol. Neurosurg. Psychiatry **29:**310-314, 1966.
14. Aschoff, J. C., Conrad, B., and Kornhuber, H. H.: Acquired pendular nystagmus with oscillopsia in multiple sclerosis: a sign of cerebellar nuclei disease, J. Neurol. Neurosurg. Psychiatry **37:**570-577, 1974.
15. Daroff, R. B., and Hoyt, W. F.: Supranuclear disorders of ocular control systems in man: clinical, anatomical and physiological correlations. In Bach-Y-Rita, P., Collins, C. C., and Hyde, J. E., editors: The control of eye movements, New York, 1971, Academic Press, Inc., pp. 175-235.
16. Keller, E. L.: Participation of medial pontine reticular formation in eye movement generation in monkey, J. Neurophysiol. **37:**316-332, 1974.

17. Cohen, B.: Komatsuzaki, A., and Bender, M. B.: Electrooculographic syndrome in monkeys after pontine reticular formation lesions, Arch. Neurol. **18:**78-92, 1968.
18. Sharpe, J. A., Rosenberg, M. A., Hoyt, W. F., and Daroff, R. B.: Paralytic pontine exotropia, Neurology (Minneap.) **24:** 1076-1081, 1974.
19. Burian, H. M., Van Allen, M. W., Sexton, R. R., and Baller, R. S.: Substitution phenomena in congenital and acquired supranucuear disorders of eye movement, Trans. Am. Acad. Ophthalmol. Otolaryngol. **69:**1105-1114, 1965.
20. Kestenbaum, A.: Clinical methods of neuro-ophthalmologic examination, New York, 1961, Grune & Stratton, Inc., p. 330.
21. Neumann, M. A.: Pathology of the reticular formation. In Minkler, J., editor: Pathology of the nervous system, vol. 1, New York, 1968, McGraw-Hill Book Company, pp. 696-707.
22. Steele, J. C., Richardson, J. C., and Olszewski, J.: Progressive supranuclear palsy, Arch. Neurol. **10:**333-359, 1964.
23. Daroff, R. B.: Chronic progressive external ophthalmoplegia. A critical review, Arch. Ophthalmol. **82:**845-850, 1969.
24. Drachman, D. A.: Ophthalmoplegia plus, Arch. Neurol. **18:**654-674, 1968.

Drug testing in Horner's syndrome

Baird S. Grimson
H. Stanley Thompson

During the last seven years 67 patients with unilateral Horner's syndrome have had documented drug tests performed at the University of Iowa.

Pupillary diameters were measured from photographs taken in clinic light before and 45 minutes after the drops were placed in the conjunctival sac. The drugs used were 5% cocaine and 1% hydroxyamphetamine (Paredine). The average pupillary dilations obtained with these drugs are shown in Fig. 13-5.

Cocaine was used in 37 patients. In each case the Horner's pupil dilated poorly while the normal pupil dilated fully. Ordinarily the diagnosis of Horner's syndrome can be made from the ocular signs (Table 16), but sometimes these are inconclusive and the diagnosis remains in doubt. In this situation cocaine is useful. Cocaine does not help to *localize* the lesion; it simply confirms the diagnosis of Horner's syndrome.

Considering the pharmacologic action of cocaine, it is not surprising that all Horner's pupils dilate poorly in response to it. Cocaine enhances the action of the transmitter substance in the neuroeffector junction by blocking the reuptake of norepinephrine into the sympathetic nerve ending. If norepinephrine is not being released, cocaine will have no effect. Any lesion, whether central, preganglionic, or postganglionic, that interferes with the passage of the nervous impulse along the oculosympathetic pathway will impair norepinephrine release and result in a diminished cocaine mydriasis.[1]

The level of interruption of the oculosympathetic pathway can usually be localized from the clinical history and associated physical signs. For example, a patient with occlusion of the posterior inferior cerebellar artery has suffered

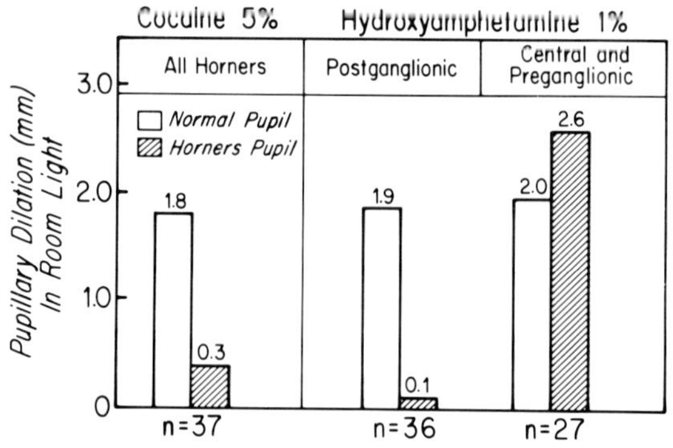

Fig. 13-5. Thirty-seven patients were tested with cocaine. All Horner's pupils dilated poorly. No statistical difference in the mydriasis to cocaine was found between the central, preganglionic, and postganglionic Horner's pupils; therefore, all these patients were grouped together. The average dilation of the Horner's pupil was 0.3 mm; the average dilation of the normal pupil was 1.8 mm. Sixty-three patients were tested with hydroxy-amphetamine. No statistical difference was found between the patients with preganglionic Horner's pupils and those with central Horner's pupils. These 27 patients were grouped together. A significant difference did exist between this group and the patients with post-ganglionic Horner's pupils; the 36 patients with postganglionic Horner's pupils were recorded separately. The average dilation of the postganglionic Horner's pupil was 0.1 mm; that of the normal pupil was 1.9 mm. The average dilation of the preganglionic and central Horner's pupils was 2.6 mm; that of the normal pupils was 2.0.

Table 16. Ocular signs of Horner's syndrome

Ptosis, minimal	"Upside-down" ptosis (elevation of lower lid)
Miosis, moderate	Congestion of conjunctiva
Anhidrosis, sometimes	Ocular hypotony, transient
Narrowed palpebral fissure (not enophthalmos)	Heterochromia (in congenital Horner's syndrome)

a lesion of the *central* oculosympathetic pathway. A brachial plexus injury involves oculosympathetic fibers in the *preganglionic* pathway. A patient with a history of cluster headaches may have damaged fibers of the *post-ganglionic* pathway.[2-5] Sometimes, however, the site of the lesion is not suggested by the clinical history. This was the case in 7 of our 67 patients and in 52 of 216 patients with Horner's syndrome evaluated by Giles and Henderson.[6] It is in patients such as these that the hydroxyamphetamine test has been especially useful.

A lesion of the postganglionic oculosympathetic pathway causes death of the sympathetic fibers in the iris dilator muscle and loss of norepinephrine stores. Poor dilation of the pupil in response to an indirectly acting sympa-

Table 17. Results of hydroxyamphetamine testing in 63 patients with Horner's syndrome

Site of lesion based on clinical story	*Number of patients*	*Site of lesion based on hydroxyamphetamine test*	*Number of patients*
Central	4	Central or preganglionic (pupil dilated)	27
Preganglionic	21		
Postganglionic	31	Postganglionic (pupil failed to dilate)	36
Subtotal	56		
Doubtful	7		
Total	63	Total	63

thomimetic drug such as hydroxyamphetamine would be expected in such a lesion.[1, 3, 4, 7-10] When the postganglionic neuron has been "decentralized" by a lesion in the preganglionic or central pathway, it still retains normal stores of norepinephrine in its nerve endings. These stores are available for release by hydroxyamphetamine, and full dilation of the pupil is observed in preganglionic and central Horner's syndrome (Fig. 13-5).

In the 56 patients localized on clinical grounds, the hydroxyamphetamine test accurately confirmed the site of the lesion (Table 17).* We thus felt justified in using this drug to separate the seven cases of Horner's syndrome in which the site of the lesion could not be determined clinically. Of these seven patients, five failed to dilate to hydroxyamphetamine and two dilated. Both "preganglionic" patients had severe cervical arthritic disease. In the other five, apparently postganglionic patients, there were no other findings, and a recent check 10 to 36 months later revealed no new symptoms.

Dividing all Horner's syndromes into two groups according to the response to hydroxyamphetamine is of definite clinical value because postganglionic Horner's syndrome is most frequently due to benign vascular headache syndromes, whereas the single most common cause of preganglionic Horner's syndrome is a metastatic lung or breast carcinoma. This is not evident in Table 18, but it should be remembered that the 63 patients recorded were ones studied with drugs by the neuro-ophthalmology service in a university hospital where contacts were closer with the neurology department than with the thoracic surgery department and in which a special interest in vascular headache syndromes had been expressed. A less biased selection of Horner's syndrome patients was obtained by reviewing all cases of Horner's syndrome recorded in the coding system at the University of Iowa hospitals during the same seven-year period. In this series the incidence of *preganglionic* Horner's syndrome associated with malignant neoplasm ap-

*The one exception (MM) has been discussed previously[6] and may well have had two lesions in the oculosympathetic pathway.

Table 18. Causes of Horner's syndrome in 63 patients

Site and nature of lesion	*Number of patients*
Central	
Brainstem vascular accident	4
Preganglionic	
Surgical trauma	11
Nonsurgical trauma	5
Malignant neoplasm	5
Cause unknown (? cervical arthritis)	2
Postganglionic	
Vascular headache syndromes	23
Cranial trauma	6
Carotid aneurysm	1
Metastasis to cavernous sinus	1
Cause unknown	5
Total	63

proached 50%. In the patients with *postganglionic* Horner's syndrome, the incidence of neoplasia was less than 2%.

Hydroxyamphetamine has replaced epinephrine and phenylephrine in our clinic as the preferred drug for identifying lesions of the postganglionic oculosympathetic pathway.[3] Other authors have also noted the clinical advantages of hydroxyamphetamine,[4, 7, 10] and the limited usefulness of supersensitivity testing with epinephrine and phenylephrine in the clinical investigation of postganglionic Horner's syndrome.[1, 6, 11-16]

Because no large series of postganglionic Horner's syndrome tested with hydroxyamphetamine has been reported in the literature, the 36 patients in this series (Table 18) will be discussed briefly.

Twenty-three of these patients had unilateral vascular headache syndromes. Nine of these had classical cluster headaches.[5, 17] In all the other 14 headache cases, results of neurologic examination were normal, with the exception of occasional trigeminal nerve involvement, as were skull films and brain scans. Arteriography was not performed due to the spontaneous resolution of these headaches and the lack of associated neurologic signs. Although the headaches in patients such as these usually are considered to have a benign cause,[13-15, 18, 19] these cases should be suspected of harboring an internal carotid aneurysm,[12, 20] especially if the headache does not resolve spontaneously.

In one patient in this series, the unilateral headache did not resolve. An angiogram revealed an intracavernous carotid aneurysm.

There were six patients with postganglionic Horner's syndrome following severe head trauma that resulted in skull fractures. Another patient, with widespread metastatic breast carcinoma, had a lesion in the cavernous sinus that was presumably metastatic.

Patients with the above causes of postganglionic oculosympathetic palsy have at one time or another been described as having "Raeder's paratrigeminal syndrome."[13-15, 18, 19, 21] However, this term cannot be used for our final five patients, each of whom suddenly developed a postganglionic Horner's syndrome without history of headache, head trauma, or neoplasia. Results of neurologic examination were otherwise normal, and evidence of known causes of postganglionic Horner's syndrome, such as middle ear infection or surgery, intraoral trauma, herpes zoster, or thrombosis of the internal carotid artery, could not be found.[11, 16, 22, 23] Because of the typical postganglionic response of the Horner's pupil to hydroxyamphetamine, the patients were not hospitalized, nor were extensive investigations for an underlying malignancy performed. So far these five patients have been followed for periods ranging from ten months to three years, and they have remained in good health with no signs or symptoms of malignancy.

It should be emphasized that all 36 patients with postganglionic Horner's syndrome were readily identified with the hydroxyamphetamine test. This drug can identify any interruption of the postganglionic oculosympathetic fibers from their origin in the superior cervical ganglion at the level of the angle of the mandible, along their course in the carotid plexus and through the cavernous sinus, to the eye. The most common cause of postganglionic Horner's syndrome in this series was benign vascular headache. Only one case was due to a malignancy.

SUMMARY

A large series of patients with Horner's syndrome have been reviewed and the following points have been emphasized:

1. All Horner's pupils dilate poorly to cocaine.
2. Cocaine does not help localize the lesion causing the Horner's syndrome.
3. Postganglionic lesions can be recognized by their failure to dilate to hydroxyamphetamine.
4. A head Horner's (postganglionic) syndrome is often benign, but a chest or neck Horner's (preganglionic) syndrome can be dangerous.

REFERENCES

1. Thompson, H. S.: Diagnostic pupillary drug tests. In Blodi, F. C., editor: Current concepts in ophthalmology, vol. 3, St. Louis, 1972, The C. V. Mosby Co.
2. Jaffe, N. S.: Localization of lesions causing Horner's syndrome, Arch. Ophthalmol. **44:**710, 1950.
3. Thompson, H. S., and Mensher, J. H.: Adrenergic mydriasis in Horner's syndrome, Am. J. Ophthalmol. **72:**472, 1971.
4. Riley, F. C., and Moyer, N. J.: Oculosympathetic paresis associated with cluster headache, Am. J. Ophthalmol. **72:** 763, 1971.
5. Ekbom, K.: A clinical comparison of cluster headache and migraine, Acta Neurol. Scand (Suppl.) **41:**1, 1970.
6. Giles, C. L., and Henderson, J. W.: Horner's syndrome: an analysis of 216 cases, Am. J. Ophthalmol. **46:**289, 1958.
7. Holland, M. G.: Treatment of glaucoma by chemical sympathectomy with 6-hydroxydopamine, Trans. Am. Acad. Ophthalmol. Otolaryngol. **76:**437, 1972.

8. Riley, R. C., and Moyer, N. J.: Experimental Horner's syndrome: a pupillographic evaluation of guanethidine-induced adrenergic blockade in human, Am. J. Ophthalmol. **69**:442, 1970.
9. Sneddon, J. M., and Turner, P.: The interactions of local guanethidine and sympathomimetic amines in the human eye, Arch. Ophthalmol. **81**:662, 1969.
10. Hitazawa, Y., Nosé, H., and Horie, T.: Chemical sympathectomy with 6-hydroxydopamine in the treatment of primary open-angle glaucoma, Am. J. Ophthalmol. **79**:98, 1975.
11. Hoffnagel, D., and Joseph, J. B.: Oculosympathetic paralysis in otitis media, N. Engl. J. Med. **265**:475, 1961.
12. Davis, R. H., Daroff, R. B., and Hoyt, W. F.: Hemicrania, oculosympathetic paresis, and subcranial carotid aneurysms: Raeder's paratrigeminal syndrome (Group 2), J. Neurosurg. **29**:94, 1968.
13. Smith, J. L.: Raeder's paratrigeminal syndrome, Am. J. Ophthalmol. **46**:194, 1958.
14. Minton, L. R., and Bounds, G. W.: Raeder's paratrigeminal syndrome, Am. J. Ophthalmol. **58**:271, 1964.
15. Boniuk, M., and Schlezinger, N. S.: Raeder's paratrigeminal syndrome, Am. J. Ophthalmol. **54**:1074, 1962.
16. Jarret, W. H.: Horner's syndrome with geniculate zoster, Am. J. Ophthalmol. **63**:326, 1967.
17. Harris, W.: Neuritis and neuralgia, London, 1926, Oxford University Press.
18. Ford, F. R., and Walsh, F. B.: Raeder's paratrigeminal syndrome, Johns Hopkins Med. J. **103**:296, 1958.
19. Klington, G. H., and Smith, W. M.: Raeder's paratrigeminal syndrome, Neurology (Minneap.) **6**:750, 1956.
20. Law, W. R., and Nelson, E. R.: Internal carotid aneurysm as a cause of Raeder's paratrigeminal syndrome, Neurology (Minneap.) **18**:43, 1968.
21. Raeder, J. G.: 'Paratrigeminal' paralysis of oculo-pupillary sympathetic, Brain **47**: 149, 1924.
22. O'Doherty, D. S., and Green, J. B.: Diagnostic value of Horner's syndrome in thrombosis of the carotid artery, Neurology (Minneap.) **8**:842, 1958.
23. Pruett, R. C.: Horner's syndrome following intra-oral trauma, Arch. Ophthalmol. **78**:420, 1967.

Demonstration of Tensilon responsiveness with infrared optokinetic nystagmography

Robert H. Spector
Robert B. Daroff
James E. Birkett

The diagnosis of myasthenia gravis (MG) depends heavily on the patient's responsiveness to intravenously administered edrophonium chloride (Tensilon). Falsely negative or equivocal edrophonium chloride tests are common and represent a distinct problem in the diagnosis and subsequent treatment of MG. In an effort to improve the objectivity, sensitivity, and specificity of the response, we have studied the effect of Tensilon on optokinetic nystagmus (OKN). Previous authors have utilized ocular electromyography,[1, 2] tonography,[3, 4] Lancaster red-green glasses,[5] and electrooculography (EOG)[6-9] for myasthenic testing and have reported variable results. We have applied infrared reflection rather than EOG as the eye movement recording technique and clearly have demonstrated that an OKN is an ideal motor substrate for objectively evaluating Tensilon responsiveness.

Table 19. Clinical data of patients with myasthenia gravis

Case	*Age*	*Sex*	*Myasthenic involvement*	*Ophthalmoparesis*	*Previous Tensilon testing* *Routine*	*EP-EMG**	*Tonography*
1	68	M	Ocular	Left inferior rectus paresis	–	+	–
2	18	F	Ocular and general	Bilateral ptosis and lateral recti pareses	+	–	
3	64	M	Ocular and general	Total external ophthalmoparesis	+	–	
4	45	F	Ocular and general	Left lateral rectus paresis	+	+	
5	68	F	Ocular and general	Left lateral rectus paresis	+	–	
6	23	F	Ocular and general	None	+	–	–
7	69	M	Complete remission	None	+	–	–
8	77	M	Ocular and general	Bilateral ptosis	+	–	+
9	27	F	Ocular	Right lateral rectus paresis	+	–	+
10	83	M	Ocular and general	Total external ophthalmoparesis	–	+	+
11	28	F	Ocular	Right superior rectus paresis	+	–	–
12	75	M	Ocular and general	None	+	–	
13	62	F	Ocular and general	None	+	–	
14	39	F	Ocular and general	Bilateral ptosis and lateral recti pareses	–	+	
15	74	F	Ocular and general	Left lateral rectus paresis	–	+	–
16	50	M	Ocular and general	Total external ophthalmoparesis	+	–	
17	70	F	Ocular and general	Bilateral ptosis and pseudo INO†	+	–	+
18	45	M	Ocular and general	Total external ophthalmoparesis	+	+	+
19	32	F	Ocular and general	Bilateral medial recti pareses	+	–	+
20	71	F	Ocular	Right medial and lateral recti pareses and bilateral upgaze pareses	–	+	–
21	46	M	Complete remission	None	+	+	

*Evoked potential electromyography.
†Internuclear ophthalmoplegia.

Table 20. Clinical data of controls and suspects

Case	*Age*	*Sex*	*Ophthalmoparesis*	*Diagnosis*
1	45	F	None	Hypothyroidism
2	65	F	Bilateral ptosis	Hypothyroidism
3	52	M	None	Polymyositis
4	65	M	Total external ophthalmoplegia	Chronic progressive external ophthalmoplegia
5	67	F	Left lateral rectus paresis	Intracavernous carotid aneurysm
6	44	M	None	Cervical spondylosis
7	32	M	Left lateral rectus and right superior oblique pareses	Nasopharyngeal cancer
8	40	F	Bilateral INO*	Multiple sclerosis
9	32	M	None	Normal control
10	48	M	Left superior rectus and inferior oblique pareses	Fractured floor of orbit
11	60	M	Bilateral horizontal gaze pareses	Charcot-Marie-Tooth disease
12	45	M	Bilateral INO and gaze pareses	Multiple sclerosis
13	68	M	Bilateral ptosis	Suspected myasthenia gravis
14	44	M	Bilateral INO	Suspected myasthenia gravis
15	74	F	Left medial rectus paresis	Suspected myasthenia gravis
16	32	F	Convergence spasms and neurasthenia	Suspected myasthenia gravis
17	28	F	Right superior rectus paresis	Suspected myasthenia gravis
18	25	F	Left ptosis and inferior rectus paresis	Suspected myasthenia gravis
19	55	M	Third nerve paresis sparing pupil	Diabetes mellitus
20	25	M	Left superior oblique paresis	Posttraumatic IV nerve palsy
21	22	F	None	Normal control
22	31	M	None	Normal control
23	23	M	None	Normal control
24	28	F	Bilateral sixth nerve paresis	Pseudotumor cerebri
25	34	F	Right fourth nerve paresis	Trauma
26	44	M	Left sixth nerve paresis	Wernicke's disease
27	46	M	Right lateral and medial recti pareses	Suspected myasthenia gravis

*Internuclear ophthalmoplegia.

METHODS

OKN was measured by infrared detectors and a recording system previously described.[10] We induced horizontal OKN by an array of constant velocity vertical bars moving across a 7 by 7 foot screen situated 44 inches in front of the subject. The head was immobilized, and movements of both eyes were recorded simultaneously after careful calibration with a 10° saccadic movement to the right and left of primary position. Isotonic saline was infused intravenously through a 20-gauge scalp-vein needle. The velocities of the OKN targets were individually adjusted to obtain the optimal nystagmus response, and the speed thereafter was kept constant throughout the testing period. The size of the screen and reduction of ambient light compelled the subjects to attend the usual OKN stimulus. We measured and compared the amplitude, frequency, and fast-phase velocity of the nystagmus before and after the intravenous infusion of 10 mg of Tensilon. For the purpose of evaluating the test, we divided the subjects into three groups (Tables 19 and 20): (1) those in whom the diagnosis of myasthenia gravis had been established previously, (2) controls, and (3) suspects.

SUBJECTS

The ages of the 21 patients with myasthenia gravis ranged from 18 to 83 years. There were 9 male and 12 female subjects in this group. All had prior diagnostic documentation with traditional Tensilon tests or electromyographic responses to repetitive stimulation (Harvey-Masland test). Four had purely ocular myasthenia, 15 had generalized involvement, and 2 were in complete remission. The extent of ophthalmoparesis ranged from isolated ptosis to total external ophthalmoplegia. Thirteen patients had no clinical weakness of either medial or lateral recti at the time they were subjected to the horizontal OKN stimulus. Explanations for the lack of horizontal diplopia included the following: (1) six had only levator or vertical muscle involvement or both, (2) five were effectively controlled with anticholinesterase or corticosteroid medication or both, and (3) two patients were in complete remission.

Two myasthenia gravis patients were studied on several occasions months apart to evaluate the reproducibility of the test.

The control group consisted of 20 subjects, 13 of whom had ophthalmoparesis of nonmyasthenic origin.

The suspect group consisted of seven patients (Table 22) six of whom had extraocular motor paresis clinically resembling MG but lacking consistent Tensilon responsivity. The other patient was clearly hysterical without objective weakness but had carried the diagnosis of MG because of equivocally positive Tensilon tests.

RESULTS

The amplitude, velocity, and frequency of OKN before and after intravenous administration of Tensilon in the myasthenic group are listed in Table 21. The medication caused an increase in amplitude in every case, varying from 24% to 130%. The velocity of the fast phase also increased in every subject. Frequency was the least sensitive parameter, with six falsely negative responses. Myasthenic response is demonstrated in Fig. 13-6.

None of the control subjects demonstrated an increased OKN amplitude

Table 21. Tensilon reponsiveness in myasthenia gravis patients

	Amplitude (degrees)			*Velocity (degrees/second)*			*Frequency (saccades/10 seconds)*		
Patient	*Pre*	*Post*	*Percent increase*	*Pre*	*Post*	*Percent increase*	*Pre*	*Post*	*Percent increase*
1	3.3	5.0	+ 52	120	163	+ 26	26	26	0
2	6.5	10.0	+ 54	270	340	+ 26	21	27	+ 29
3	6.8	14.0	+ 106	315	360	+ 14	22	30	+ 36
4	6.9	9.6	+ 39	135	163	+ 21	23	20	− 13
5	4.7	7.5	+ 59	138	206	+ 49	23	19	− 17
6A	4.5	5.6	+ 24	157	300	+ 91	19	24	+ 26
6B	5.2	12	+ 130	156	180	+ 15	22	19	− 14
7	5.0	8.2	+ 64	100	234	+ 134	21	21	0
8	4.0	6.7	+ 68	140	190	+ 36	17	18	+ 6
9A	6.3	12.5	+ 98	140	188	+ 34	14	21	+ 50
9B	2.2	3.3	+ 50	115	143	+ 24	24	26	+ 8
10	5.1	8.5	+ 67	213	263	+ 23	17	26	+ 53
11	3.8	7.8	+ 105	123	170	+ 38	28	32	+ 14
12	4.4	6.7	+ 52	160	207	+ 29	28	30	+ 7
13	4.8	9.5	+ 98	157	245	+ 56	21	19	+ 10
14	5.6	7.6	+ 36	186	240	+ 29	32	25	+ 22
15	4.0	6.8	+ 70	100	220	+ 220	18	18	0
16	9.8	16	+ 63	180	296	+ 64	19	26	+ 37
17	4.0	9.0	+ 120	140	280	+ 100	20	31	+ 52
18	3.9	6.8	+ 74	130	190	+ 46	20	20	0
19	4.5	7.5	+ 66	160	240	+ 50	18	23	+ 28
20	3.5	7.0	+ 100	115	200	+ 74	15	21	+ 40
21	4.5	8.1	+ 80	150	240	+ 60	12	16	+ 33
Mean %			80			60			
Median %			64			34			

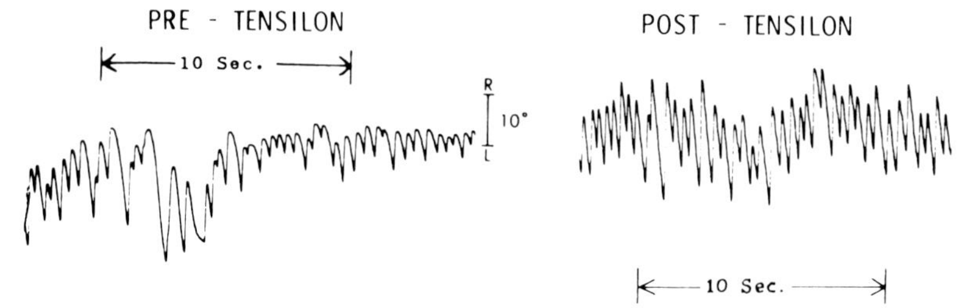

Fig. 13-6. Infrared optokinetic nystagmogram of myasthenic patient. Targets rotated toward patient's left. Note fatigue of amplitude in pre-Tensilon tracing and enhanced amplitude following intravenous Tensilon administration.

Table 22. Tensilon responsiveness in controls and suspects

Patient	*Amplitude (degrees)*			*Velocity (degrees/second)*			*Frequency (saccades/10 seconds)*		
	Pre	*Post*	*Percent increase*	*Pre*	*Post*	*Percent increase*	*Pre*	*Post*	*Percent increase*
1	10	9	– 10	320	300	– 6	23	32	+ 39
2	7	5.5	– 21	170	200	+ 18	24	26	+ 8
3	18	12	– 33	290	210	– 28	18	17	– 6
4	5.2	2.5	– 52	130	120	– 8	22	21	– 5
5	5.3	4.8	– 9	190	125	– 34	17	15	– 12
6	3.5	3.4	– 3	140	140	0	27	27	0
7	3.7	2.9	– 22	100	73	– 27	32	35	+ 9
8	4.2	4.0	– 5	80	60	25	20	18	– 10
9	6.0	5.3	– 12	160	120	– 25	27	22	– 19
10	6.0	5.4	– 10	200	180	– 5	27	25	– 7
11	6.0	5.0	– 17	190	140	– 26	18	15	– 17
12	3.5	2.0	– 42	110	80	– 27	20	18	– 10
13	4.5	5.5	+ 28	124	140	+ 13	21	17	– 19
14A	2.3	4.3	+ 87	50	70	+ 40	8	12	+ 50
14B	5.0	9.0	+ 80	202	245	+ 21	29	20	– 31
15	3.5	10.0	+ 180	120	300	+ 150	15	21	+ 40
16	5.2	3.0	– 42	180	70	– 60	15	10	– 33
17	3.5	8.5	+ 243	120	170	+ 41	27	33	+ 18
18	4.0	8.0	+ 100	120	190	+ 58	25	21	– 16
19	8	5.1	– 36	180	140	– 22	17	15	– 12
20	5.0	4.0	– 20	140	110	– 21	14	16	+ 14
21	6.0	4.1	– 31	160	130	– 19	23	13	– 43
22	7.0	5.0	– 29	170	140	– 18	18	15	– 17
23	6.2	4.1	– 34	170	125	– 26	23	20	– 13
24	6.0	3.0	– 50	160	110	– 31	24	22	– 8
25	5.0	4.1	– 18	140	125	– 11	20	12	– 40
26	5.4	4.1	– 24	150	120	– 20	15	10	– 33
27	3.0	7.0	+ 133	180	280	+ 55	10	18	+ 20

following administration of Tensilon (Table 22). The fast-phase velocity did increase in one of the controls (case 2). Again, the frequency response was variable and unpredictable.

The six MG suspects with ophthalmoparesis demonstrated amplitude increase ranging from 28% to 243% above predrug level. In patient 16, who had no objective neurologic signs, the amplitude decreased as a result of Tensilon administration.

DISCUSSION

Our study demonstrated the sensitivity and specificity of Tensilon infrared optokinetic nystagmography for the diagnosis of myasthenia gravis. All the myasthenic patients and none of the controls manifested increased OKN amplitude following intravenous Tensilon administration. All the myasthenics also manifested increased velocity of the OKN fast phase after Tensilon administration, but one control also had increased velocity. Amplitude, therefore, seemed the most reliable parameter for diagnosing myasthenia. OKN frequency proved to be totally unpredictable.

Thirteen of the 21 myasthenic patients had no clinical paresis of their horizontal recti at the time of testing, yet all had positive Tensilon responses to horizontal optokinetic targets. The test was obviously sufficiently sensitive to uncover even subclinical myasthenic weakness of extraocular muscles.

Of the six ocular myasthenic suspects with positive responses, five have since developed generalized myasthenia. In the other the disorder has remained purely ocular, with partial anticholinesterase responsiveness.

Four previous studies of edrophonium chloride OKN utilized EOG as the eye movement recording technique.[6-9] A total of 25 myasthenics were studied, and 30% had false negative responses despite the examiners' intentional sampling of patients with horizontal recti paresis. All thirteen patients tested in three of the reports had positive edrophonium chloride OKN responses.[6, 7, 9] However, half of the twelve patients studied by Campbell and co-workers[8] had falsely negative tests. This indicated either a specific methodologic fault in the examiners' technique or a relative insensitivity of EOG for recording edrophonium chloride responsiveness, at least as compared to infrared. We studied one of our proven myasthenics with both recording techniques simultaneously and found that the infrared nystagmogram was unequivocally positive while the concomitant EOG showed no change after the administration of Tensilon.

We attempted to explain the disparity between infrared and EOG as follows. EOG is a recording technique that measures changes in corneoretinal potentials. Skin electrodes applied around the orbit are required to convert these voltage potentials into recordable electric deflections. We theorized that the accumulation of an electrolyte-rich film of sweat at the skin-electrode interface might interfere with accurate conduction. This hypothesis was tested by placing two skin electrodes on a control subject and measuring resistance changes before and after intravenously administering Tensilon. The resistance dropped 50%, which would have been reflected as an equivalent depression of nystagmus amplitude. We therefore demonstrated that the relative insensitivity of EOG resulted from the potent diaphoretic effect of Tensilon. This could reduce and possibly mask an actual amplitude increase. Such a problem does not occur with infrared OKN because skin electrodes are not used.

In conclusion, Tensilon infrared optokinetic nystagmography is a sensitive and specific test for myasthenic weakness in extraocular muscles and is not limited to patients with clinically apparent ophthalmoparesis. To date, we have had no falsely negative or falsely positive responses.

REFERENCES

1. Breinin, G.: Electromyography: a tool in ocular and neurologic diagnosis, Arch. Ophthalmol. **57**:161-164, 1957.
2. Sears, M. L., Walsh, F. B., and Teasdale, R. D.: The electromyogram from ocular muscles in myasthenia gravis, Arch. Ophthalmol. **63**:791-798, 1960.
3. Glaser, J. S., Miller, G. R., and Gass, J. D. M.: The edrophonium tonogram test in myasthenia gravis, Arch. Ophthalmol. **76**:368-373, 1966.
4. Wray, S. H., and Pavan-Langston, D.: A re-evaluation of edrophonium chloride (Tensilon) tonography in the diagnosis of myasthenia gravis, Neurology (Minneap.) **21**:586-588, 1971.
5. Retzlaff, J. A., Kearns, T. P., Howard, F. M., and Cronin, M. L.: Lancaster red-green test in evaluation of edrophonium effect in myasthenia gravis, Am. J. Ophthalmol. **67**:13, 1969.
6. Blomberg, L. H., and Persson, T.: A new test for myasthenia gravis, Acta Neurol. Scand. **41**(suppl. 13): 363-364, 1965.
7. Stella, S.: Optokinetic nystagmus in patients with occular myasthenia, Invest. Ophthalmol. **6**:668, 1967.
8. Campbell, J. J., Simpson, E., and Cronbie, A. L.: Ocular myasthenia. Evaluation of tensilon tonography and electromyography as diagnostic tests, J. Neurol. Neurosurg. Psychiatry **33**:639-646, 1970.
9. Metz, H. S., Scott, A. B., and O'Meara, D. M.: Saccadic eye movement in myasthenia gravis, Arch. Ophthalmol. **88**:9-11, 1972.
10. Young, L. R.: Measuring eye movements, Am. J. Med. Electronics **4**:300-307, 1963.
11. Dell'Osso, L. F., Flynn, J. T., and Daroff, R. B.: Hereditary congenital nystagmus: an intrafamilial study, Arch. Ophthalmol. **92**:366-374, 1974.

Binasal field loss and prefixation blindness

Sydney F. J. Pilley
H. Stanley Thompson

Binasal field loss has been described by a number of authors since von Graefe first recognized this type of defect in 1858.[1] It is a relatively rare ophthalmologic finding.

The usually accepted causes include retinal degenerative lesions—in particular, bilateral retinoschisis—glaucoma, drusen of the optic disc, fracture of the base of the skull, neurosyphilis, chiasmal arachnoiditis, intracranial tumor, and hysteria.[2]

The nature of pure binasal field loss requires that damage be present bilaterally and anterior to the chiasm, since lesions of the lateral chiasm or optic tracts will necessarily involve crossing or crossed fibres from the nasal retinas resulting in additional temporal field loss.

The main sites of involvement are thus: (1) the retina, (2) the optic disc, and (3) the prechiasmal optic nerve (Fig. 13-7). In addition, a number of cases have a hysterical basis.

Clinically, cases fall into three major groupings (Fig. 13-8): (1) those

Dr. Pilley's work was supported in part by the Fulbright Hayes Scholarship program and the Ernest Hart Scholarship (British Medical Association).

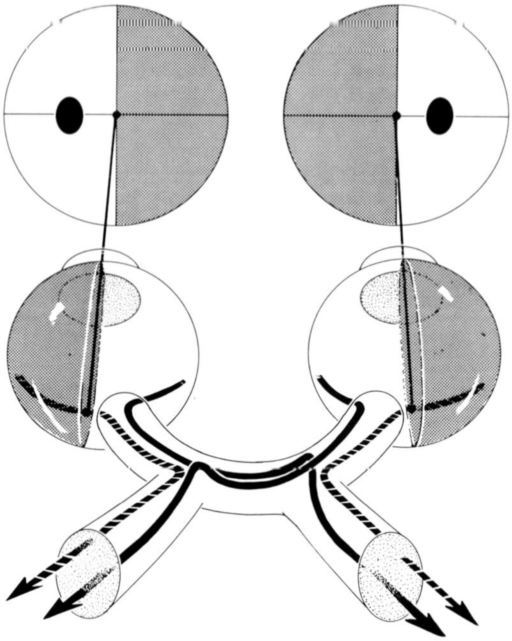

Fig. 13-7. Two lesions are required to produce binasal field loss. These may be (1) in both retinas, (2) in both optic discs, or (3) in both optic nerves. Lesions farther back cause either bitemporal or homonymous field loss.

presenting with *peripheral* loss in both nasal fields; (2) those presenting with asymmetric and incomplete binasal field loss; such defects often extend across the midline and show evidence of *disc-related* character on careful perimetry; and (3) those presenting with dense and clearly *vertically delineated* binasal field loss.

SECTORIAL FIELD LOSS

The major causes for sectorial loss of peripheral binasal field are retinoschisis and other rarer forms of chorioretinal degeneration such as sectorial retinitis pigmentosa. It is also possible for glaucoma to cause such patterns of loss in early stages. On careful ophthalmic examination, cases with field loss in this group usually show clinical signs of retinoschisis, cupped discs, or increased intraocular pressure.

DISC-RELATED FIELD LOSS

The second clinical group consists of patients with irregular binasal defects due to lesions of the optic disc.

The pathogenesis of these disc lesions involves ischemia of the optic nerve head due to occlusion of the small vessels in this region. This process prob-

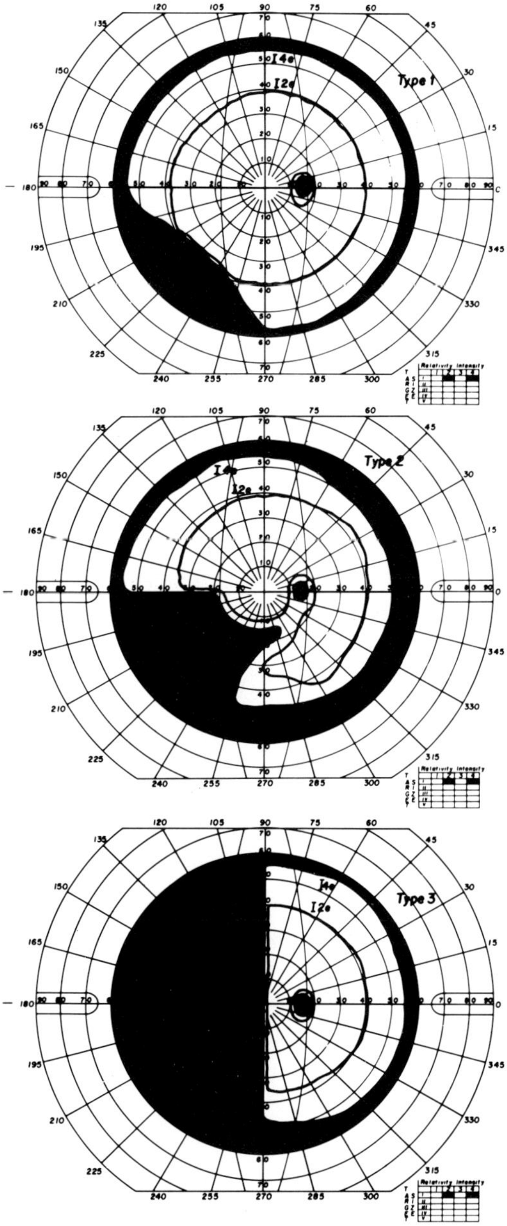

Fig. 13-8. Three different types of nasal field loss, each suggesting a different area of involvement within the visual system.

ably causes the binasal field defects found in glaucoma and intrapapillary drusen.

Papilledema may result in similar ischemic changes at the optic nerve head and will progress to complete optic atrophy if long-standing. Field loss in long-standing papilledema tends to occur as peripheral constriction, with more rapid progression in the nasal field.[3, 4] Frequently, arcuate defects develop so that there may be a markedly binasal character to the early field loss.

Progressive intracranial space-occupying lesions are well documented causes of binasal field loss and almost invariably show evidence of associated papilledema or optic atrophy.[5]

The classically accepted cause of binasal field loss occurring with progressive intracranial mass lesions involves pressure on the lateral angles of the prechiasmatic optic nerves by the anterior vessels of the circle of Willis.[5-8]

Some authors have cited pressure from dilation of the third ventricle as a cause of chiasmal distortion and compression resulting in binasal hemianopia,[9] but dilation of the third ventricle is most frequently associated with bitemporal rather than binasal loss.

Compressive ischemia of the prechiasmatic optic nerves has been suggested as the cause of binasal hemianopia,[10] but it has recently been shown that chiasmal and prechiasmal vasculature is good, especially on the lateral aspects.[11, 12]

Descriptions of cases with massive distortion of the chiasm,[13] and with marked notching of the chiasm by vessels[14] have been notable in failing to show convincing nasal field loss in general.

A case was reported in 1971 of binasal hemianopia with recovery of field following intracranial decompression, and this was regarded as evidence supporting the concept of ischemic damage to the prechiasmatic optic nerves.[15] Neurosurgical decompression also led to rapid resolution of the coexistent papilledema, so that recovery of nasal field could equally well have been due to improved perfusion at the optic disc.

We would suggest that the evidence for acceptance of the classical pathogenesis in binasal field loss associated with intracranial mass lesions is poor and unconvincing and that most of these patients develop binasal field loss as a result of ischemic changes at the optic disc due to coexistent papilledema. This concept is not new but needs reemphasis since it was so tentatively considered by earlier authors[7, 16] that it has failed to achieve general acceptance.

It must be conceded that there may be exceptional cases in which binasal field loss results from damage to both optic nerves, and within this group probably fall the rare cases described as a result of opticochiasmal arachnoiditis, neurosyphilis, and closed head trauma.[5] These cases are less frequently associated with papilledema, but most of the reported cases have not had detailed fields described, and some of these patients may have proved to be hysterical on more careful testing.

HEMIANOPIC FIELD LOSS

Most cases of binasal hemianopic field loss fail to show any other abnormality despite careful and complete ophthalmic and neurologic examinations. In such patients the alternative diagnoses include small but progressive intracranial mass lesion, chiasmal arachnoiditis, and hysteria. Since the diagnoses of chiasmal arachnoiditis and hysteria are so notoriously dangerous and made only by exclusion of all other causes, patients are frequently subjected to contrast-study radiography before either of these diagnoses is accepted.

Within this group, and as an aid in separating organic causes of binasal field loss from those of hysterical origin, testing for the presence of "hemifield phenomena" is of use.

Hemifield phenomena

Hemifield phenomena have been described by Nachtgäller and Hoyt[17] and Kirkham.[18] These authors concern themselves with such phenomena in cases of *bitemporal* field loss, although similar phenomena would be expected in complete hemianopic binasal field loss. Hemifield phenomena may be described as (1) hemifield slide phenomena and (2) binocular prefixation blindness.

Here we are interested in prefixation blindness. Patients with complete hemianopic binasal loss are necessarily blind in the prefixation binocular field (Fig. 13-9). It is our experience in two cases that patients with hysterical binasal field loss will fail to show this expected area of blindness on binocular confrontation field testing.

Patient 1. J. McL., a 34-year-old nurse, sought medical attention in July 1974 because of an intermittent fever over a 9-month period. During this time she had had several short episodes of loss of consciousness. She was found to be anemic.

Neurologic examination showed a dense binasal hemianopia and vague abnormalities of deep sensation in both legs, but skull x-ray films, EEG, and brain scan were normal.

Visual acuity was 20/20 OD and 20/200 OS due to an old anisometropia, exotropia, and amblyopia. The exotropia had been treated surgically in 1972 with a good cosmetic result.

Dense nasal field loss was found in each eye on monocular confrontation testing with hand movement targets. At the Goldmann perimeter there was a consistent dense binasal hemianopia falling accurately along the entire vertical meridian through fixation.

The binocular prefixation field was tested, as described below. It could be demonstrated repeatedly that the patient was able to see small objects in her nasal fields when both eyes were open.

Invasive neurologic tests were not performed. The patient was discharged and has not developed any new neurologic symptoms or signs.

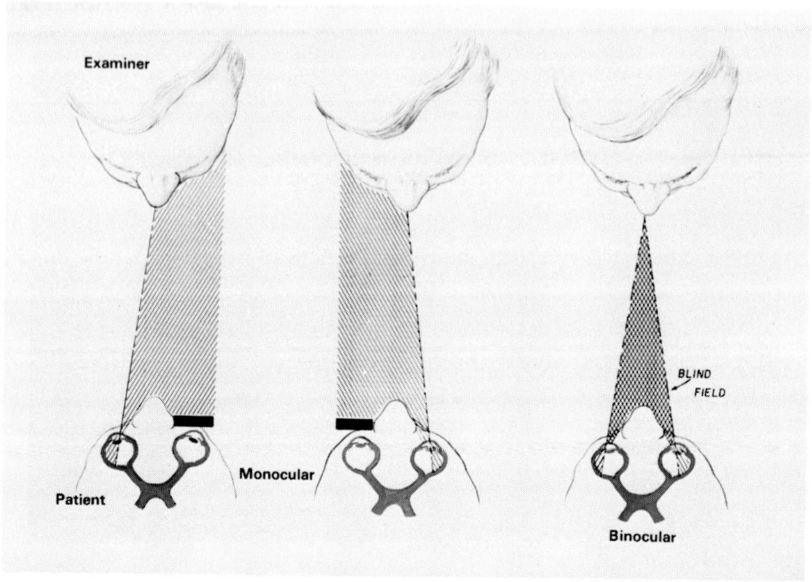

Fig. 13-9. Monocular confrontation field testing confirms binasal field loss. In the binocular field there is an area temporal to the left visual axis perceived with the left eye and an area temporal to the right visual axis perceived with the right eye. The area nasal to each visual axis cannot be seen with either eye, and there is thus an area of blindness in the prefixation field. Binocular confrontation testing in organic binasal hemianopia confirms the presence of prefixation blindness.

Patient 2. B. W., a 24-year-old woman, first came for eye examination in November 1971 with vague complaints of ocular irritation. Examination was within normal limits except for inconstant binasal field defects.

Neurologic examination four days later showed reduced acuity of 20/200 OU, complete right anosmia, and definite binasal field defects on confrontation.

Repeat examination after three weeks confirmed dense binasal field defects by confrontation and on Goldmann perimetry using a variety of targets including V-4_e, but otherwise full ophthalmic examination was normal. Visual acuities had returned to 6/7.5 OU. Skull films and polytomograms were normal.

Examination findings remained static for three months, following which reexamination of the cerebrospinal fluid, brain scan, and pneumoencephalography were undertaken. All results were normal.

Binocular prefixation field testing at this time consistently demonstrated physiologic diplopia even with small targets, while complete nasal hemianopia was present in each visual field when tested separately with large targets.

Further neurosurgical studies were postponed.

From this time visual field defects began to resolve, and on the latest review fields were completely full. There were no residual or new neurologic signs.

When the test for binocular prefixation blindness is applied, it is most important that fixation be firmly held. This is best accomplished in a confrontation situation with the patient seated facing the examiner. The patient is requested to fixate on the examiner's nose, for example, and targets may then be introduced into the space between the patient and the examiner from below. The targets should be of a size that the patient denies seeing in the previously charted uniocular nasal field. The patient is asked to state whether he sees one or two objects as the target enters the prefixation field below, and only a statement of blindness is consistent with organic field loss, assuming that fixation has been maintained as instructed. This test is then repeated using varied targets.

The test appears to give remarkably consistent results, clearly differentiating hysterical from organic binasal field loss. The patient is, of course, being placed in a novel test situation and is not aware that the nasal fields are being tested because both eyes are open throughout the test.

Binocular prefixation field testing provides useful information in cases of binasal field loss when the field loss is of the third clinical type, showing definite vertical delineation, and when there are no other signs on ophthalmic or neurologic examination, thus making the diagnosis of hysteria a possibility. By using this test one can distinguish positively the cases of hysterical origin in this group and thereby avoid invasive and contrast study investigations and all of their associated morbidity.

SUMMARY

1. Look for the causes of genuine binasal field loss anterior to the chiasm, because everything from the lateral chiasm back causes homonymous loss.

2. Most real binasal loss is disc related, but occasionally one encounters a case due to a retinal lesion (schisis) or to an optic nerve lesion (trauma, dilated third ventricle, neurosyphilis, arachnoiditis, etc.—all rare and all hard to prove).

3. If a clear-cut, complete binasal hemianopia is seen, suspect hysteria.

4. A case can be confirmed as hysterical with binocular prefixation field testing.

REFERENCES

1. von Graefe, A.: Ueber die untersuchung des Gesichtsfeldes bei amblyopischen Affectionen, Albrecht von Graefes Arch. Klin. Ophthalmol. **2**:258-298, 1858.
2. Duke-Elder, S.: System of Ophthalmology, vol. 12: Neuro-ophthalmology, St. Louis, 1971, The C. V. Mosby Co., pp. 292-293.
3. Huber, A.: Eye symptoms in brain tumours, edited and translated by F. C. Blodi, St. Louis, 1971, The C. V. Mosby Co.
4. Bynke, H. G.: On early diagnosis and prevention of secondary optic atrophy in papilloedema, Acta Ophthalmol. (Kbh.) **44**:801-813, 1966.
5. Francois, J.: L'hemianopsic binasalc, Ophthalmologica **113**:321-343, 1947.
6. Knapp, H.: Defects in the fields of vision and their connection with diseases of the heart and brain, Arch. Scient. Pract. Med. Surg. p. 293, 1873.
7. Cushing, H., and Walker, C. B.: Distortions of the visual fields in cases of brain tumors—binasal hemianopsia, Arch. Ophthalmol. **61**:559-598, 1912.
8. Polyak, S.: The vertebrate visual system, Chicago, 1957, University of Chicago Press, pp. 340-342.
9. Dubois-Poulsen, A.: Le champ visuel. Topographie normale et pathologique de ses sensibilitees, Paris, 1952, Masson & Cie.
10. Hoyt, W. F.: Correlative functional anatomy of the optic chiasm, Clin. Neurosurg. **17**:189-208, 1969.

11. Wollschlaeger, P. D., et al.: Arterial blood supply of the human optic chiasm and surrounding structures, Ann. Ophthalmol. pp. 862-869, 1971.
12. Bergland, R., and Ray, B. S.: The arterial supply of the human optic chiasm, J. Neurosurg. **31**:327-334, 1969.
13. Page, L. K.: Developmental tumors about the optic chiasm. In Smith, J. L., and Glaser, J. S., editors: Neuro-ophthalmology, vol. 7, St. Louis, 1973, The C. V. Mosby Co.
14. Rucker, C. W., and Kernohan, J. W.: Notching of the optic chiasm by overlying arteries in pituitary tumors, Arch. Ophthalmol. **5**:161-170, 1954.
15. Frisen, L.: Genuine, relative, binasal hemianopia, Acta Ophthalmol. **49**:734-740, 1971.
16. Shelden, W. D., and Lillie, W. I.: Importance of visual fields as an aid in localization of brain tumours, J.A.M.A. **94**:677, 1930.
17. Nachtigäller, H., and Hoyt, W. F.: Storungen des Seheindruckes bei bitemporaler Hemianopsie und Verschiebung der Sehachsen, Klin. Monatsbl. Augenheilkd. **156**:821-836, 1970.
18. Kirkham, T. H.: The ocular symptomatology of pituitary tumours, Proc. R. Soc. Med. **65**:517-518, 1972.

Periodic alternating nystagmus: clinicopathologic correlation

John O. Susac
James M. Henry

Periodic alternating nystagmus (PAN) is an unusual form of horizontal jerk nystagmus in which the phases repeatedly change direction in a cyclic fashion. In primary position, a jerk nystagmus to one side will be followed by a short, quiet interlude and then be replaced by a jerk nystagmus to the opposite side. This cycling repeats constantly, with the duration of the jerk nystagmus varying from one to six minutes.

Davis and Smith[1] have recently reviewed the many different clinical conditions that have been associated with periodic alternating nystagmus. These include cerebral trauma, encephalitis, syphilis, vertebrobasilar insufficiency, multiple sclerosis, spinocerebellar degeneration, posterior fossa tumors, and Arnold-Chiari malformations. Although usually acquired, PAN may rarely be congenital.

Only three cases of PAN have been studied with morphologic correlation. Towle[2, 3] briefly reported two of them. His first patient had an arachnoid cyst that compressed the medulla, and an Arnold-Chiari malformation was present in the other. Keane[4] recently published a detailed neuropathologic analysis of a 54-year-old woman with multiple sclerosis who had periodic alternating nystagmus and downbeat nystagmus.* The following case, the clinical aspects of which were previously reported (case 1),[5] details the

*EDITOR'S NOTE. Recently a fourth case of PAN with pathologic findings has been published (Karp, J. S., and Rorke, L. B.: Arch. Neurol. **32**:422, 1975). It is noted that in all cases of PAN studied histologically, lesions have been found at the pontomedullary level, involving the vestibular nuclear complex. J. S. G.

neuro-ophthalmologic and pathologic findings in a middle-aged woman with neurosyphilis.

CASE REPORT

This 42-year-old black woman was first seen in neuro-ophthalmologic consultation in December 1970 because of abnormal eye movements. Examination revealed classic PAN that had a cycle of 110 seconds of nystagmus to either side with a quiet phase of 20 seconds. A right-beating horizontal nystagmus for 110 seconds was followed by 20 seconds of rest and then a left-beating horizontal nystagmus for 110 seconds. The patient experienced oscillopsia and reduced acuity during the height of the oscillations. Visual acuity during the quiet phase was 20/25 in both eyes, and visual fields were normal. The pupils reacted 2+ to light and 4+ to near. Ophthalmoscopy revealed mild pallor of the optic discs and sheathing of the arterioles.

Past history revealed that the patient had delivered a stillborn fetus when 16 years old and several months later had had a positive reaction to a serologic test for syphilis. She was treated with penicillin twice, at age 16 and again at 20 years. In 1961, at the age of 30 years, an unremitting, progressive neurologic disorder began. Her initial complaints were shooting pains in her legs and difficulty seeing. An optician told her that she had "jumping eyes." She subsequently began having difficulty in walking and developed paresthesias in the lower extremities. Hearing loss occurred on the left. She was hospitalized at Jackson Memorial Hospital in 1963 and was thought to have multiple sclerosis. Her gait steadily worsened so that by 1967 she required a walker. By 1970 she was confined to a wheelchair and had bowel and bladder incontinence.

Neurologic examination revealed a severe spastic paraparesis with bilateral extensor plantar responses. There was mild finger to nose ataxia, decreased hearing on the left, and normal sensation.

Laboratory findings included normal hemogram and urinalysis, a weekly reactive VDRL test, and a 2+ reactive FTA-ABS test. Chest, skull, and cervical spine x-ray films were normal. A complete myelogram up to the foramen magnum level was normal. Study of the cerebrospinal fluid revealed the following: lymphocytes, 5/cu mm; protein, 40 mg/100 ml; and a nonreactive VDRL test. The gamma globulin was elevated at 25%.

A presumptive diagnosis of neurosyphilis was made. The patient received ampicillin and probenecid (Benemid) for three months with no significant change in clinical course.

On November 24, 1972, the patient was hospitalized for rectal bleeding. She had had melena and diarrhea for two weeks prior to admission. She denied abdominal pain. No cause for the bleeding was discovered. There was marked anemia for which she received four units of whole blood. She subsequently developed a urinary tract infection and was treated with gentamicin and Keflin. A febrile course, which was attributed to infected sacral decubiti, continued. The diarrhea also persisted, and over the next few weeks she developed protracted nausea and vomiting.

On December 10, 1972, she became unresponsive, hypotensive, and stopped breathing. Resuscitation was instituted, and she was placed on a respirator. Her pupils were 2.5 mm in diameter and poorly responsive to light. The PAN was no longer present. Vestibuloocular movements were absent horizontally but intact vertically. She was flaccid, areflexic, and unresponsive to pain. She died three days later.

General autopsy findings revealed ulcers in the gastroesophageal region, fatty metamorphosis of the liver, chronic passive congestion of the spleen, chronic pyelonephritis, and bilateral hydronephrosis.

EYE PATHOLOGY. On gross examination there was bilateral optic disc pallor. Microscopic examination of the optic nerves revealed loss of nerve fibers and a round cell infiltrate within the pial septa (Fig. 13-10). Loss of ganglion cells in the retina reflected

A

B

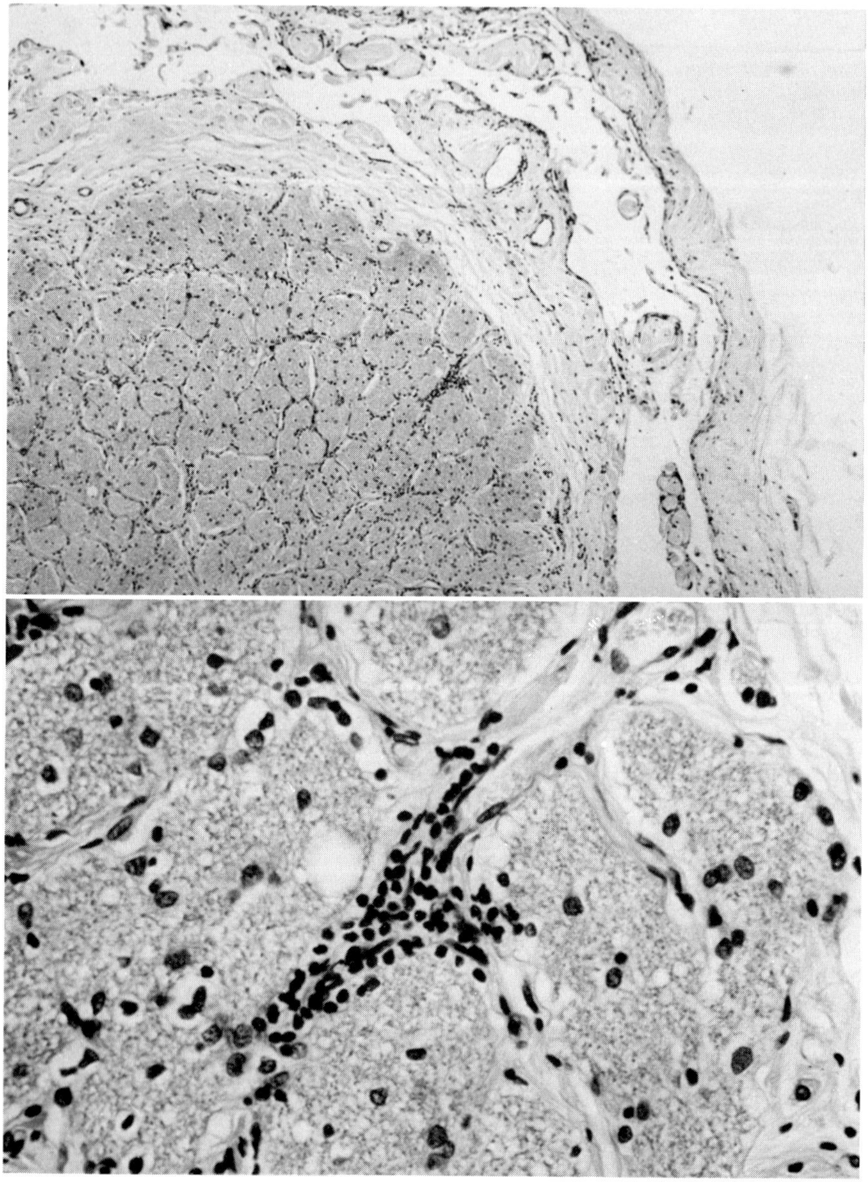

Fig. 13-10. A, Round cell infiltrate of pial septa within nerve and thickening of leptomeninges, right optic nerve. **B,** Round cell infiltrate of pial septa, right optic nerve. (**A,** H&E, ×100; **B,** H&E, ×400.)

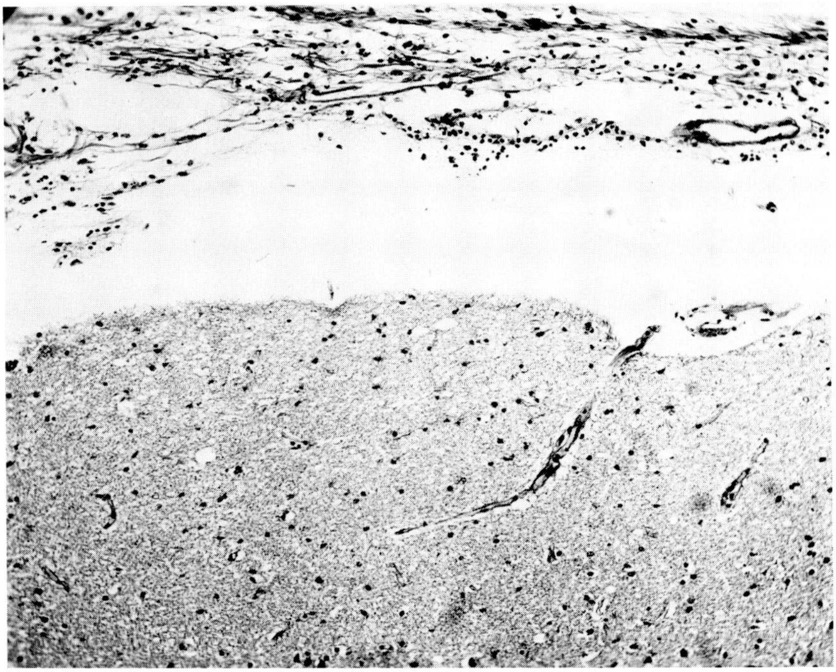

Fig. 13-11. Cerebral leptomeninges, illustrating round cell infiltrate. (H&E, ×100.)

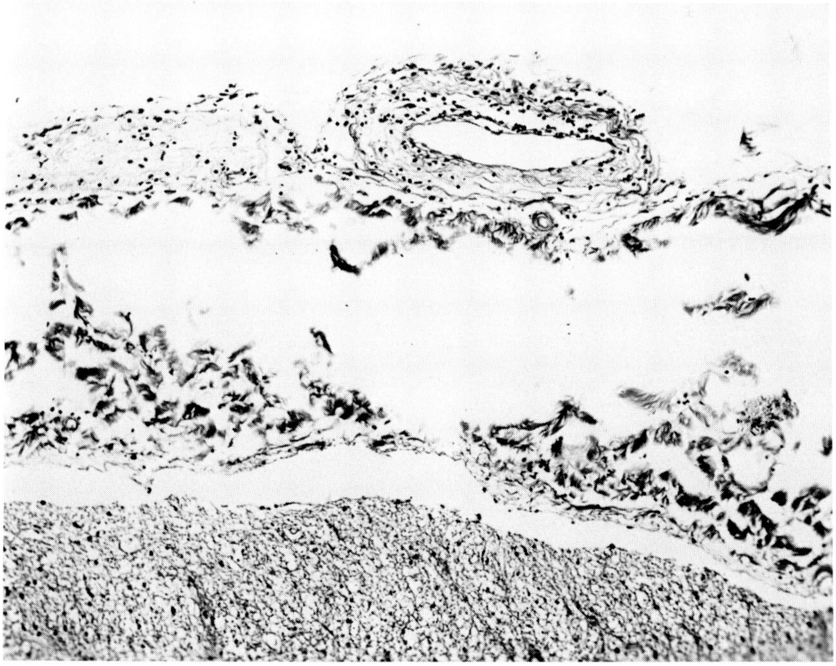

Fig. 13-12. Cerebral vessel, illustrating vasculitis. (H&E, ×100.)

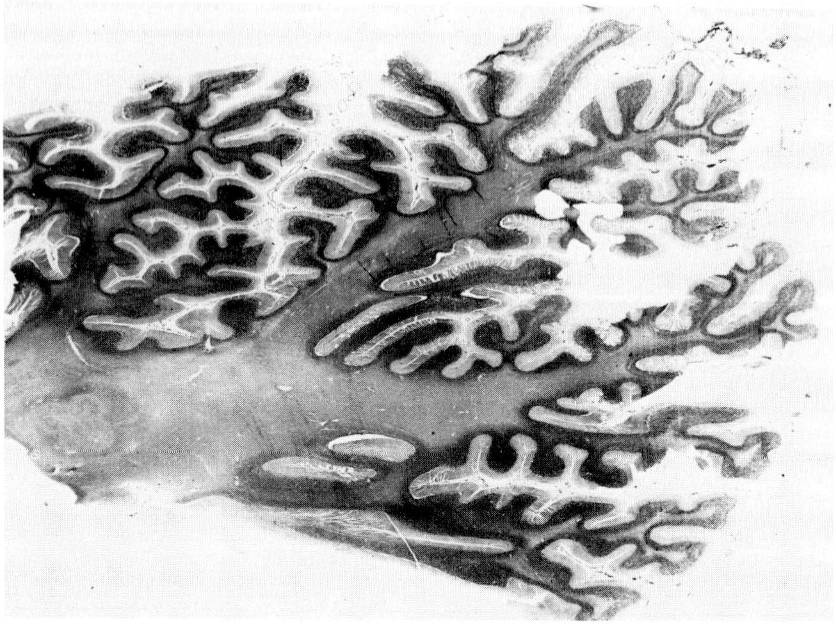

Fig. 13-13. Cerebellum, illustrating atrophy. (H&E, ×4.)

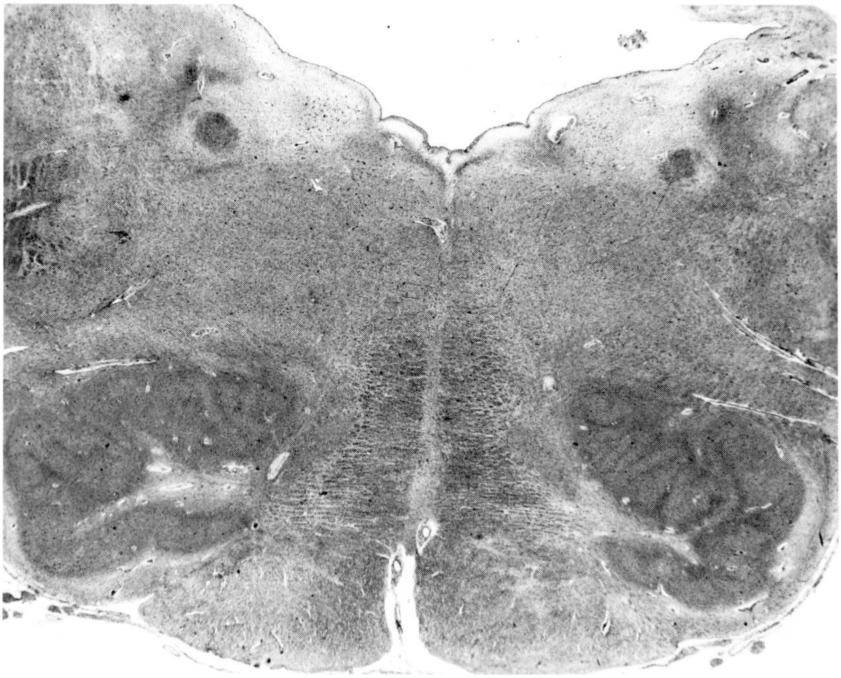

Fig. 13-14. Medulla, illustrating normal architecture of nuclear structures with minimal gliosis of vestibular nuclei and inferior olivary nuclei. (LFB-PAS, ×10.)

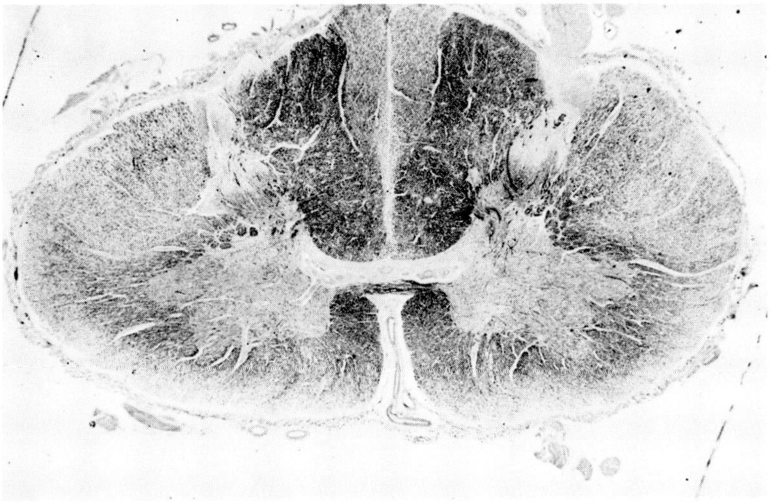

Fig. 13-15. Spinal cord, showing atrophy of ascending and descending tracts. (H&E, ×9.)

retrograde degeneration. Mild pial thickening was associated with a chronic inflammatory response indicative of a chronic meningitis. Additionally there was a mild inflammatory infiltrate in the choroid and atrophy of the ciliary muscles. In summary, the pathologic conditions in the eye included (1) mild optic neuritis and optic atrophy, (2) loss of ganglion cells, (3) ciliary atrophy, (4) mild uveitis, and (5) chronic meningitis.

NEUROPATHOLOGY. Gross examination of the brain revealed mild thickening of the leptomeninges. Microscopic examination showed thickening and fibrosis of the leptomeninges throughout the neuraxis associated with scattered small round cell infiltrates (Fig. 13-11) that were also present in the Virchow-Robin spaces of the parenchyma. Adjacent cerebral vessels displayed thickening of the adventitia with frequent invasion of the vessel walls by round cells, indicative of a chronic vasculitis (Fig. 13-12). Multiple microfoci of lymphocytes with occasional admixed macrophages were found throughout the brain. Although there was little evidence of recent granular ependymitis, there were extensive areas of remote neuronal loss and gliosis in the subependymal region of the third ventricle and midbrain.

All sections of the CNS showed recent coagulation necrosis and neuronal loss consistent with generalized terminal hypoxia. These changes, which were most severe in the cerebral cortex, precluded interpretation of possible chronic neuronal loss secondary to syphilis.

Marked atrophy of the cerebellum with loss of Purkinje's cells and gliosis of Bergmann's layer was noted (Fig. 13-13). Rarefaction of cerebellar white matter was associated with severe loss of neurons and gliosis of the cerebellar nuclei, especially the dentate. The brainstem showed diffuse rarefaction of the long tracts with scattered foci of round cells within the roots of occasional cranial nerves. At the level of the medulla, the vestibular nuclei and inferior olivary nuclei showed mild neuronal loss and gliosis (Fig. 13-14). Marked atrophy of both pyramids was also noted.

Sections of the spinal cord revealed marked atrophy of descending and ascending tracts (Fig. 13-15). The fasciculus gracilis and the corticospinal tracts were most severely involved. The spinocerebellar and vestibulospinal tracts were also involved, while the anterior funiculus was relatively spared.

DISCUSSION

The pathologic findings of optic neuritis and optic atrophy, chronic leptomeningitis with vasculitis of cerebral vessels, and diffuse nervous-system involvement corroborated the clinical impression of neurosyphilis in this patient. There was marked degeneration of the ascending and descending tracts in the spinal cord. Severe involvement of the fasciculus gracilis with sparing of the cuneate fasciculus, which is typical of tabes, was observed. Diffuse cerebral and cerebellar degeneration manifested by neuronal loss and gliosis were noted. There was marked involvement of long tracts within the brainstem. Brainstem nuclear structures were relatively spared, although there was mild gliosis of the inferior olivary and the vestibular nuclei.

Since the neuropathologic changes were so extensive, it is impossible to determine the pathologic substrate for the nystagmus in this case. In Keane's[4] patient, bilateral rather symmetric demyelination in the region of the vestibular nuclei was found, and he suggested that these lesions were most likely related to the production of the nystagmus. In contrast, the vestibular nuclei in our case were minimally involved in comparison to the vestibular connections with the cerebellum and spinal cord, suggesting that sufficient disruption of the vestibular connections might induce PAN in the presence of relatively normal vestibular nuclei. From the available pathologic material, no actual critical site or sites necessary for induction of PAN can be determined. PAN probably requires a combination of lesions and cannot be understood by a structure-bound theory.

The pathophysiologic mechanisms involved in the production of this extraordinary nystagmus remain unknown. Kornhuber[6] has postulated a central vestibular hyperresponsiveness. One of his patients with multiple sclerosis showed a central vestibular hyperexcitability for eight years and then developed typical PAN. He suggested that loss of inhibition to the vestibular nuclei most likely resulted from bilateral lesions in the paramedian reticular formation of the pontomesencephalic tegmentum. This region was minimally involved in the present case.

Like downbeat nystagmus, PAN should suggest a lower brainstem lesion. Cogan[7] has shown that downbeat nystagmus is usually associated with lesions in the caudal end of the brainstem, such as Arnold-Chiari malformations, basilar impressions, and foramen magnum meningiomas. All the pathologically verified cases of PAN to date have shown involvement of the lower brainstem. Keane's[4] patient was especially interesting because both downbeat nystagmus and PAN were present. Schatz[8] has recently described a patient with downbeat nystagmus in association with an Arnold-Chiari malformation who developed PAN following surgery.

The diagnosis of PAN is often overlooked during the clinical examination. One should suspect PAN in a nonvertiginous patient who has nystagmus in the primary position. This nystagmus should be watched over a two- to three-minute period to determine changes of direction. If there are no direction changes and the nystagmus remains horizontal on upgaze, congenital nystagmus is most likely, but an acquired central vestibulopathy may also be responsible. One should also suspect PAN when reviewing a hospital chart in which a right beating nystagmus has been described by one resident and a left beating nystagmus by another.

Periodic alternating gaze deviation seems closely related to PAN. This rare condition in which the eyes periodically deviate to either side is associated with contralateral head movements but not nystagmus. The well-documented patient of Goldberg and associates,[9] had a basilar artery aneurysm and basilar insufficiency. Kestenbaum[10] interpreted his case as actually having PAN with the fast phases obliterated by a bilateral horizontal gaze palsy.

Periodic alternation of null point in congenital nystagmus[11] shows striking similarities to both PAN and to periodic alternating gaze deviations. In this condition there is a periodic alternation of gaze to either side as well as nystagmus with a shifting null point. When the null point is shifted to the right, a left-beating nystagmus is seen in primary position, and *vice versa.* This phenomenon is very closely related to PAN. Daroff and Dell'Osso[5] have suggested that one can conceptualize PAN as being a horizontal jerk nystagmus with an omnipresent shifting of the null.

Rebound nystagmus[12] should not be confused with PAN.[5] Rebound nystagmus is usually a first degree horizontal jerk nystagmus that is initially noted during lateral gaze to one side. If the eyes are maintained in lateral gaze for a prolonged period (10 to 20 seconds) or if the eyes are promptly returned to primary position, a brief rebound nystagmus occurs in the opposite direction. Although rebound nystagmus may be unidirectional and occur only after lateral gaze to one side, it is usually bidirectional and elicited after gaze deviations to either side.[12] Daroff and Dell'Osso[5] described one patient who had primary position jerk nystagmus that shifted direction irregularly and without definite periodicity. They initially thought that he had "atypical" PAN, but electronystagmography recordings showed that the directional shifts resulted from rebounding. They have suggested that rebound nystagmus be ruled out in patients with nystagmus resembling PAN but with asymmetric or irregular periodicity.

Hood and co-workers[12] reported that the pathologic condition underlying rebound nystagmus was a chronic, progressive cerebellar degeneration of varied cause. They consistently found the following constellation of signs and symptoms: (1) rebound nystagmus, either unilateral or bilateral, (2) neurologic evidence of cerebellar involvement, (3) ataxia of gait, (4) complaint of feeling unsteady, (5) impaired pursuit eye movements, (6) deranged optokinetic responses, and (7) markedly enhanced caloric responsiveness. The hyperresponsiveness of the calorics was felt to be secondary to the release of the inhibitory influence of the cerebellum itself or of the cerebellovestibular connections.

REFERENCES

1. Davis, D. G., and Smith, J. L.: Periodic alternating nystagmus: A report of eight cases, Am. J. Ophthalmol. **72:**757-762, 1971.
2. Towle, P. A., and Romanul, F.: Periodic alternating nystagmus: First pathologically studied case, abstracted, Neurology (Minneap.) **20:**408, 1970.
3. Towle, P. A. Cited in Davis, D. G., and Smith, J. L.[1]
4. Keane, J. R.: Periodic alternating nystagmus with downward beating nystagmus, Arch. Neurol. **30:**399-402, 1974.
5. Daroff, R. B., and Dell'Osso, L. F.: Periodic alternating nystagmus and the shifting null, Can. J. Otolaryngol. **3:**3, 367-371, 1974.
6. Kornhuber, H. H.: Der periodisch altermerende Nystagmus (Nystagmus Alternans) und die Enthemmung des Vestibularen Systems, Arch. Ohr. Nas. Kehlkopfheilk. **174:**182-209, 1959.
7. Cogan, D. G.: Downbeat nystagmus, Arch. Ophthalmol. **80:**757-768, 1968.
8. Schatz, N. J.: Vestibular aspects of nystagmus, Audio-Dig. Ophthalmol. **11:**1, 1973.
9. Goldberg, R. T., Gonzalez, C., Breinin, G. M., and Reuben, R. N.: Periodic alternating gaze deviation with dissociation of head movement, Arch. Ophthalmol. **73:**324-330, 1965.
10. Kestenbaum, A.: Clinical methods of neuro-ophthalmologic examination, New York, 1961, Grune and Stratton, Inc., p. 383.
11. Robb, R. M.: Periodic alternation of null point in congenital nystagmus, Arch. Ophthalmol. **87:**169-173, 1972.
12. Hood, J. D., Kayan, A., and Leech, J.: Rebound nystagmus, Brain **96:**507-526, 1973.

Ocular perforation in pulseless disease

Henry M. Clayman
Joel S. Sandberg
Roy D. Altman

Pulseless disease, also known as Takayasu's disease and aortic arch syndrome, was described in 1908 by Takayasu, a Japanese ophthalmologist. The syndrome is based on retinal changes compatible with chronic hypoxia and absent radial pulses and is seen predominantly in female patients 9 to 40 years old. A nonspecific arteritis produces an obliterative process in the brachiocephalic aorta and its branches, with protean clinical cerebrovascular and ocular manifestations.[1] The following case presents the association of ocular perforation in a patient with this syndrome.

A 44-year-old Cuban-born white housewife had reported the onset of dizziness 15 years previously, concomitant with migratory muscle and joint pains. Medical evaluation at that time had revealed absent peripheral pulses. Pulseless disease was confirmed

Supported in part by Public Health Service Training Grant No. EY00028 from the National Eye Institute, National Institutes of Health, Bethesda, Maryland, and by the Florida Lions Eye Bank, Inc., Miami, Florida.

eight years later by an arteriogram that showed obstruction of the right subclavian artery at its axillary portion, with considerable collateral circulation. An intermittent regimen of prednisone was begun. While off steroids in 1968, the patient required hospitalization for pulmonary infiltrates, abdominal pain, pericardial friction rub, and temperature of 103° F. Skin tests for blastomycosis, coccidioidomycosis, histoplasmosis and an intermediate PPD were negative. Second strength PPD had a 16-mm induration. Sputum and cultures for tuberculosis were negative. The patient improved after prednisone therapy (80 mg per day) was begun.

One month later while medically in remission, the patient was first examined by the ophthalmology service of the University of Miami, for refraction. Visual acuity was 20/30 OD and 20/40 OS. There was no active intraocular inflammation, but the pupils dilated irregularly and there was pigment on the anterior lens capsules bilaterally.

The amount of prednisone the patient was taking was decreased over the next three months to 30 mg every other day, resulting only in some blurring of vision. The patient then presented with a bilateral anterior and posterior uveitis, more severe in the left eye. Further medical examination, radiologic exam, and laboratory and skin tests failed to reveal a treatable cause for the uveitis. The patient was treated with corticosteroids by infra-Tenon's injection,[2] topical steroid, and atropine drops. Over subsequent visits during the next six months, the vision in the left eye relentlessly decreased due to anterior and posterior uveitis. The left anterior chamber revealed a marked cellular reaction, anterior and posterior synechiae, rubeosis iridis, and eventually seclusion of the pupil. The posterior segment showed a 3+ vitreous reaction and was poorly visualized. The right eye had a visual acuity of 20/70 with a low grade uveitis and cystoid macular edema.

In July 1969, six months after the initial visit, an elevation and thinning of the sclera of the left eye was first noted, just distal to the limbus inferiorly, and visual acuity was reduced to light perception. About one year after the patient's initial presentation, the

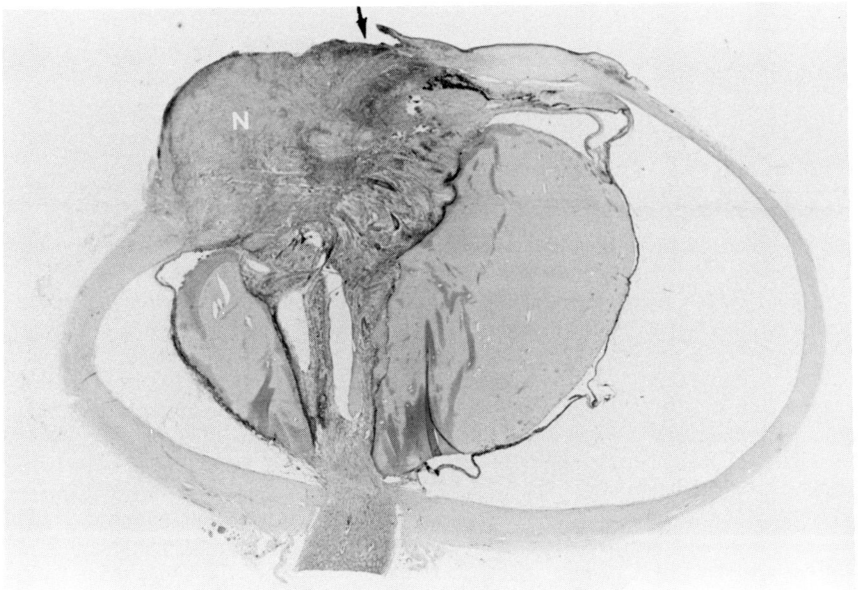

Fig. 13-16. A large inflammatory nodule *(N)* is immediately posterior to the ocular perforation (arrow). (Original magnification ×8.)

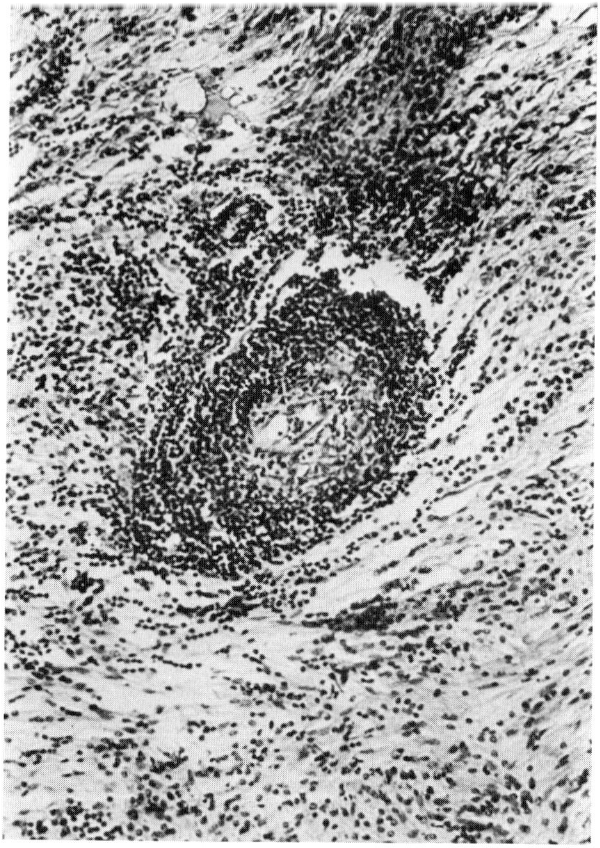

Fig. 13-17. Perivascular infiltration with chronic inflammatory cells in area of ocular perforation. (Original magnification ×500.)

left eye was without light perception, chronically irritated, painful, and cosmetically distasteful. An uneventful enucleation of the left eye was performed in December 1971. In the interim the patient has been medically stable on prednisone therapy of 10 mg every other day. Visual acuity in the right eye decreased to 20/400 with a significant lens opacity. A cataract extraction was performed in August 1972, but the postoperative vision was no better than 20/80 due to persistent cystoid macular edema.

PATHOLOGIC FINDINGS. On gross examination there was a corneoscleral perforation at the limbus in the 5 o'clock position. The retina was totally detached and adherent to the limbal scar. Microscopic examination showed a large inflammatory nodule involving cornea and sclera extending to the corneoscleral perforation (Fig. 13-16). The nodule contained considerable connective tissue necrosis with a prominent chronic inflammatory cell response. The small blood vessels showed a marked perivascular lymphocytic and plasma cell infiltration (Fig. 13-17). Some multinucleated giant cells were present. Pigmented precipitates were found on the corneal endothelium. A membrane occluded the pupillary space, and rubeosis iridis was prominent on the anterior surface of the iris. Peripheral anterior synechiae were present and the lens was cataractous. The detached disorganized retina showed pronounced perivascular cuffing by inflammatory cells with occasional obliteration of the lumen of blood vessels.

There was segmental atrophy of the optic nerve, but the arteries and veins were normal. The principal pathologic diagnosis was corneoscleral perforation with loss of intraocular contents secondary to necrotizing granulomatous keratoscleritis. Specimens submitted to the Armed Forces Institute of Pathology confirmed this diagnosis (A.F.I.P. Accession No. 1469402), and special staining techniques demonstrated neither fungal nor bacterial agents.

DISCUSSION

A chronic inflammatory process involving the cornea and sclera has not been reported in pulseless disease to our knowledge. Ocular manifestations that have been described include amaurosis fugax, pigmentary corneal precipitates, cataracts, iris atrophy, mydriasis, obliteration of peripheral retinal arterioles, retinal hemorrhage, and microaneurysms.[1, 3] Scleromalacia perforans does occur in rheumatoid arthritis, an entity which has been reported in association with pulseless disease.[4] A vasculitis can be seen in rheumatoid arthritis, and conversely, pulseless disease can present in its early phase as a rheumatic syndrome,[5] which occurred in this case. Our patient showed neither clinical nor laboratory evidence of rheumatoid arthritis.

The relationship of the underlying illness to the ocular findings is presumed on the basis of the similarity of the ocular changes to a closely related collagen vascular disease, rheumatoid arthritis, and the bilaterality of symptoms. In addition, the symptoms presented during the rapid decrease in the patient's steroid dose.

Our patient fulfilled the criteria for the diagnosis of pulseless disease,[6] including radiologic findings. There was neither clinical nor pathologic evidence for an infectious cause. Knox[7] has stressed that interference with the vascular supply to the eye can produce a picture of ocular inflammation. Thus, the pathogenesis of the uveitis and subsequent ocular perforation was probably ischemic necrosis of the ocular anterior segment.

REFERENCES

1. Jain, I. S., and Grove, A. D.: Pulseless disease, Br. J. Ophthalmol. **47:**304-307, 1963.
2. Smith, J. L., McCrary, J. A., Bird, A. C., et al.: Sub-Tenon steroid injection for optic neuritis, Trans. Am. Acad. Ophthalmol. Otolaryngol. **74:**1249-1253, 1970.
3. Dowling, J. L., and Smith, T. R.: An ocular study of pulseless disease, Arch. Ophthalmol. **64:**236-243, 1960.
4. Falicov, R. E., and Cooney, R. E.: Takayasu's arteritis and rheumatoid arthritis, Arch. Intern. Med. **114:**594-600, 1964.
5. Strachan, R. W., Wigzell, F. W., and Anderson, J. R.: Locomotor manifestations and serum studies in Takayasu's arteriopathy, Am. J. Med. **40:**560-568, 1966.
6. Riehl, J.: Paradoxes of Takayasu's disease, Calif. Med. **102:**185-192, 1965.
7. Knox, D. L.: Ischemic ocular inflammation, Am. J. Ophthalmol. **60:**995-1002, 1965.

Index

C

D

L

M

N

O

P